Fairbank's Atlas of General Affections of the Skeleton

Fairbank's Atlas of General Affections of the Skeleton

RUTH WYNNE-DAVIES, M.B., B.S.(Lond.),
Ph.D.(Edin.), F.R.C.S.
Reader, Department of Orthopaedic Surgery (Genetics
Research), University of Edinburgh; Honorary Consultant
Orthopaedic Surgeon, The Lothian Health Board, Edinburgh.

T. J. FAIRBANK, M.A., M.B., B.Chir.(Camb.),
F.R.C.S.
Senior Consultant Orthopaedic Surgeon, Cambridgeshire
Area Health Authority (T), East Anglian Regional Health
Authority.

SECOND EDITION

CHURCHILL LIVINGSTONE
EDINBURGH LONDON AND NEW YORK 1976

CHURCHILL LIVINGSTONE
Medical Division of Longman Group Limited

Distributed in the United States of America by
Longman Inc., 19 West 44th Street, New York,
N.Y. 10036 and by associated companies,
branches and representatives throughout
the world.

First Edition 1951
Second Edition 1976

ISBN 0 443 01399 3

Library of Congress Cataloging in Publication Data

Fairbank, Harold Arthur Thomas, Sir, 1876–1961.
  Fairbank's Atlas of general affections of the
skeleton.

  1. Bones—Radiography—Atlases. I. Wynne-Davies,
Ruth. II. Fairbank, Thomas John. III. Title.
IV. Title: Atlas of general affections of the skeleton.
[DNLM: 1. Bone diseases. WE200 F164a]
RC930.F3 1976   616.7′1′07572   76-25820

Printed in Great Britain by
William Clowes & Sons, Limited
London, Beccles and Colchester.

Preface I

It is now 25 years since the first edition of this Atlas appeared, and perhaps there should be some explanation for the long delay. Sir Thomas Fairbank was aged 75 in 1951, and for several years thereafter eagerly continued to collect material for a further edition. This was drawn from cases generously supplied by his many friends seeking an opinion on problems in the field he had made so very much his own, particularly in his latter years. When the first edition was all sold he was advised against a further printing even though there was a continued demand for this book, so uniquely filling a gap amongst orthopaedic text books. His declining health made the task of preparation of a second edition matching his meticulous standards beyond him, and at his invitation, and with his guidance and help, I started the task. However, my other heavy commitments limited the speed of progress so much that this too proved impracticable.

Since Sir Thomas's death in 1961 nobody in Great Britain has quite taken his place as the oracle to whom problems relating to the rare skeletal dysplasias could gravitate. However, in the last few years Miss Ruth Wynne-Davies, Reader in the Department of Orthopaedic Surgery (Genetics Research), University of Edinburgh, has been led by her own studies to develop increasingly an interest in the field of general diseases of the skeleton, and has set up special Skeletal Dysplasia Clinics in Edinburgh, London, Harlow Wood and Oswestry, in which patients with the rare bone dysplasias can be further studied.

Believing as I do that the need for a second edition remains no less cogent than before I have been fortunate indeed in persuading her to join me in this task which was beyond my ability to do alone. I must make it clear that much the greater part of the organisation, research and hard work put into the second edition has been done by R.W-D. and to her I express my deepest gratitude.

1976   T. J. Fairbank

Preface II

In planning the second edition it rapidly became obvious to us that no mere revision of the first would be appropriate. Firstly, many 'new' dysplasias of the skeleton have been described during the last 25 years; secondly, our understanding of a number of conditions described by H.A.T.F. (such as some of the mucopolysaccharidoses) has radically changed; thirdly, we are now able to define more clearly such conditions as the spondylo-epiphyseal dysplasias and metaphyseal chondrodysplasias, many of them in the past having just been called 'osteochondrodystrophy'. Furthermore, it became apparent that with the much increased number of disorders to be described it would be impossible to deal with each one in the detailed manner employed by H.A.T.F.

We therefore decided to change both the style as well as the content while still trying to maintain the original author's object—to provide an atlas helping towards the diagnosis of those rare conditions in which there was major skeletal involvement. The choice of which of the more recently reported dysplasias should be included has been a difficult one; we have aimed to include those that have been established as an entity and in which the opinion of an orthopaedic surgeon is most likely to be sought. We have specifically avoided including a host of so-called 'malformation syndromes' except in so far as they may be of particular orthopaedic interest, and accepting that the dividing line is not always clear cut. Sections on metabolic bone disease and some acquired disorders are included for completeness and to aid in the differential diagnosis of the general affections of the skeleton.

The descriptions of clinical and radiographic appearances have been considerably shortened, particularly in those conditions with which the better trained orthopaedic surgeon of today is already familiar, and we have not gone into the minutiae of occasional variations and associations which have only rarely been reported. The case histories which took up a considerable part of the first edition have been abandoned. Although they perhaps added interest, we did not feel that they contributed to the object of the book as an aid to diagnosis, nor did they add information to that already presented in the text. Comments regarding treatment are included, but only in very general terms: this is in no sense a book on orthopaedic therapeutics.

We have included genetic information where it is available, an aspect that was prominent by its absence in the first edition, the subject of clinical genetics being still in its infancy at that time.

In general, the nomenclature recommended by the group under sponsorship of the European Society of Paediatric Radiology has been followed (McKusick & Scott, 1971, *Journal of Bone and Joint Surgery*, **53A,** 978). The study of the constitutional disorders of bone has been confused not least by the host of synonyms and eponyms that have grown up and we have deliberately avoided giving more than those still in general use. It is hoped that the section on 'Diagnosis' which follows will be of help in the initial stages of investigation.

References are selected, and include the original ones describing the disorder, significant contributions since and the latest review articles where the subject has been dealt with in detail.

The source of the illustrations is manifold. Because of the long time interval all the original blocks of the first edition had been destroyed, but the whole of H.A.T.F.'s collection of clinical photographs was left, with T.J.F.'s approval, to the Institute of Orthopaedics, Great Portland Street, London, where, under the supervision of Dr Ronald O. Murray it remains available for study. With his kind agreement, R.W-D. has worked through the entire collection, selecting material suitable for illustration, often being able to place under the correct diagnosis patients whom H.A.T.F. had marked 'atypical' but which in his day fell into no recognised group. (*Marked 'H.A.T.F.' in the text.*)

Another prolific source of illustrations has been the X-Ray Museum in the Orthopaedic Department at Addenbrooke's Hospital, Cambridge. This collection has been built up largely through the work of Mr R. Weeden Butler who started to accumulate material shortly after his appointment at Addenbrooke's Hospital in 1932 and whose careful work we acknowledge with great gratitude. (*Marked 'A.H.' in the text.*)

Some further illustrations have been obtained from the teaching collection at the Princess Margaret Rose Orthopaedic Hospital, Edinburgh and our thanks are due to the numerous clinicians who have helped to build this up. (*Marked 'P.M.R.' in the text.*)

We were extremely fortunate in having the assistance of Dr John Sutcliffe and Dr Christine Hall of the Radiology Department at the Hospital for Sick Children, Great Ormond Street, London in selecting some of the material from the teaching collection at that hospital. (*Marked 'G.O.S.' in the text.*)

Many other clinicians have helped us with individual cases and to all of them we are deeply grateful. Wherever possible personal acknowledgment is made with each illustration, but where material has been duplicated, used for teaching purposes and kept in departmental museums, the original 'owner', or clinician in charge, can often no longer be identified and we extend our humble apologies if any mistakes have arisen. Furthermore we realise the possibility that some, particularly of the H.A.T.F. illustrations, may have been published elsewhere without our knowledge; we can only ask that our ignorance and discourtesy may be forgiven.

Certain illustrations are known to have been previously published and acknowledgment is due to the Editor of the *British Journal of Bone and Joint Surgery* for those in Chapter 9 (Metaphyseal dysostosis type Jansen), Chapter 19 (parastremmatic dwarfism) and Chapter 51 (homocystinuria). The illustrations in Chapter 27 (sclerosteosis) have appeared in the *Annals of Internal Medicine,* the *British Journal of Radiology* and in *Clinical Genetics,* and acknowledgment is made to the Editors of these journals. Figure 54.2 has appeared in *Metabolic Disorders of Bone* by C. R. Paterson, published by Blackwell Scientific Publications, and acknowledgment is made here to them. Finally, many of the illustrations loaned by Mr A. G. Apley (noted in the text) have appeared in his *System of Orthopaedics and Fractures,* and acknowledgment is made here to Butterworth.

Much of the research carried out by R.W-D. would not have been possible without a travel grant from the Carnegie Trust for the Universities of Scotland, to whom grateful thanks are due.

We have had a great deal of background assistance in the preparation of this book and our thanks are due to Mrs C. Darlington and Mrs K. Fyfe (Edinburgh) and to Mrs O. L. Challis (Cambridge) for the secretarial work. They have assisted also with the interminable reference checking, together with Mrs A. Littlejohn and Mrs J. Gormley and with much help from the staff of the Central Medical Library, Edinburgh. We are also indebted to Mrs E. M. Thoday of the Orthopaedic Department of Addenbrooke's Hospital for help in searching out records and radiographs. The very considerable amount of work relating to the index has been done by Mrs Ruby Davies and we are most grateful to her for this. Finally we should like to record with much appreciation the unfailing courtesy and friendly assistance we have had from all members of the staff at Churchill Livingstone's.

The difficulties of producing a work worthy of H.A.T.F.'s original book are very great and we have been very conscious of this, but we hope that this second edition may be of use to our orthopaedic colleagues, and if members of other specialties in the field of medicine find it helpful then we shall thereby be the more gratified.

Ruth Wynne-Davies, Edinburgh
T. J. Fairbank, Cambridge

June, 1976

Contents

Preface I   v
Preface II   vi
Diagnosis   xi

Section I: Bone Dysplasias

A. With predominantly epiphyseal involvement
1. Multiple epiphyseal dysplasia   2
2. Chondrodysplasia punctata   10
3. Dysplasia epiphysealis hemimelica   14
4. Hereditary arthro-ophthalmopathy   16

B. With predominantly metaphyseal involvement
5. Achondroplasia (classical type)   20
6. Hypochondroplasia   24
7. Lethal forms of short-limbed dwarfism   26
    Thanatophoric dwarfism   26
    Achondrogenesis   26
    Asphyxiating thoracic dystrophy   27
    Short rib-polydactyly syndromes   27
8. Chondro-ectodermal dysplasia   30
9. The metaphyseal chondrodysplasias   32
    Congenita (Jansen)   32
    Tarda   (Schmid)   34
    Tarda   (McKusick)   38
    With malabsorption and neutropenia   40
    With thymolymphopenia   42
    Others   42
10. The hypophosphatasias   44

C. With vertebral involvement only
11. Brachyolmia   48

D. With predominantly vertebral and epiphyseal involvement
12. The spondyloepiphyseal dysplasias   50

E. With predominantly vertebral and metaphyseal involvement
13. Spondylometaphyseal dysplasia Kozlowski type   53

F. Vertebral, epiphyseal and metaphyseal involvement
14. Pseudoachondroplasia   54
15. Spondyloepiphyseal dysplasia congenita   60
16. Metatropic dwarfism   64
17. Kniest disease   67
18. Diastrophic dwarfism   68
19. Parastremmatic dwarfism   72
20. Dyggve–Melchior–Clausen disease   74

G. Disorders with decreased bone density
21. Osteogenesis imperfecta   78
22. Idiopathic juvenile osteoporosis   86
23. The osteolyses   88
    Hereditary, of hands and feet   88
    Multicentric   88

H. Disorders involving the skull and long bones with increased bone density
24. Osteopetrosis   90

25. Dysosteosclerosis   95
26. Pycnodysostosis   96
27. Sclerosteosis   100
28. Craniometaphyseal dysplasia   104
29. Familial metaphyseal dysplasia   106
30. Craniodiaphyseal dysplasia   109
31. Progressive diaphyseal dysplasia   110
32. Osteodysplasty   113
33. The hyperphosphatasias   114
34. Pachydermoperiostitis   118
35. Paget's disease   120

J. Anarchic development of bone
36. Diaphyseal aclasis   126
37. Ollier's enchondromatosis and Maffucci's disease   130
38. Melorheostosis   134
39. Polyostotic fibrous dysplasia   138
40. Osteopoikilosis   142
41. Osteopathia striata   144

Section II: Miscellaneous Dysplasias and Malformation Syndromes with Major Bony Involvement

42. Neurofibromatosis   148
43. The Marfan syndrome   152
44. Cleido-cranio-dysplasia   156
45. Nail-patella syndrome   158
46. Fibrodysplasia ossificans progressiva   160
47. Tricho-rhino-phalangeal syndrome   163

Section III: Inborn Errors of Metabolism

48. The mucopolysaccharidoses   166
    Hurler   166
    Scheie   167
    Hunter   167
    Sanfilippo   168
    Maroteaux–Lamy   168
    Morquio   168
49. The mucolipidoses   178
    GM_1 gangliosidosis type 1   178
    I-cell disease   178
    Others   178
50. The sphingolipidoses   180
    Gaucher   180
51. Homocystinuria   182
52. Histiocytosis X   186

Section IV: Metabolic Bone Disease

53. Metabolic bone disease with hypercalcaemia   192
    Hyperparathyroidism   192
    Vitamin D poisoning   197
    Vitamin A poisoning   197
    Idiopathic hypercalcaemia of infancy   198

54. Metabolic bone disease with hypocalcaemia: 200
    Rickets and osteomalacia 200
        Vitamin D deficiency 200
        Renal tubular disease 201
        Uraemic osteodystrophy 201
    Hypoparathyroidism and pseudohypopara-
    thyroidism 208
    Tubular stenosis with periodic hypocalcaemia
    (Kenny–Caffey) 209
55. Metabolic bone disease with bone loss 210
    Osteoporosis 210
    Vitamin C deficiency 212

Section V: Endocrine Disorders
56. Pituitary 216
    Hypopituitarism 216
    Gigantism 216
    Acromegaly 216
57. Thyroid 220
    Hypothyroidism 220
58. Adrenals 222
    Glucocorticoid excess 222

Section VI: Infections, Toxins, Blood Dyscrasias, Neoplasia and Trauma
59. Infections 226
60. Infantile cortical hyperostosis 230
61. Toxins 232
62. The haemoglobinopathies 234
63. The reticuloses 238
    Leukaemia 238
    Hodgkin's disease 242
    Myelomatosis 244
    Myelofibrosis 246
64. Generalised neoplasia of bone 248
    Cystic angiomatosis 248
    Metastatic bone disease 248
65. Hypertrophic osteoarthropathy 254
66. The battered baby 256

Index 258

Diagnosis

The object of an atlas is to enable the reader to locate the place he is looking for, or in the present context to identify the disorder of the patient with whom he is concerned. While some of the conditions described here are commonplace, the majority are rare, some so rare that a clinician may not see one example in a medical lifetime. Furthermore, the boundary between one dysplasia and another may not be clear cut and each itself may be liable to wide variations. This is a developing field of rapid change and thus the groupings we have made will no doubt in due course become outdated and require alteration.

There is no infallible and easy way to reach a diagnosis, since in most of the skeletal dysplasias biochemical tests are not available. The essential preliminaries are a complete history, family history and clinical examination, together with a radiographic survey of the skeleton. Laboratory investigations are sometimes diagnostic, but this section is mainly concerned with those disorders in which only clinical, perhaps genetic, and radiographic data are available—and it is the latter which provides the main evidence.

GROUPING OF DISEASES IN SECTIONS
(See Contents list)

This is the first stage in the clinical diagnosis of a skeletal dysplasia and the groupings used in this Atlas provide a valuable starting point. The main section headings, together with additional diseases described elsewhere in the Atlas, are here noted. Individual dysplasias in these sections are listed in the Contents (pages ix to x).

Section I: Bone Dysplasias

(a) with predominantly epiphyseal involvement (*note also cretinism*).

(b) with predominantly metaphyseal involvement (*note also rickets, whether nutritional, renal tubular or associated with uraemic osteodystrophy*).

(c) with vertebral involvement only.

(d) with predominantly vertebral and epiphyseal involvement.

(e) vertebral, epiphyseal and metaphyseal involvement (*note also the mucopolysaccharidoses, mucolipidoses and other inborn errors of metabolism*).

(f) disorders with decreased bone density.

(g) disorders involving the skull and long bones with increased bone density.

(h) anarchic development of bone (*i.e. irregular and often asymmetrical disorders of bone growth*).

Section II: Miscellaneous Dysplasias and Malformation Syndromes with Major Bony Involvement
(*not fitting clearly into Section I*)

Section III: Inborn Errors of Metabolism
(*the storage diseases, homocystinuria and histiocytosis X; in many cases there is a known enzyme defect, see also I(e) above*)

Section IV: Metabolic Bone Disease
(*Usually with a known disturbance of the Calcium–Phosphorus balance, and grouped as those with hypercalcaemia, with hypocalcaemia and with bone loss*)

Section V: Endocrine Disorders

Section VI: Infections, Toxins, Blood Dyscrasias, Neoplasia and Trauma

USE OF THE INDEX AS AN AID TO DIAGNOSIS

The index is as full as possible and includes physical and radiographic signs as well as laboratory findings. Thus, for example, under 'scoliosis' or 'epiphyses, cone-shaped' or 'hypercalcaemia' will be found the main diseases in which these are characteristic findings, but not those in which they only occasionally occur.

AGE OF DIAGNOSIS

The age of onset of a disorder can be a useful guide to diagnosis, though in some cases (particularly of the less severe disorders) there is wide variation, to the point of some bone lesions only being discovered incidentally on radiography· for some unrelated reason in adult life.

The Table which follows (on page xiii) lists the typical age of presenting signs (noting those with a wide range). In general, the more severe and lethal disorders are congenital (that is, clinically obvious at birth).

If the clinician has prior knowledge of a possibly affected child (perhaps because a parent or previous sib is affected), then earlier diagnosis than noted here can be made. For example, Hurler's disease is not clinically apparent at birth, but the enzyme defect can be demonstrated then (or pre-natally) if looked for specifically. Similarly, diaphyseal aclasis is rarely diagnosed at birth, but exostoses may indeed be present at this time, and would be found if radiographic examination was carried out then.

GENETICS AND GENETIC ADVICE

The inheritance of a disorder may provide a clue as to its diagnosis, or at least a strong family history of the condition puts it among the 'constitutional' disorders, rather than those that are acquired. Warning is due here, in that our present-day ignorance of patterns of inheritance in the rare skeletal dysplasias is very great, and secondly, disorders which appear identical clinically may not invariably present with the same mode of inheritance—or indeed may be non-genetic (sporadic).

Basic genetics are not dealt with, and the reader is referred to the many textbooks on the subject. Briefly, the chromosomal anomalies (which give rise to some of the multitude of malformation syndromes) are not discussed; there is no disorder described in this book of proven multifactorial inheritance, thus, these skeletal dysplasias, if a pattern of inheritance is present at all, are unifactorial (dominant or recessive, either autosomal or X-linked). Those disorders which, so far as is known, are without genetic factors, are noted in the text as sporadic.

In the simplest possible terms the patterns of inheritance likely to be encountered in clinical practice are as follows:

1. *Autosomal dominant inheritance, established in two or more generations.* The risk to an affected individual (married to a normal one) is that up to 1 in 2 (half) his children will also be affected.

2. *Autosomal dominant inheritance, new mutation.* Here *normal* parents have had an affected child (e.g. achondroplasia, which is known to be of dominant inheritance). The mutation must have occurred in only one sperm (or ovum) and there is only the remotest possibility that another mutation will occur in these parents. Thus there is virtually no risk to them of having a second affected child. However, the affected child himself, once adult, has the same 1 in 2 risk described in (1) above.

(To make things more difficult, in some disorders there may be skipped generations and in very rare instances normal parents have had more than one child affected with a known dominant mutation. In such cases it is presumed there is a gonadal mosaic, that is, a whole section of a gonad has been affected by the mutation.)

3. *Autosomal recessive inheritance.* Here parents appear clinically normal but each is carrying the same 'bad' gene, and their children homozygous for this gene (i.e. carrying one from each parent) will exhibit the disease. An affected individual will thus have normal parents, and, provided he marries a normal individual, his own children will also appear normal. The risk that any subsequent sib of his will be affected is up to 1 in 4 (25 per cent). Many of these autosomal recessive disorders are due to enzyme deficiencies (e.g. homocystinuria) and it may be possible to detect this in the apparently normal heterozygotes (i.e. those individuals carrying only one 'bad' gene). This subject is becoming increasingly important in the field of ante-natal diagnosis where in some instances (e.g. Hurler's disease) the enzyme disorder can be diagnosed on amniocentesis followed by cell culture, and abortion offered to the mother before the 20th week of pregnancy.

4. *X-linked recessive inheritance.* This has the well-known pattern of a disease limited to males, and in which affected individuals pass the gene to their daughters only. In the next generation up to half *their* sons are affected.

5. *X-linked dominant inheritance.* This is much less common, but again, affected males can only pass the gene to their daughters—who this time will exhibit the disease—and pass it on to up to half their own children (e.g. familial hypophosphataemia). A characteristic point is that twice as many females as males will be affected, since the female has two X chromosomes and will exhibit the disease if either is involved.

In no case of X-linked inheritance, dominant or recessive, is it possible for an affected male to pass the disease to his son, who necessarily carries his father's Y chromosome.

Giving genetic advice to patients, parents or other members of the family is extremely difficult in many of the rare skeletal dysplasias. Where the genetics are known for certain this is noted in the text. However, many disorders which seem clinically to be similar have been reported as of varying patterns of inheritance and it is often not possible to give accurate genetic advice. In these cases, until biochemical tests are available, it is better to admit lack of precise genetic knowledge and avoid giving specific 'risk' figures to the family.

Constitutional disorders of the skeleton: typical age of presenting signs

Birth
- Achondroplasia (classical)
- Chondrodysplasia punctata (severe rhizomelic form)
- Chondroectodermal dysplasia
- Diastrophic dwarfism
- Fibrodysplasia ossificans progressiva (short hallux)
- Gaucher's (acute)
- GM_1 gangliosidosis Type I
- Hypercalcaemia, severe idiopathic
- Hyperphosphatasia (severe)
- Hypophosphatasia (severe)
- Lethal forms of short-limbed dwarfism
- Metaphyseal chondrodysplasia—Jansen
- Metaphyseal chondrodysplasia—McKusick
- Metatropic dwarfism
- Mucolipidosis II
- Nail-patella syndrome (nail defects)
- Neurofibromatosis* (pseudoarthrosis)
- Osteogenesis imperfecta (severe)
- Osteopetrosis (severe)
- Spondyloepiphyseal dysplasia congenita

Infancy
- Chondrodysplasia punctata (mild form)
- Craniocleidodysostosis*
- Craniodiaphyseal dysplasia
- Diaphyseal aclasis*
- Dyggve–Melchior–Clausen disease
- Engelmann's
- Familial hypophosphataemia
- Hurler's (MPS)
- Hunter's (MPS)
- Hypophosphatasia tarda
- Infantile cortical hyperostosis
- Kenny–Caffey syndrome
- Letterer Siwe
- Metaphyseal chondrodysplasia-Schmid
- Metaphyseal chondrodysplasia + malabsorption and neutropenia
- Metaphyseal chondrodysplasia and thymolymphopenia
- Morquio's (MPS)
- Mucolipidosis III
- Osteodysplasty
- Osteogenesis imperfecta tarda
- Parastremmatic dwarfism
- Pycnodysostosis*
- Scheie (MPS)

Childhood
- Craniometaphyseal dysplasia
- Dysosteosclerosis
- Dysplasia epiphysealis hemimelica
- Eosinophilic granuloma
- Fibrodysplasia ossificans progressiva*
- Gigantism
- Haemoglobinopathies
- Hand–Schüller–Christian disease
- Hereditary arthro-ophthalmopathy
- Hyperphosphatasia tarda
- Hypochondroplasia*
- Homocystinuria*
- Idiopathic juvenile osteoporosis
- Maffucci's
- Marfan's*
- Maroteaux–Lamy (MPS)
- Melorheostosis*
- Multiple epiphyseal dysplasia
- Neurofibromatosis (café au lait patches and scoliosis)
- Ollier's
- Osteolysis of hands and feet
- Osteopathia striata*
- Osteopetrosis tarda*
- Osteopoikilosis*
- Pituitary insufficiency
- Polyostotic fibrous dysplasia*
- Pseudoachondroplasia
- Pyle's*
- Sanfilippo (MPS)
- Sclerosteosis
- Spondyloepiphyseal dysplasia (X-linked)
- Spondylometaphyseal dysplasia (Kozlowski)

Adolescence
- Nail-patella syndrome* (main defects)
- Pachydermoperiostitis*

Adult life
- Acromegaly
- Gaucher's
- Hyperparathyroidism
- Hypertrophic osteo-arthropathy (secondary)
- Hypophosphatasia (mild)
- Osteoporosis, primary
- Paget's
- Pseudohypoparathyroidism

* or at any age thereafter

SECTION I

BONE DYSPLASIAS

1 Multiple Epiphyseal Dysplasia
Dysplasia Epiphysealis Multiplex

Multiple epiphyseal dysplasia is one of the commoner of the skeletal dysplasias and is characterised by irregular epiphyseal growth with little or no vertebral involvement and mild shortness of stature.

It is probable there is more than one type, that described by Fairbank (1935, 1947) which is a severe disorder with small, late-appearing epiphyses and considerable involvement of the wrist and hand, and a second type described by Ribbing (1937) which appears to be milder, with flattened epiphyses and only minimal involvement of the wrists and hands.

Inheritance. Multiple epiphyseal dysplasia is clearly of unifactorial inheritance, the most usual form being of autosomal dominant inheritance (Fairbank, 1935; Barrie, Carter and Sutcliffe, 1958; Hoefnagel et al, 1967; Kozlowski and Lipska, 1967). There is also evidence in some cases for a pattern of autosomal recessive inheritance (Ribbing, 1937; Juberg and Holt, 1968) with families in whom several affected sibs and unaffected consanguineous parents have been noted. However, clinical delineation of genetic types is not yet possible.

Frequency. Population incidence figures are not available but it is not a rare dysplasia. The sexes are equally affected. The disorder is not apparent at birth, there probably being little disability until the child is over two years of age or more.

Clinical and radiographic features. Apart from some shortness of stature, these individuals are of normal appearance and have normal intelligence. The presenting sign is usually of pain and stiffness in the knees and hips, and when the onset is in infancy there is delay in learning to walk. Sometimes enlargement of the joints is noticed, or flexion contractures particularly of the knees and elbows. The fingers and toes are short and stubby, but apart from this and the (not invariably present) short stature, there is no marked deformity.

On radiography the principal abnormalities are seen in the limb epiphyses. The vertebrae show only minimal changes with perhaps some blunting of the vertebral margins with flattening and irregularity.

The main defect is of the limb epiphyses where the centres of ossification are late in appearing, small, mottled and irregular. There is no true stippling, the appearances are more those of subsidiary ossification centres, which may indeed be present. Radiographs of the hand and wrist are characteristic with stumpy metacarpals, late ossifying carpal bones and with all epiphyses affected although in the milder Ribbing type of multiple epiphyseal dysplasia the hands are normal.

The femoral capital epiphyses are nearly always involved, and it also seems that a true Perthes' disease may occur in hips which are relatively unaffected by the epiphyseal dysplasia disease process. The acetabulum is not usually irregular in outline, a point of diagnostic importance in differentiating this from some of the spondylo-epiphyseal dysplasias, though in later life it may alter to conform to the shape of the deformed head of femur.

Hunt et al (1967) have reported coincidental slipped upper femoral epiphyses. Juberg and Holt (1968) noted double patellae in several sibs. Fairbank's original papers and Murphy, Shine and Stevens (1973) have pointed out that a slanting mortice, lower tibial epiphysis diminishing in depth from within outwards with the ankle joint is common.

The degree of severity of this disease is very variable, some epiphyses merely flattening slightly, or having a somewhat square outline. In others, they appear grossly irregular, fragmented and dense even in adult life. It is likely that multiple epiphyseal dysplasia is a heterogeneous collection of disorders which have not yet been delineated clinically or genetically.

Pathology. Rubin (1964) has reported on the histology and Hunt and colleagues (1967) were able to examine an affected limb amputated for osteosarcoma in one of two brothers with multiple epiphyseal dysplasia. There is non-specific irregularity of epiphyseal cartilage cells with disordered columns and areas of degeneration. Enchondral ossification is in disarray, whereas modelling appears normal.

Differential diagnosis. This is from the spondylo-epiphyseal dysplasias, which are differentiated by their severe vertebral changes, acetabular involvement and absence of major band changes. In pseudo-achondroplasia the dwarfing is severe, there are marked metaphyseal as well as epiphyseal changes, and in childhood the vertebral bodies are characteristic with a central protruding tongue seen on the lateral radiographs. Untreated hypothyroidism is differentiated by the general clinical and biochemical features. The changes in the femoral capital epiphyses in multiple epiphyseal dysplasia may be identical with those seen in Perthes' disease but this is a disorder which is confined to the head of the femur and is probably of multifactorial inheritance.

The more usual diagnostic problem is that patients with multiple epiphyseal dysplasia when adult, are simply thought to have osteoarthritis, which is indeed present, but the multiple joints affected and a family history of the condition differentiate this disease from primary osteoarthritis.

Progress and complications. There is little disability in the first years of infancy and childhood but it gradually becomes apparent that the child is rather shorter than average and has difficulty in running and

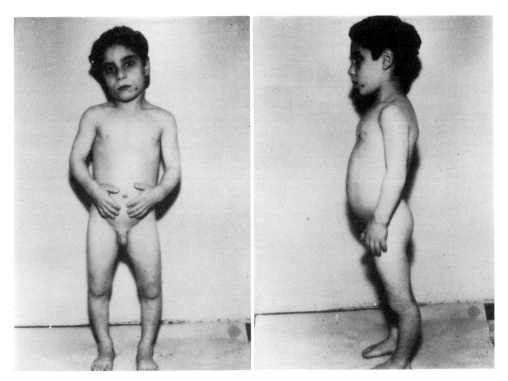

Fig. 1.1 (R.S. aged 8 years.) Some shortening of limbs and mild genu varum, but there is no marked deformity. (H.A.T.F.)

climbing stairs. The final height is between 145 and 170 cm (approximately 4′6″ to 5′6″). The chief problem is the early onset of osteoarthritis, perhaps even during childhood. Life expectancy is normal.

Treatment. This is directed to care of the osteoarthritis.

REFERENCES

Barrie, H., Carter, C. & Sutcliffe, J. (1958). Multiple epiphyseal dysplasia. *British Medical Journal*, **ii**, 133.

Fairbank, H. A. T. (1935). Generalised diseases of the skeleton. *Proceedings of the Royal Society of Medicine*, **28**, 1611.

Fairbank, H. A. T. (1947) Dysplasia epiphysialis multiplex. *British Journal of Surgery*, **34**, 225.

Hoefnagel, D., Sycamore, L. K., Russell, S. W. & Bucknall, W. E. (1967). Hereditary multiple epiphyseal dysplasia. *Annals of Human Genetics*, **30**, 201.

Hunt, D. D., Ponseti, I. V., Pedrini-Mille, A. & Pedrini, V. (1967). Multiple epiphyseal dysplasia in two siblings. *Journal of Bone & Joint Surgery*, **49A**, 1611.

Juberg, R. C. & Holt, J. F. (1968). Inheritance of multiple epiphyseal dysplasia, tarda. *American Journal of Human Genetics*, **20**, 549.

Kozlowski, K. & Lipska, E. (1967). Hereditary dysplasia epiphysealis multiplex. *Clinical Radiology*, **18**, 330.

Murphy, M. C., Shine, I. B. & Stevens, D. B. (1973). Multiple epiphyseal dysplasia: Report of a pedigree. *Journal of Bone & Joint Surgery*, **55A**, 814.

Ribbing, S. (1937). Studien über hereditäre multiple epiphysenstörungen. *Acta Radiologica (Stockholm)*, Supplement 34.

Rubin, P. (1964). *Dynamic Classification of Bone Dysplasias*. Yearbook Medical Publishers.

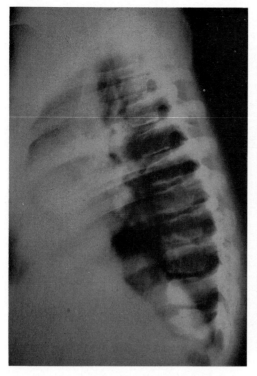 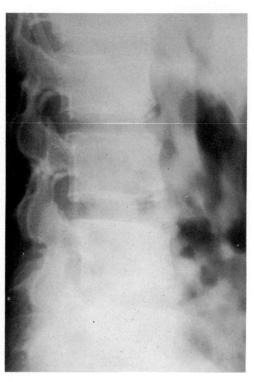

Fig. 1.2 (L.C.) 16 year old female with some irregularity of epiphyseal plates. (H.A.T.F.)

Fig. 1.3 (E.C.) 18 year old female, less severely affected. (Courtesy of Mr A. G. Apley, Pyrford.)

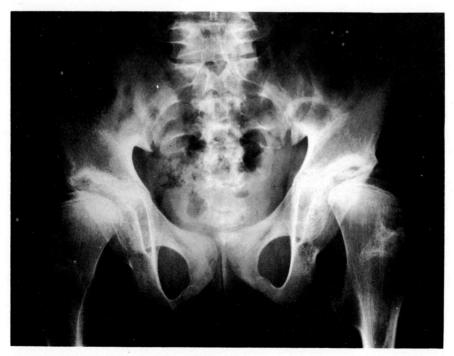

Fig. 1.4 (E.C.) Deformity of femoral heads and early osteoarthritis. (Courtesy of Mr A. G. Apley, Pyrford.)

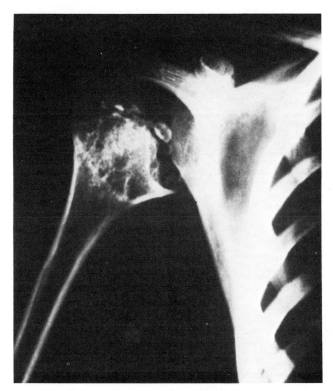

Fig. 1.5 (J.S.) 13 year old female with severe dysplasia of humeral head. (H.A.T.F.)

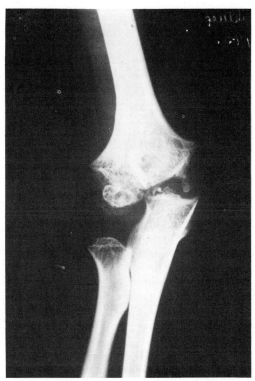

Fig. 1.6 (J.S.) All epiphyses at the elbow are involved. (H.A.T.F.)

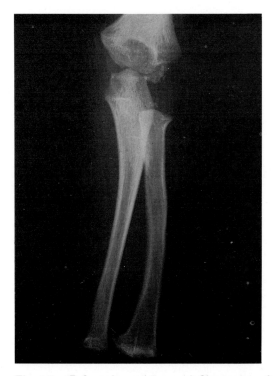

Fig. 1.7 (R.S. male aged 8 years.) Shortening of the forearm and retarded epiphyseal growth at the elbow and wrist. (H.A.T.F.)

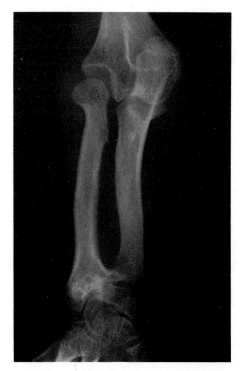

Fig. 1.8 (D.W.) Adult with much shortened forearm and deformity at the elbow and wrist. (H.A.T.F.)

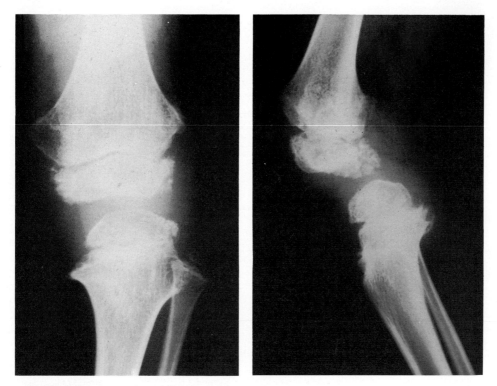

Figs 1.9 and 1.10   Severe involvement of all epiphyses at the knee. (H.A.T.F.)

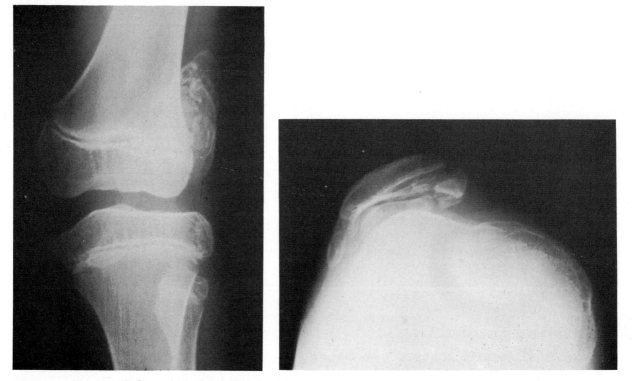

Figs 1.11 and 1.12   (E.C. aged 18 years.) Female with a mosaic patella, an unusual feature of this disease. (Courtesy of Mr A. G. Apley, Pyrford.)

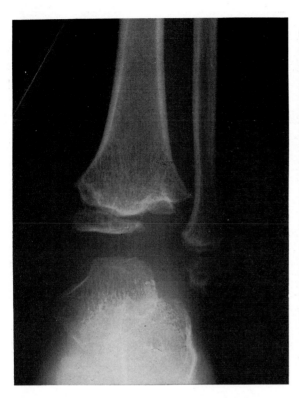
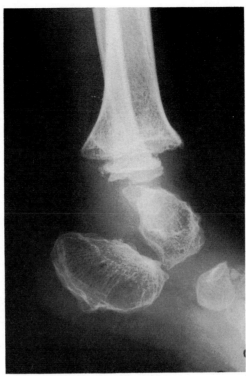

Figs 1.13 and 1.14 (R.S.) 8 year old male with severe involvement of the ankle and tarsus, and a deficiency of the lower lateral tibial epiphysis. (H.A.T.F.)

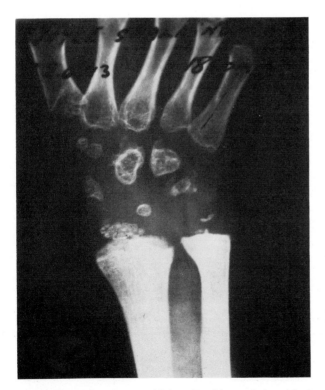
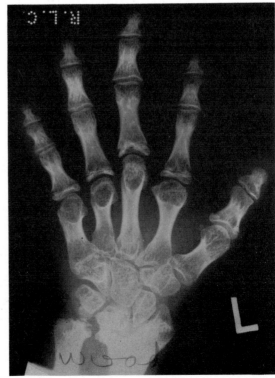

Fig. 1.15 (J.S.) 13 year old female with much irregularity and delay in ossification of the carpal bones and the lower radial and ulnar epiphyses. (H.A.T.F.)

Fig. 1.16 (D.W.) Stubby hands, particularly with shortening of the metacarpals. (H.A.T.F.)

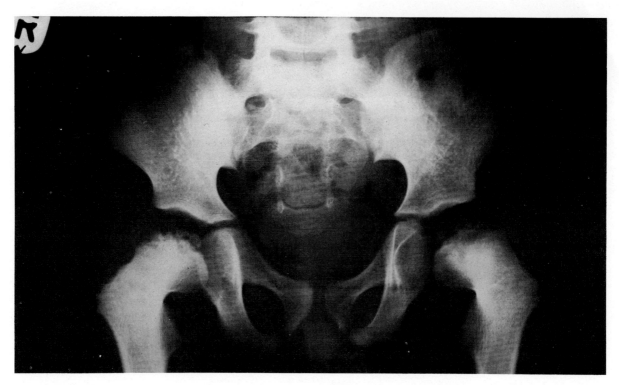

Fig. 1.17 (M.R. male aged 5 years.) The pelvis is normal in shape and the changes in the femoral heads are similar to Perthes' disease. (A.H.) (Patient M.R. Figs 1.17 to 1.21, has the less severe Ribbing form of the disease.)

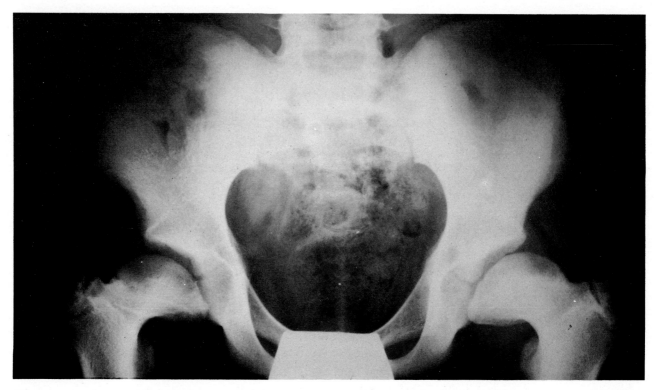

Fig. 1.18 (M.R. aged 14 years.) There is considerable flattening and deformity of the femoral heads but the acetabulum is not involved. (A.H.)

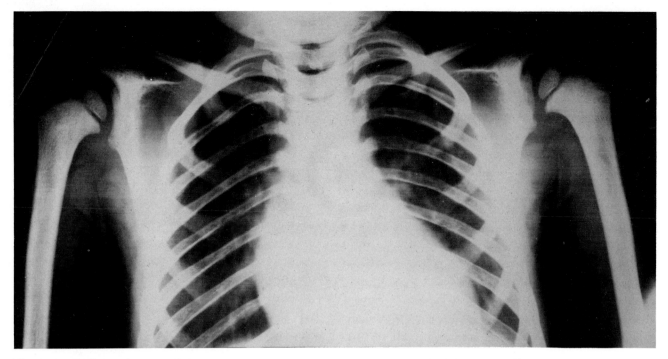

Fig. 1.19 (M.R. aged 14 years.) The humeral epiphyses are small but not unduly deformed. (A.H.)

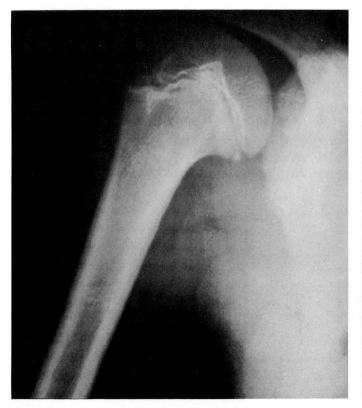

Fig. 1.20 (M.R. aged 14 years.) There is some flattening of the humeral head but no marked deformity. (A.H.)

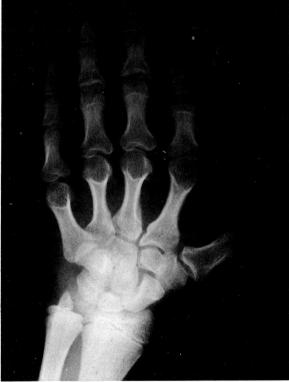

Fig. 1.21 (M.R. aged 14 years.) Apart from some shortening of the metacarpals the hand and wrist is little involved. (A.H.)

2 Chondrodysplasia Punctata
Conradi Disease

Conradi disease is probably a heterogeneous group of conditions, all characterised by stippling of epiphyses and extra-epiphyseal calcification (in infancy only) and accompanied either by a short-limb type of dwarfism or by asymmetrical shortening of a limb. Skin lesions, congenital cataracts and mental retardation are frequently associated.

Spranger, Opitz and Bidder (1971) suggested there are at least two clear entities; first a severe rhizomelic form in which the limbs are extremely short, bilateral cataracts and psychomotor retardation usual, and death occurs in the perinatal period or during the first year of life. The second, milder form they designated Conradi–Hünermann disease, the limbs here being only slightly short and often asymmetrically so. Mental retardation and cataracts are less usual. This type was described by Conradi (1914), Fairbank (1927) and Hünermann (1931). The distinction between the two is not always clear cut and probably yet more types distinguishable both clinically and genetically will be delineated in the future. However, the two extremes can be differentiated and are described here separately.

SEVERE RHIZOMELIC FORM

Inheritance. This form is of autosomal recessive inheritance, kindreds with affected sibs being reported and also parental consanguinity in several cases.

Frequency. The condition is extremely rare. Spranger *et al* (1971) were able to report on 6 personal cases and 94 from the literature. Since then Mason and Kozlowski (1973) have reported on a further 10. The sexes are equally affected and the condition is apparent at birth.

Clinical and radiographic features. The appearance of these infants is characteristic with their very short limbs, flat face and depressed bridge of nose. Bilateral cataracts are present in about three-quarters of cases. A variety of skin disorders may be present, ranging from mild erythema and a dry scaly skin to seborrhoeic dermatitis, ichthotic hyperkeratosis and cicatricial alopecia (Melnick, 1965; Comings, Papazian and Schoene, 1968). Mental retardation is usual, and optic atrophy may develop. Congenital heart disease or other internal congenital anomalies such as tracheo-oesophageal fistula or imperforate anus may be present, as well as multiple contractures of joints and congenital dislocation of the hip.

On radiography the typical sign is stippling of the epiphyses, and there may also be extra-cartilaginous calcification, often in relation to the vertebral column. Craniostenosis is a feature and the proximal limb bones (humerus and femur) are extremely short. All long bones show metaphyseal cupping and splaying.

Congenital vertebral anomalies and irregularities result in scoliosis. Lateral radiographs of the spine may show separate centres of ossification for the vertebral bodies, one anteriorly and the other posteriorly, separated by a wide translucent band.

Pathology. Enchondral bone formation is grossly abnormal and there is reduced vascularity and little calcification. The stippling is caused by circumscribed, polymorphous, chalky deposits in cartilage (Selakovich and Warren White, 1955).

Differential diagnosis. Congenital stippling of epiphyses is seen in many conditions, for example pre-natal infections, sometimes in chromosomal anomalies and in the cerebro-hepato renal syndrome. However, in these cases calcification is rarely seen in the region of the vertebral column. In multiple epiphyseal dysplasia there are often multiple ossification centres in the epiphyses of limb bones but these areas are larger and not usually confused with true stippling (Silverman, 1969).

Progress and complications. The prognosis is poor in the severe rhizomelic form and only a few infants survive the first year of life, most of them dying from respiratory infection.

CONRADI–HÜNERMANN FORM

This is a milder disorder than the rhizomelic type and although many of the same features are apparent, there is much wider variation between individuals.

Inheritance. Certainly in some cases this disorder is of autosomal dominant inheritance, though most cases are sporadic. There are also reports of clearly autosomal recessive inheritance, with related parents and more than one affected sib. The genetic pattern is difficult to determine without more detailed surveys being available, because in mild cases there may be no obvious defect in adult life; thus autosomal dominance is difficult to exclude.

Clinical and radiographic features. The disease appears to be two or three times more common in females than in males. Individuals have a flat face with depressed nasal bridge. Congenital cataracts are present only in about one-fifth of cases. The skin may be affected, being dry and scaly. Contractures of shoulder, hip and knee occur and shortening of only one limb may be a feature—though shortening of all proximal limb bones also occurs. In milder cases the condition may not be recognised at birth.

Radiographic changes include craniostenosis, punctate calcification at the ends of long bones, mostly within the area of the epiphysis, and both in and adjacent to the vertebrae and pelvis. Irregular congenital deformities of the vertebrae are associated with unequal bone growth and developing scoliosis.

Pathology. Enchondral bone formation seems to be little affected but the epiphyseal cartilage shows cysts as well as areas of calcification.

Differential diagnosis. This is as for the severe rhizomelic type.

Progress and complications. The epiphyseal stippling usually vanishes by the age of four years (Tasker, Mastri and Gold, 1970), but there may be later epiphyseal changes in those areas previously affected by stippling.

There is wide variation in the prognosis: some of these children may be stillborn or die in the perinatal period, but if they survive this time then life expectancy is likely to be normal. Complications which may require treatment relate to the developing scoliosis, skin condition and leg inequality.

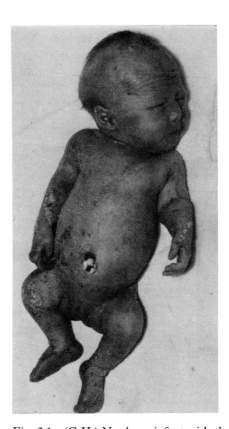

Fig. 2.1 (G.H.) Newborn infant with the milder form of the disease showing the dry scaling skin. (H.A.T.F.)

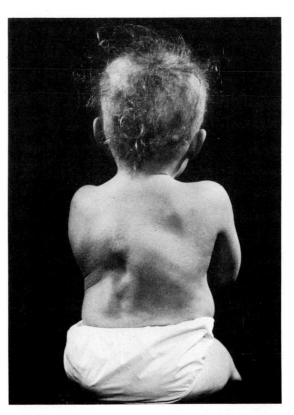

Fig. 2.2 (L.S.) Female aged 18 months with a mild form of the disease but showing marked structural scoliosis. (Courtesy of Professor J. I. P. James, Edinburgh.)

REFERENCES

Comings, D. E., Papazian, C. & Schoene, H. R. (1968). Conradi's disease. *Journal of Pediatrics*, **72**, 63.

Conradi, E. (1914). Verzeitiges Auftreten von Knochen und eigenartigen Verkalkungskernen bei Chondrodystrophia foetalis hypoplastica. *Zeitschrift für Kinderheilkunde*, **80**, 86.

Fairbank, H. A. T. (1927). Some general diseases of the skeleton. *British Journal of Surgery*, **15**, 120.

Hünermann, C. (1931). Chondrodystrophia calcificans congenita als abortive Form der chondrodystrophie. *Zeitschrift für Kinderheilkunde*, **51**, 1.

Mason, R. C. & Kozlowski, K. (1973). Chondrodysplasia punctata: A report of 10 cases. *Radiology*, **109**, 145.

Melnick, J. C. (1965). Chondrodystrophia calcificans congenita. *American Journal of Diseases of Children*, **110**, 218.

Selakovich, W. G. & Warren White, J. (1955). Chondrodystrophia calcificans congenita. *Journal of Bone & Joint Surgery*, **37A**, 1271.

Silverman, F. N. (1969). Discussion on the relation between stippled epiphyses and the multiplex form of epiphyseal dysplasia. *Birth Defects Original Article Series 5*, Part 4, 68.

Spranger, J. W., Opitz, J. M. & Bidder, U. (1971). Heterogeneity of chondrodysplasia punctata. *Human Genetics*, **11**, 190.

Tasker, W. G., Mastri, A. R. & Gold, A. P. (1970). Chondrodystrophia calcificans congenita. (Dysplasia epiphysalis punctata.) Recognition of the clinical picture. *American Journal of Diseases of Children*, **119**, 122.

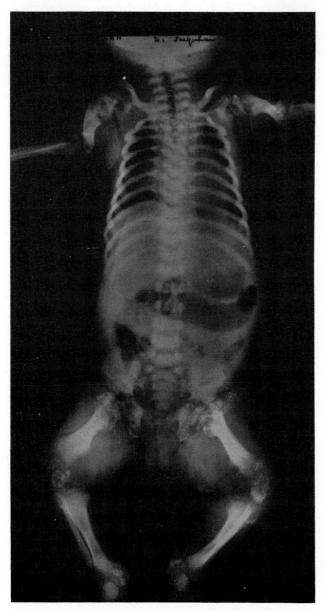

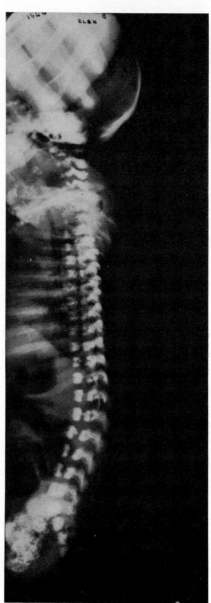

Fig. 2.3 (M.W.) Female infant (perinatal death) with severe rhizomelic form. The limb bones, particularly the humeri, are short and deformed and there is stippling around all joint areas and in the pelvis. (H.A.T.F.)

Fig. 2.4 (M.W.) Stippling in the region of the pelvis. The anterior and posterior ossification of the vertebral bodies with a clear space between, is well shown in the lumbar region. (H.A.T.F.)

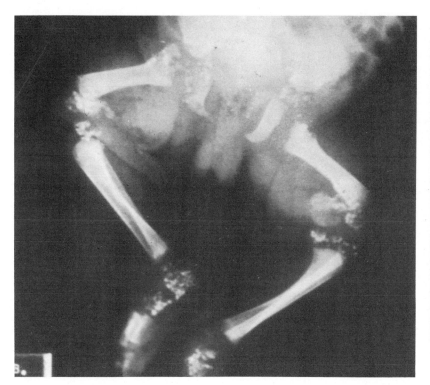

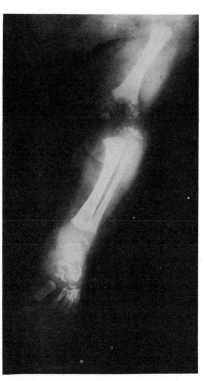

Fig. 2.5 (G.H.) Stippling around the lower limb joint areas. (H.A.T.F.)

Fig. 2.6 (L.J.) Stippling around the elbow, wrist and hand and some metaphyseal splaying. (H.A.T.F.)

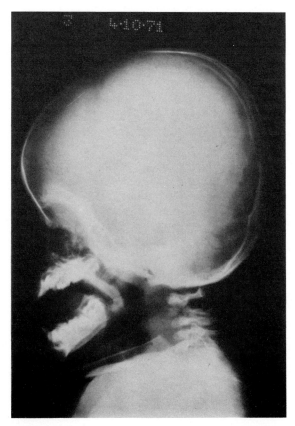

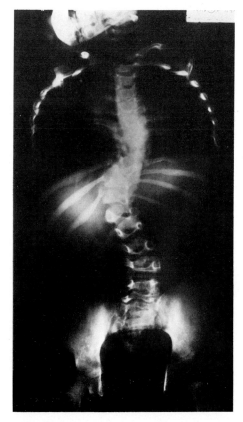

Fig. 2.7 (L.S.) An 18 month old female with the milder form of the disease. The nasal bridge is depressed and the skull round in shape, with premature fusion of sutures. (Courtesy of Professor J. I. P. James, Edinburgh.)

Fig. 2.8 (L.S.) A severe scoliosis for a child of eighteen months, associated with congenital vertebral anomalies. (Courtesy of Professor J. I. P. James, Edinburgh.)

3 Dysplasia Epiphysialis Hemimelica

In this disorder osteocartilaginous outgrowths are usually confined to the lateral or medial half of a single limb.

It was described by Trevor (1950) who called it tarso-epiphyseal aclasis and Fairbank (1956) who gave it the present title. A more recent review was by Kettlecamp, Campbell and Bonfiglio (1966). The first case was probably reported by Mouchet and Belot (1926), the condition being referred to by them as 'tarsomegaly'.

Aetiology. The cause is unknown. All cases appear to be sporadic.

Frequency. The population incidence is not known but the disorder is rare. Males are affected three times more commonly than females. The age of onset is usually in early childhood though cases as early as three months of age have been reported.

Clinical and radiographic features. The usual symptoms are of pain, deformity and swelling in the region of a joint, perhaps with restricted movement and locking. The commonest sites are in the region of the lower femoral epiphysis, the tarsus (particularly the talus) and the lower tibia, though many other areas have been reported, including the carpus. The exostoses project from sites normally occupied by epiphyseal cartilage and they can also protrude into the adjacent joint, producing secondary distortion of the opposing joint surface and later osteoarthritis. In two-thirds of cases lesions are multiple.

Frequently the outgrowth is confined to the lateral or medial half of a single limb but Luck and Smith (1972) point out that, particularly in the lower limb, there may be total involvement of an epiphysis. The medial side is involved twice as commonly as the lateral. In severe cases there may be some streaking of the metaphysis, reminiscent of Ollier's disease but this appears to be secondary to the epiphyseal distortion. There may also be local reduction of the rate of growth of the epiphyseal plate.

Pathology. The lesion is essentially one of abnormal cartilage proliferation in the region of an epiphysis, tarsal or carpal bone, with associated enchondral ossification. Microscopically it is indistinguishable from an osteocartilaginous exostosis with both a base and cap of hyaline cartilage. Within the affected area there may be multiple centres of ossification.

Differential diagnosis. The diagnosis is not usually in doubt, but in severe cases a disorder having some similarity is Ollier's disease though here the metaphyseal involvement is clear, and the epiphysis only involved if the adjacent metaphysis is severely affected. Multiple hereditary exostoses (diaphyseal aclasis) should be differentiated by the multiplicity of sites, normal epiphyses, frequently symmetrical involvement, and the family history of the condition.

Progress and complications. In dysplasia epiphysealis hemimelica the length of the limb is unaffected and the lesion usually stops growing when the child ceases growth, though there are some reports of increase in size during adult life. Fracture of the exostosis may occur and intra-articular loose bodies have been reported as well as secondary osteoarthritis, when an exostosis damages the adjacent articular cartilage. There have been no reports of malignant change but clearly there is a potential danger of this, and also the danger of 'over diagnosis' of malignant change.

Treatment. Surgery is required if the lesion is troublesome or is increasing in size during adult life, and repeated local excision is often needed.

REFERENCES

Fairbank, T. J. (1956). Dysplasia epiphysialis hemimelica (Tarso-epiphysial aclasis). *Journal of Bone & Joint Surgery*, **38B,** 237.

Kettlekamp, D. B., Campbell, C. J. & Bonfiglio, M. (1966). Dysplasia epiphsealis hemimelica. *Journal of Bone & Joint Surgery*, **48A,** 746.

Luck, V. J. & Smith, C. F. (1972). Dysplasia epiphysialis osteochondromata: 22 cases correlated with 70 cases in medical literature. *Journal of Bone & Joint Surgery*, **54A,** 1351.

Mouchet, A. & Belot, J. (1926). La tarsomégalie. *Journal de Radiologie et d'Electrologie*, **10,** 289.

Trevor, D. (1950). Tarso-epiphyseal aclasis: a congenital error of epiphysial development. *Journal of Bone & Joint Surgery*, **32B,** 204.

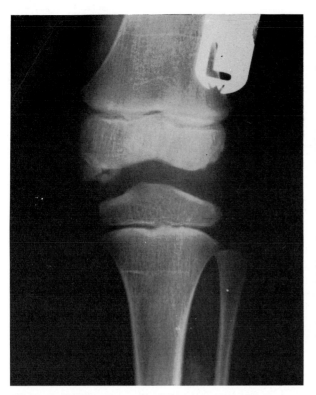

Fig. 3.1 (N.D.) An osteocartilaginous exostosis is developing on the inner side of the lower femoral epiphysis. (A.H.)

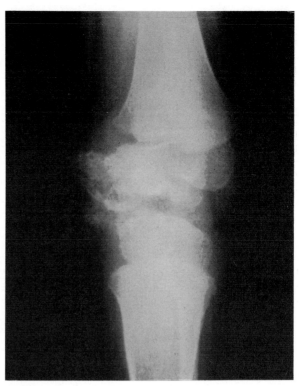

Fig. 3.2 (L.V.) A more severe lesion in an older child. (A.H.)

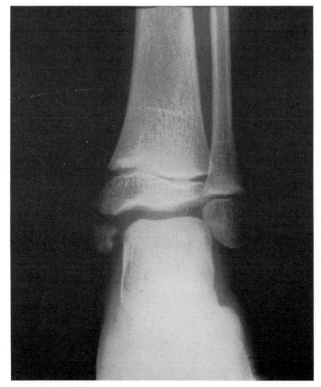

Fig. 3.3 (B.) Male aged 6 years with a lesion associated with medial side of lower tibial epiphysis. (A.H.)

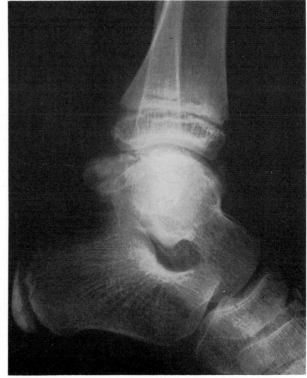

Fig. 3.4 (R.S.) Male aged 9 years with a lesion associated with the talus. (A.H.)

4 Hereditary Progressive Arthro-Ophthalmopathy

This condition is characterised by enlargement of joints with epiphyseal irregularity, together with progressive myopia leading to retinal detachment and blindness.

The disease was first described by Stickler *et al* (1965); and Stickler and Pugh (1967), who traced five generations of a family with 11 affected members.

Inheritance. It is of autosomal dominant inheritance.

Frequency. The population incidence is not known but Opitz *et al* (1972) stated that it was 'more common than the Marfan syndrome', and noted that the disorder is sometimes associated with the Pierre Robin syndrome and should be suspected in all such cases. The sexes are equally affected and the age of onset is during childhood.

Clinical and radiographic features. The presenting features to be seen in early childhood are enlargement of joints, particularly the knees, ankles and wrists, together with a high degree of myopia. This is progressive and leads to complete retinal detachment and associated chorioretinal degenerative changes. Associated features may be a cleft palate and conductive hearing loss.

Radiographic changes include enlarged and irregular epiphyses and the carpal and tarsal bones are also irregular though this is not specifically related to their joints. The vertebrae are a little flat with uneven epiphyseal surfaces, chiefly in the thoracic and upper lumbar region. Anterior wedging may be present causing thoracic kyphosis. The vertebral appearances are reminiscent of Scheuermann disease and also of Morquio disease.

Differential diagnosis. Multiple epiphyseal dysplasia is distinguished by its lack of eye signs and by the fact that the epiphyses are usually more severely affected at an earlier age. Spondyloepiphyseal dysplasia congenita is differentiated by the more severe spinal involvement, delayed ossification and dwarfism.

Progress and complications. The eye symptoms in progressive arthro-ophthalmopathy can be severe and it should be noted that this is a form of blindness which can be treated if diagnosed early. If severe secondary changes develop then enucleation may be required for the severe intractable pain of glaucoma. So far as the epiphyseal changes are concerned, this is not a very severe disorder, though premature osteoarthritis is to be expected.

Treatment. This relates to the eye complications and to the osteoarthritis.

REFERENCES

Opitz, J. M., France, T., Herrmann, J. & Spranger, J. W. (1972). The Stickler Syndrome. *New England Journal of Medicine*, **286**, 546.

Stickler, G. B., Belau, P. G., Farrell, F. J., Jones, J. D., Pugh, D. G., Steinberg, A. G. & Ward, L. M. (1965). Hereditary progressive arthro-ophthalmopathy. *Mayo Clinic Proceedings*, **40**, 433.

Stickler, G. B. & Pugh, D. G. (1967). Hereditary progressive arthro-ophthalmopathy. II. Additional observations on vertebral anomalies, a hearing defect, and a report of a similar case. *Mayo Clinic Proceedings*, **42**, 495.

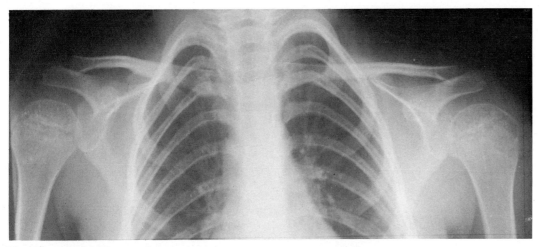

Fig. 4.1 (K.M.) Narrow chest and mild epiphyseal dysplasia. (G.O.S.)

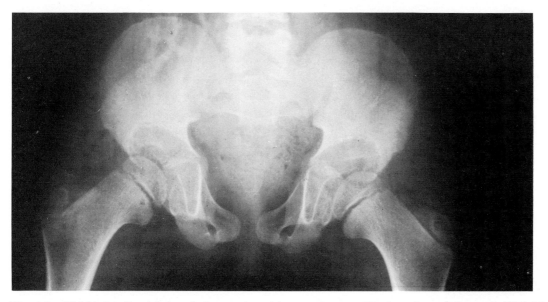

Fig. 4.2 (K.M.) Small pelvis in relation to size of femora. Poor ossification of acetabular roof. (G.O.S.)

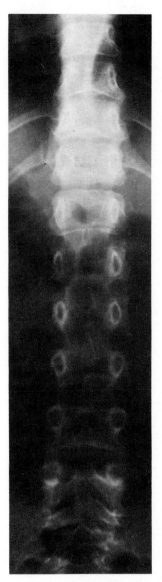

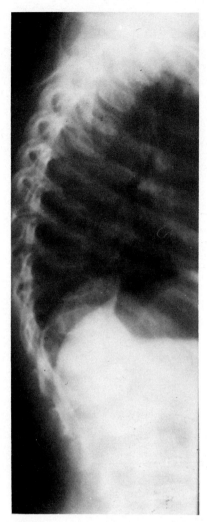

Fig. 4.4 (K.M.) Some flattening and irregularity of end plates. Thoracic kyphosis. (G.O.S.)

Fig. 4.3 (K.M.) Mild flattening of several vertebral bodies. (G.O.S.)

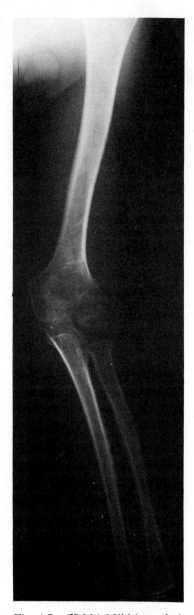

Fig. 4.5 (K.M.) Mild irregularity of articular surfaces and poor musculature, particularly in upper arm. (G.O.S.)

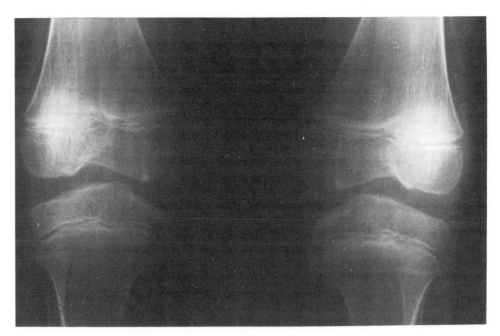

Fig. 4.6 (K.M.) Irregular defects of the articular surfaces. (G.O.S.)

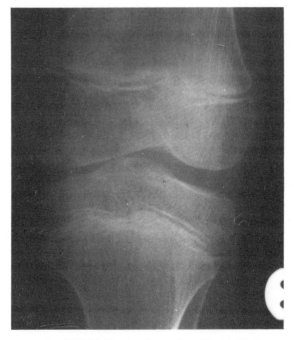

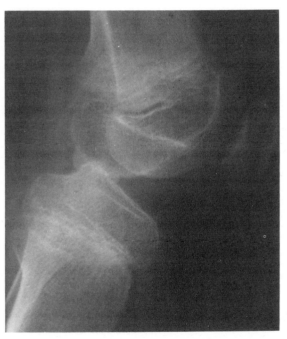

Fig. 4.7 (K.M.) (2 years later than Fig. 4.6.) Osteo-chondritis dissecans-like lesion. (G.O.S.)

Fig. 4.8 (K.M.) Marked irregularity of posterior surface of patella. (G.O.S.)

5 Achondroplasia
Classical Type

True achondroplasia is characterised by short limbs, a bulging cranium, low nasal bridge, narrowed spinal canal in the lumbar region and distinctive pelvic changes.

The term 'achondroplasia' has been used over the past century for a number of conditions with severely affected metaphyses and dwarfing and it is only recently that the true classical type of achondroplasia has been delineated.

Inheritance. Classical achondroplasia is of autosomal dominant inheritance but since most individuals with the disorder do not reproduce, most cases in the population are the outcome of new mutations. It is very rare for there to be more than two generations of a family affected. The condition shows a paternal age effect, fathers being older than average, the assumption being that there has been a spontaneous mutation in the sperm (Mørch 1941; Grebe 1955; Stevenson 1957 and Murdoch *et al*, 1970).

Hall *et al* (1969) have reported two possible cases of homozygosity for the achondroplasia gene: the infants born to parents who were both achondroplastic were a great deal more severely affected than usual and died soon after birth in respiratory failure. The histological report noted a failure of chondroblasts to proliferate, line up in columns or hypertrophy, and fibrotic tissue had been laid down instead of bone.

Frequency. The population prevalence of classical achondroplasia is thought to be between 2 and 3 per 100,000 in Europe. Surveys have been reported by Mørch (1941) from Denmark, Stevenson (1957) from Northern Ireland and Gardner (1975) from Edinburgh.

The sexes are equally affected. The condition can usually be diagnosed at birth and always becomes apparent during the first year of life.

Clinical and radiographic features. The short-limbed dwarf with a bulging forehead and lumbar lordosis is well known. These individuals are usually bright and intelligent. The head is disproportionately large and the depressed nasal bridge with a prominent frontal area is characteristic. The limb shortness is chiefly in the proximal segments and this is particularly obvious in the upper limb where the fingertips reach only to the iliac crest. There appears to be too much skin and soft tissue for the length of the limb bones, with resultant skin folds. The hands are podgy with short fingers and the so-called 'trident' appearance. There is frequently lack of full elbow extension and the marked lumbar lordosis is associated with flexion contracture of the hips. There is bowing of the lower limbs and a characteristic rolling gait.

On radiography the vault of the skull is enlarged and the base shortened. This results from continuing development of the vault without comparable growth of the base. Mild dilatation of the ventricles is usual but there is no other evidence of a raised intracranial pressure. The head growth curves parallel the normal, though at a higher level (Cohen, Rosenthal and Matson, 1967). There is sometimes significant hydrocephalus in classical achondroplasia and this is probably due to the reduced size of the foramen magnum leading to local obstruction here. The mandible is somewhat large compared with the other facial bones.

The cervical spine is often abnormal with occipitalisation of the first cervical vertebra and there may be instability at the atlanto-axial level. The lumbar spine is characteristic in that the interpedicular distances diminish from the first to last lumbar vertebrae. This sign is usually apparent at birth, though not invariably. The anteroposterior diameter of the spinal canal is reduced as a result of shortness of the pedicles, this becomes more marked as the child grows. On lateral radiographs of the spine the posterior border of the vertebral bodies is concave. Anterior wedging of the vertebrae at the thoracolumbar junction gives a characteristic kyphus at this level in infancy, but the sign does not persist. The thoracic cage is flattened in its anteroposterior diameter as a result of the ribs being shortened and the scapula appears 'cut off' at its inferior angle.

The characteristic shape of the pelvis is diagnostic in classical achondroplasia. The inferior margin of the ilium is horizontal rather than slanting and the iliac wings are almost square. The pelvic inlet is wide from side to side but with a narrowed anteroposterior diameter and the greater sciatic notch appears as only a slit. There is increased pelvic tilt with posterior displacement of the acetabulae—thus leading to the distinctive lumbar lordosis of these individuals, which is accentuated by the acute angulation between the lumbar spine and sacrum.

The long bones are short and thick, particularly the humerus, and the metaphyses flared with a V-shaped notch into which the epiphyseal plate fits. The proximal end of the femur is characteristic in the newborn child, being square with a radiolucent, oval-shaped area on anteroposterior view (Langer, Baumann and Gorlin, 1967). Coxa valga is often present, coxa vara never. In general, epiphyses are not affected nor is osteoarthritis of peripheral joints a feature.

Pathology. Most histological reports of supposed achondroplasia are likely to be autopsy reports of other short-limbed dwarfs suffering from unrelated lethal dysplasias. However Ponseti (1970) studied classical achondroplasia from biopsies of cartilage from the iliac crest and upper fibular epiphyseal plates. Iliac crest cartilage and its growth plate were nearly normal. The fibular growth plate had cartilage cell clusters separated by wide septa of fibrous matrix which appeared to be very slowly resorbed. Bone was formed normally in the iliac wings, in the fibula head at the insertions of tendons and ligaments, and in the periosteal region. The abnormalities were associated with the *metaphyseal* area only.

Differential diagnosis. At birth, classical achondroplasia must be distinguished from lethal forms of short-limbed dwarfism. Thanatophoric dwarfism and achondrogenesis are more severe with extremely short limbs and short ribs. During childhood, achondroplasia can be confused with hypochondroplasia, but this condition is less severe and patients do not have the characteristic skull and pelvic changes. Pseudo-achondroplasia is superficially similar but here the skull is normal: there is severely disordered epiphyseal as well as metaphyseal ossification and the shape of the vertebral bodies is distinctive.

Progress and complications. The average adult height in classical achondroplasia is: males 131 cms (4′3½″) and females 124 cms (4′1″), or even less. This is the standing height. The sitting height, however, is in or above the 10th percentile value for normal children (Ponseti, 1970). Life expectancy is normal.

The complications of achondroplasia arise chiefly from the abnormalities of skeletal growth in the vertebral column. Bailey (1970) has reported spinal malalignment in 70 per cent of cases, with serious neurological problems in 12 per cent (either spinal cord or nerve root signs). Symptoms do not usually arise until adult life although mild kyphosis and scoliosis may be noted in childhood. Prolapsed intervertebral disc occurs; the spinal stenosis in the lumbar region may give rise to serious problems, and the vertebral column is the one area in the body where degenerative arthritis is found early (Nelson, 1972). In general, osteoarthritis is not a feature of classical achondroplasia.

Obstetric complications may arise in relation to the narrowed pelvis and Caesarean section is likely to be required.

Treatment. This is related chiefly to complications which arise from the spine and to the occasional hydrocephalus.

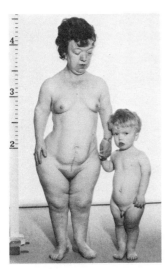

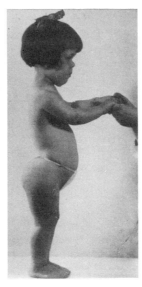

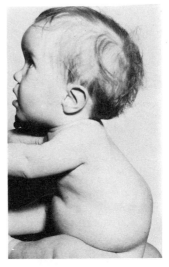

Fig. 5.1 (E. & J. McC.) Mother and son with classical achondroplasia illustrating its dominant inheritance. The upper limbs reach only just past the iliac crest. (Courtesy of Mr A. G. Apley, Pyrford.)

Fig. 5.2 (A.M.) Note the bulging forehead, depressed nasal bridge and lumbar lordosis. (H.A.T.F.)

Fig. 5.3 (H.) In the infant of a few months old there is a characteristic thoracolumbar kyphus, a sign which does not persist as the child grows. (Courtesy of Mr A. G. Apley, Pyrford.)

REFERENCES

Bailey, J. A. (1970). Orthopaedic aspects of achondroplasia. *Journal of Bone & Joint Surgery*, **52A,** 1285.

Cohen, M. E., Rosenthal, A. D. & Matson, D. D. (1967). Neurological abnormalities in achondroplastic children. *Journal of Pediatrics*, **71,** 367.

Gardner, R. J. M. (1975). Congenital chondrodysplastic short limbed dwarfism in Edinburgh. M.Sc. dissertation. University of Edinburgh.

Grebe, H. (1955). *Chondrodysplasia.* Instituto G. Mendel, Rome.

Hall, J. G., Dorst, J. P., Taybi, H., Scott, C. I., Langer, L. O. & McKusick, V. A. (1969). Two probable cases of homozygosity for the achondroplasia gene. *Birth Defects Original Article Series 5*, Part 4, 24.

Langer, L. O., Baumann, P. A. & Gorlin, R. J. (1967). Achondroplasia. *American Journal of Roentgenology*, **100,** 12.

Mørch, E. T. (1941). *Chondrodystrophic Dwarfs in Denmark*, 3, Munksgaard, Copenhagen.

Murdoch, J. L., Walker, B. A., Hall, J. G., Abbey, H., Smith, K. K. & McKusick, V. A. (1970). Achondroplasia—a genetic and statistical survey. *Annals of Human Genetics*, **33,** 227.

Ponseti, I. V. (1970). Skeletal growth in achondroplasia. *Journal of Bone & Joint Surgery*, **52A,** 701.

Stevenson, A. C. (1957). Achondroplasia: an account of the condition in Northern Ireland. *American Journal of Human Genetics*, **9,** 81.

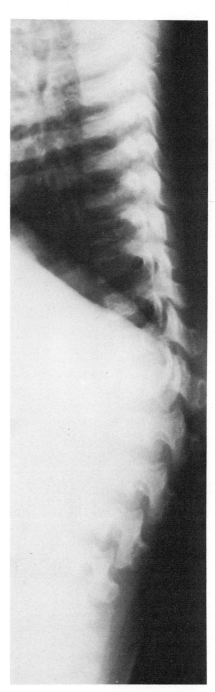

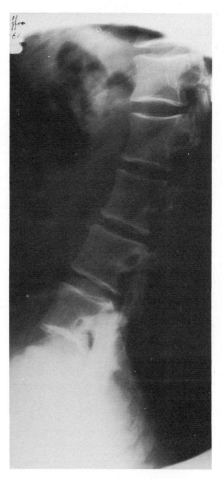

Fig. 5.5 (G.K.) In this adult the vertebrae are of normal height but there is concavity of the posterior borders associated with shortening of the pedicles. (A.H.)

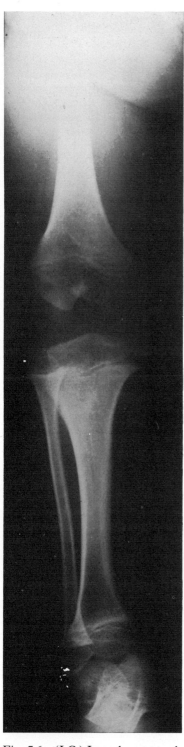

Fig. 5.4 (H.) A lumbar kyphus, shortness of pedicles with a concave posterior border of the vertebral bodies is already seen in early infancy. (Courtesy of Mr A. G. Apley, Pyrford.)

Fig. 5.6 (J.C.) Long bones are short and thick with flared metaphyses. At the lower end of the femur the V-shaped notch into which the epiphysis fits is clearly shown. (P.M.R.)

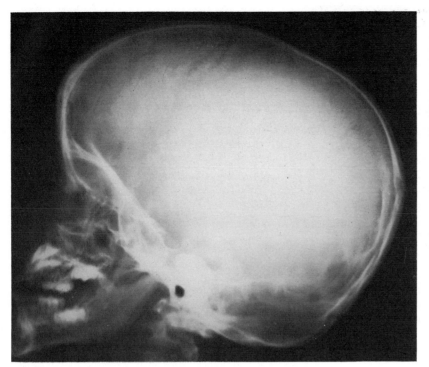

Fig. 5.7 Vault of skull enlarged in comparison with short base. (Courtesy of Mr A. G. Apley, Pyrford.)

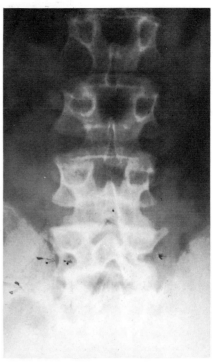

Fig. 5.8 (G.B.) The narrowing of the inter-pedicular distance from the upper to lower lumbar vertebrae is shown. This is a particularly severe example. (A.H.)

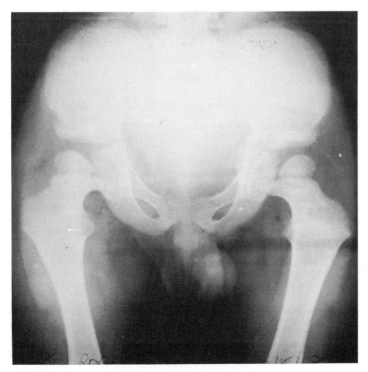

Fig. 5.9 (R.) Iliac wings are almost square and inferior margin of ilium horizontal. The greater sciatic notch appears as only a slit. The upper femoral epiphyses are normal but the neck of the femur has a beaked appearance. (H.A.T.F.)

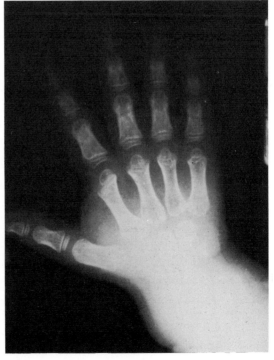

Fig. 5.10 (J.C.) The fingers are not markedly short, the most obvious changes being in the proximal and middle phalanges which are broader than normal. (P.M.R.)

6 Hypochondroplasia

This condition is similar to classical achondroplasia but less severe, particularly with regard to the skull and pelvic changes.

The term was first used by Ravenna (1913) and the condition fully described by Lamy and Maroteaux (1961).

Inheritance. It is likely to be of autosomal dominant inheritance (Beals, 1969; Hall, 1969), but not a great deal of family data is yet available. Since both achondroplasia and hypochondroplasia appear to breed true, they cannot be variations of a single disorder. McKusick, Kelly and Dorst (1973) have suggested there are two alleles at the achondroplasia locus, one for achondroplasia and the other for hypochondroplasia. Homozygosity for classical achondroplasia leads to a lethal skeletal dysplasia, but these authors have reported a child who is possibly a genetic compound of the two, her father having achondroplasia and her mother hypochondroplasia.

Frequency. The population incidence is not known but hypochondroplasia may be a fairly common disorder, individuals being regarded as merely having 'short stature'. The condition cannot be diagnosed at birth or in early infancy and the child is usually of school age before it is apparent.

Clinical and radiographic features. These individuals are short but not so markedly as those with classical achondroplasia. Slight lumbar lordosis, some generalised joint laxity and bow legs in childhood have been reported (Beals, 1969). As in achondroplasia the lumbar lordosis may be more apparent than real, the prominent buttocks being attributable to the acute angle between the sacrum and lumbar spine.

The radiographic appearances are similar to those of classical achondroplasia but less severe in degree. The skull may be normal or have a slightly prominent frontal area. The vertebral column is normal apart from a slightly reduced interpedicular distance in the lumbar region. The sacrum is inclined to be horizontal. The long bones have flared metaphyses and are somewhat short although there is no major asymmetry in relation to the trunk. Minor anomalies include limitation of elbow movement, shortening of the ulna, and an elongated distal end of the fibula. The pelvis is essentially normal, although the sciatic notches are rather small.

Differential diagnosis. This is chiefly from classical achondroplasia, the characteristic skull and pelvic changes in the latter being the best guides. The long bones in hypochondroplasia are a little similar to those seen in the Schmid type of metaphyseal chondrodysplasia but there are no vertebral changes in this condition. In dyschondrosteosis the forearm deformity is more marked.

Progress and complications. There are no symptoms and life expectancy is normal. The adult height is between 127 and 152 cms (4'2" to 5').

REFERENCES

Beals, R. K. (1969). Hypochondroplasia: report of 5 kindreds. *Journal of Bone & Joint Surgery,* **51A,** 728.
Hall, J. G. (1969). Hypochondroplasia. *Birth Defects Original Article Series 5,* part 4, 267.
Lamy, M. & Maroteaux, P. (1961). Les chondrodystrophies genotypiques. *L'Expansion scientifique française,* Paris.
McKusick, V. A., Kelly, T. E. & Dorst, J. P. (1973). Observations suggesting allelism of the achondroplasia and hypochondroplasia genes. *Journal of Medical Genetics,* **10,** 11.
Ravenna, F. (1913). Achondroplasie et chondrohypoplasie. Contribution clinique. *Nouvelle Iconographie de la Salpêtrière Clinique des Maladies du Système Nerveux,* **26,** 157.

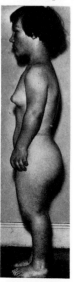

Fig. 6.1 (A.S.) The limb shortening is similar to classical achondroplasia but not so severe and the head is normal. (Courtesy of Mr A. G. Apley, Pyrford.)

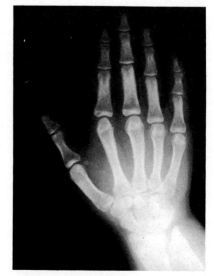

Fig. 6.2 (M.R. aged 14 years.) The wrist and hand are almost normal, though some of the proximal and middle phalanges are broad and the styloid process of the ulna is prominent. (P.M.R.)

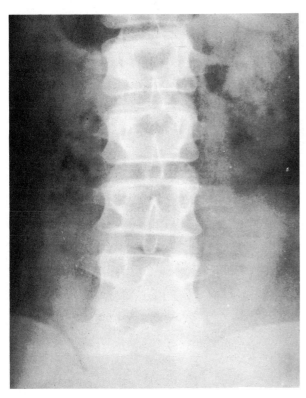

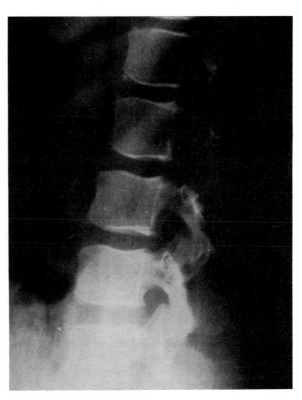

Fig. 6.3 (M.R. aged 11 years.) The interpedicular distance does not narrow from the first to last vertebra, but neither does it widen as in the normal individual. (P.M.R.)

Fig. 6.4 (M.R. aged 11 years.) Posterior borders of vertebral bodies are slightly concave and the pedicles somewhat short, though not so markedly as in achondroplasia. (P.M.R.)

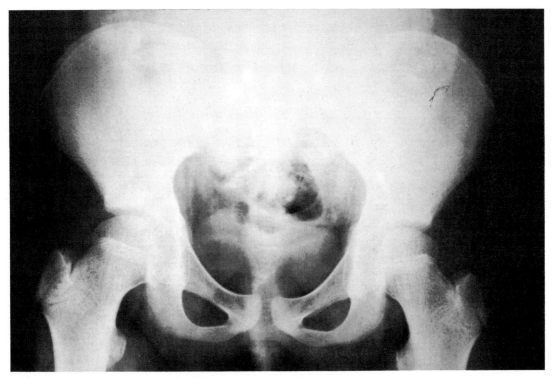

Fig. 6.5 (M.R. aged 11 years.) The pelvis is essentially normal. (P.M.R.)

7   Lethal Forms of Short-limbed Dwarfism

In the past many forms of short-limbed dwarfism were classified as 'achondroplasia', but in recent years there has been greatly increased interest and knowledge concerning these skeletal dysplasias and it is now clear that many of the suspect infants, stillborn or dying in the perinatal period, are clinically and genetically distinct from classical achondroplasia. It is important to make this distinction in view of the different prognosis and genetic counselling.

THANATOPHORIC DWARFISM

This was originally reported by Maroteaux, Lamy and Robert (1967), who collected 21 cases between 1898 and 1967. Since then a number of authors have reviewed past 'achondroplasia' records and found that the condition is not particularly rare (Langer *et al*, 1969; Keats, Riddervold and Michealis, 1970; Shah, Astley and Cameron, 1973; Cremin and Beighton, 1974).

Inheritance. Most cases described have been sporadic but it is possible the disorder is of autosomal recessive inheritance, many cases aborting early in pregnancy. There is no evidence for autosomal dominant inheritance, as in classical achondroplasia.

Frequency. The population incidence is probably about 3 per million total births which is about as common as classical achondroplasia itself (Gardner, 1975). There is a preponderance of males. The condition can be diagnosed prenatally and is immediately apparent at birth.

Clinical and radiographic features. These children have extreme shortness of limbs, much more so than in classical achondroplasia, but the trunk is of normal length. The thorax is very narrow, both in the lateral and anteroposterior diameters. Other features are similar to achondroplasia in that there is a short base to the skull with prominent frontal bones and depressed bridge of the nose.

Radiographic features include characteristically very short ribs, not extending beyond the axillary line and extreme flatness of the vertebrae with wide intervertebral spaces and a notch-like defect in the centre of both upper and lower epiphyseal plates. The interpedicular distances narrow from the first to fifth lumbar vertebrae as in classical achondroplasia.

The epiphyses of all limb bones are absent at birth and the extremely short long bones are characteristic. The femur in particular is curved as well as very short. Metaphyses are wide and irregular.

Pathology. There is gross retardation of cartilage maturation, no regular cell columns, and general disruption of enchondral ossification. There is more intercellular matrix than normal.

Differential diagnosis. This is from other forms of

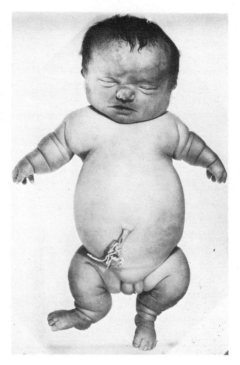

Fig. 7.1   Stillborn thanatophoric dwarf. Limbs extremely short, trunk normal length. (P.M.R.)

congenital short-limbed dwarfism. Classical achondroplasia is not invariably apparent at birth, the vertebrae are not flat and the long bones not so short, bowed or flared. Achondrogenesis is differentiated by a short trunk and absent ossification in the lower vertebral column and pelvis. The short-rib/polydactyly syndromes do not have such markedly short limbs and polydactyly is present.

Progress and complications. These infants are stillborn or die in the first few hours of life from cardiorespiratory failure, due to the extremely narrow rib cage with little space for lungs to expand.

ACHONDROGENESIS

This condition was probably first described by Parenti in 1936 and more fully by Maroteaux and Lamy (1968). Like thanatophoric dwarfism the condition is lethal, the infants being stillborn or dying very shortly after birth. It is likely that it is less common than either achondroplasia or thanatophoric dwarfism and there may be more than one type (Spranger, Langer and Wiedemann, 1974).

Inheritance. The condition is of autosomal recessive inheritance (Scott, 1972; Houston, Awen and Kent, 1972).

Clinical and radiographic features. The trunk is

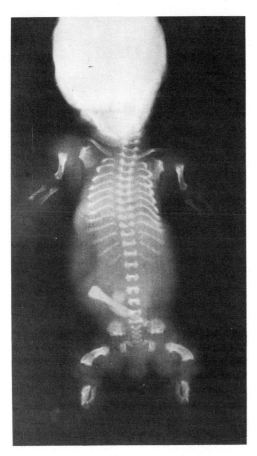

Fig. 7.2 Thanatophoric dwarf. Narrow chest with short ribs; notching of vertebral bodies with wide intervertebral space: extremely short long bones with characteristic curved femora. (Courtesy of Dr R. G. M. Gardner, Edinburgh.)

short as well as the limbs, but the thorax is not so narrow as in thanatophoric dwarfism. However, the clinical features of the two disorders do overlap and it is on radiographic examination that they are differentiated (Saldino, 1971). The most obvious feature is that the whole skeleton is poorly ossified, with complete failure of ossification in the lumbar and sacral spine and the pubic bones. The iliac bones are small but the sacro-iliac notch is not narrowed. The metaphyseal ends of the long bones are much enlarged.

Pathology. The resting cartilage appears markedly hypercellular with large hollowed chondrocytes and little matrix. There is no formation of columns and enchondral ossification is completely disorganised.

Differential diagnosis. This is from other lethal forms of short-limbed dwarfism.

Progress. All are born dead or die shortly after birth.

ASPHYXIATING THORACIC DYSTROPHY
(*Jeune Disease*)

This condition was first described by Jeune *et al* (1954); it is characterised by a narrowed thoracic cage together with some shortening of limbs, with or without post-axial polydactyly.

Inheritance. It is of autosomal recessive inheritance. The condition was first described in two sibs, and there have been subsequent reports of this (Shokeir, Houston and Awen, 1971).

Clinical and radiographic features. The chief feature is the long, narrow cylindrical thorax, small both in the transverse and anteroposterior diameters. The lower ribs may be flared. The chest is relatively immobile and there is a high incidence of death in infancy due to respiratory insufficiency. The limbs are short but not very markedly so.

Radiographic changes include enlarged epiphyses of the long bones, similar to those found in the Ellis van Creveld syndrome but the bones are of more nearly normal length. There are metaphyseal irregularities and the hands are characteristic in that there is postaxial polydactyly (with or without an extra metacarpal) and the middle and terminal phalanges are short. If the child survives infancy, then cone-shaped epiphyses of the phalanges develop.

The pelvis has short, square iliac wings, a short ischium and pubis and there are spur-like downward projections of the medial and lateral aspects of the acetabular roof.

Pathology. This is non-specific. The epiphyseal and metaphyseal changes are indistinguishable from classical achondroplasia, though milder in extent.

Differential diagnosis. This is from other lethal forms of short-limbed dwarfism, and from the Ellis van Creveld syndrome which is also characterised by post-axial polydactyly. However, in the latter condition there are ectodermal (hair, nail and teeth) changes, congenital heart defects and the capitate and hamate bones are often fused.

Progress and complications. These children frequently die in the perinatal period from respiratory failure, but if they live the thoracic size tends to improve with growth. No deaths from respiratory failure have been noted after the age of 2 years (Langer, 1969).

Shokeir and colleagues and Langer have noted that kidney defects are common and progressive renal failure with secondary hypertension may develop. This is a form of hereditary nephritis with renal interstitial fibrosis and atrophy. Kidneys with persistent foetal lobulation and bilateral polycystic disease have also been reported.

The final height of these children is probably below the third percentile.

SHORT-RIB POLYDACTYLY SYNDROMES MAJEWSKI AND SALDINO–NOONAN TYPES

These appear to be clinically distinct varieties of short-limbed dwarfs, both types being either stillborn or dying in the perinatal period. The Majewski type was described by him and colleagues in 1971 and the Saldino–Noonan type in 1972. The two syndromes have been reviewed by Spranger *et al* (1974).

Inheritance. The Saldino–Noonan type was described in two stillborn sibs and is likely to be of autosomal recessive inheritance. The aetiology of the Majewski type is not known.

Clinical and radiographic features. Both are characterised by very short ribs and a narrow thorax. The polydactyly may be pre- or post-axial, though in the Saldino–Noonan type it is usually post-axial. Cardiovascular, renal and genital anomalies are common, and in the Saldino–Noonan syndrome the short, ragged-ended long bones are characteristic, in contrast to the Majewski type where the ends of long bones are smooth and rounded.

Differential diagnosis. This is from other forms of lethal short-limbed dwarfism.

Progress and complications. Death occurs early from respiratory failure and multiple internal anomalies.

REFERENCES

Bouvet, J. P., Maroteaux, P. & Feingold, J. (1974). Étude génétique du nanisme thanatophore. *Annales de Génétique,* **17,** 181.

Cremin, B. J. & Beighton, P. (1974). Dwarfism in the newborn: the nomenclature, radiological features and genetic significance. *British Journal of Radiology,* **47,** 77.

Gardner, R. J. M. (1975). Congenital chondrodysplastic short-limbed dwarfism in Edinburgh. *MSc. Dissertation, University of Edinburgh.*

Houston, C. S., Awen, C. F. & Kent, H. P. (1972). Fatal neonatal dwarfism. *Journal of the Canadian Association of Radiologists,* **23,** 45.

Jeune, M., Carron, R., Beraud, C. & Loaec, Y. (1954). Polychondrodystrophie avec blocage thoracique d'évolution fatale. *Pédiatrie,* **9,** 390.

Keats, T. E., Riddervold, H. O. & Michaelis, L. L. (1970). Thanatophoric dwarfism. *American Journal of Roentgenology,* **108,** 473.

Langer, L. O. (1969). The thoracic-pelvic-phalangeal dystrophy. *Birth Defects Original Article Series 5,* Part 4, 55.

Langer, L. O., Spranger, J. W., Greinacher, I. & Herdman, R. C. (1969). Thanatophoric dwarfism. *Radiology,* **92,** 285.

Majewski, F., Pfeiffer, R. A., Lenz, W., Müller, R., Feil, G. & Seiler, R. (1971). Polysyndaktylie, verkürzte gliedmassen und genitalfehlbildungen: Kennzeichen eines selbständigen syndromes? *Zeitschrift für Kinderheilkunde,* **111,** 118.

Maroteaux, P., Lamy, M. & Robert, J. M. (1967). Le nanisme thanatophore. *La Presse Médicale,* **75,** 2519.

Maroteaux, P. & Lamy, M. (1968). Le diagnostic des nanismes chondrodystrophiques chez les nouveaux-nés. *Archives Françaises de Pédiatrie,* **25,** 241.

Parenti, G. C. (1936). La anosteogenesi. Una varieta della osteogenesi imperfecta. *Pathologica,* **28,** 447.

Saldino, R. M. (1971). Lethal short-limbed dwarfism: achondrogenesis and thanatophoric dwarfism. *American Journal of Roentgenology,* **112,** 185.

Saldino, R. M. & Noonan, C. D. (1972). Severe thoracic dystrophy with striking micromelia, abnormal osseus development, including the spine, and multiple visceral anomalies. *American Journal of Roentgenology,* **114,** 257.

Scott, C. I. (1972). Chapter 7 in *Progress in Medical Genetics,* eds. Steinberg, A. G. & Bearn, A. G., volume 8, Grune and Stratton, New York.

Shah, K., Astley, R. & Cameron, A. H. (1973). Thanatophoric dwarfism. *Journal of Medical Genetics,* **10,** 243.

Shokeir, M. H. K., Houston, C. S. & Awen, C. F. (1971). Asphyxiating thoracic chondrodystrophy: association with renal disease and evidence for possible heterozygous expression. *Journal of Medical Genetics,* **8,** 107.

Spranger, J., Grimm, B., Weller, M., Weissenbacher, G., Hermann, J., Gilbert, E. & Krepler, R. (1974). Short rib-polydactyly (SRP) syndromes, types Majewski and Saldino–Noonan. *Zeitschrift für Kinderheilkunde,* **116,** 73.

Spranger, J. W., Langer, L. O. & Wiedemann, H. R. (1974). *Bone Dysplasias: An Atlas of Constitutional Disorders of Skeletal Development.* W. B. Saunders Company: Philadelphia.

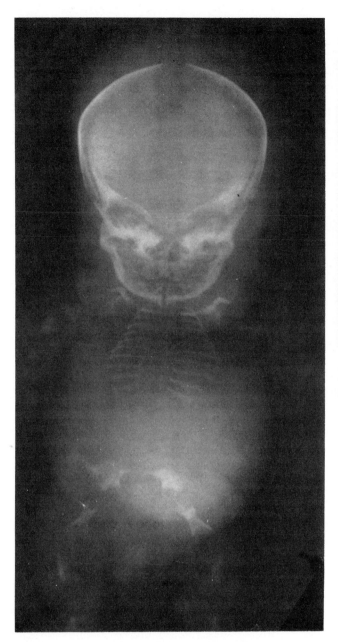

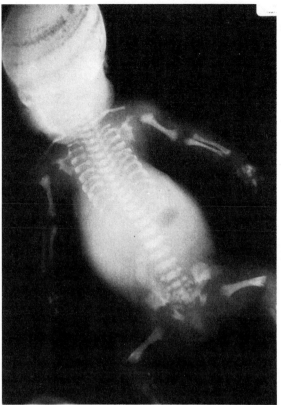

Fig. 7.4 Jeune disease. Short limbs with long narrow cylindrical thorax. (Courtesy of Dr R. G. M. Gardner, Edinburgh.)

Fig. 7.3 (K.T.) Achondrogenesis. The trunk is short and limbs even shorter than in thanatophoric dwarfism. Complete failure of ossification in lumbar and sacral spine and pubic bones. (G.O.S.)

8 Chondro-ectodermal Dysplasia
Ellis-van Creveld Syndrome

This type of short-limbed dwarfism is associated with post-axial polydactyly and disordered growth of the hair, nails and teeth and is often accompanied by congenital heart disease. The first report was by Ellis and van Creveld in 1940 and subsequently there was a review of 38 patients by Ellis and Andrew (1962). McKusick *et al* (1964) discovered an exceptionally high frequency of the condition amongst the Amish; a markedly inbred religious isolate descended from Swiss immigrants, 80 per cent of whom now live in Pennslyvania, Ohio and Indiana.

Inheritance. The condition is of autosomal recessive inheritance. In Ellis and van Creveld's first report of three cases, two had parents who were first cousins, and in the subsequent 1962 report there was consanguinity in 9 of 33 marriages. Murdoch and Walker (1969) noted 61 cases of chondro-ectodermal dysplasia amongst the Amish of Lancaster County, Pennsylvania. They were distributed amongst 33 sib-ships, 59 of the 200 children (58·5 per cent) being affected. Their figures confirm the hypothesis of autosomal recessive inheritance.

Frequency. The disorder appears to be very rare in Britain and Europe, the 61 American cases amongst the religious isolate of 9,000 individuals being quite exceptional. The disorder is apparent at birth.

Clinical and radiographic features. The shortness of the limbs is chiefly in the distal part (the forearms and legs, unlike classical achondroplasia). The polydactyly is usually only of the hand and is on the post-axial (little finger) side. There may be neonatal teeth, and other disorders such as absent or small teeth, delayed eruption, and an underdeveloped mandible. There is a characteristic minor deformity in which the upper lip is 'tied' to the alveolar ridge and a so-called partial hare lip—a small central cleft of the upper lip. Nails are small, ill-formed, perhaps ridged or even absent. The hair may be normal but has also been reported as thin and sparse. The skin is not otherwise involved and sweating is normal. Congenital heart defects may be present; usually this is an atrioseptal defect of either the ostium secundum or ostium primum.

Radiographs confirm the shortening of the distal limb segments and post-axial polydactyly (the extra digit may or may not contain bone). Metaphyseal borders are rounded and the humerus and femur may be bowed and thickened.

The pelvis is characteristic in infancy and early childhood with its decreased height of the iliac bones and a downward directed hook-like projection in the area of the medial, and sometimes lateral, aspects of the acetabulum, as in asphyxiating thoracic dysplasia.

The upper end of the tibia is characteristic with a defect in growth on the lateral side of the epiphysis and metaphysis, with the epiphysis apparently placed too far medially. The subsequent genu valgum deformity may be very severe.

The head of the radius may be dislocated, the radius flared distally, and fusion of the capitate and hamate bones is common. In the older child cone-shaped epiphyses in the middle and terminal phalanges may be seen.

Pathology. The cartilage cells maintain a parallel arrangement but are disordered and fewer than normal in number.

Differential diagnosis. In the neonatal period this is from asphyxiating thoracic dystrophy and other forms of lethal short-limbed dwarfism. The chief guide is the severe hypoplasia of the nails and the short fused upper lip which are present only in chondro-ectodermal dysplasia. In childhood the short distal limb segments, the deformity of the upper tibia and the fused capitate and hamate bones differentiate chondro-ectodermal dysplasia from other short-limbed dwarfs.

Progress and complications. About half these children die in infancy from respiratory difficulties and cardiac complications. Those that survive are not severely handicapped and may reach near normal height (107–160 cm; 3'6" to 5'3"). The chest and pelvis tend to become normal during childhood.

Treatment. This is directed to the teeth anomalies, polydactyly and the cardiac disorder.

REFERENCES

Ellis, R. W. B. & van Creveld, S. (1940). A syndrome characterised by ectodermal dysplasia, polydactyly, chondrodysplasia and congenital morbus cordis. *Archives of Diseases in Childhood,* **15,** 65.

Ellis, R. W. B. & Andrew, J. D. (1962). Chondro-ectodermal dysplasia. *Journal of Bone & Joint Surgery,* **44B,** 626.

McKusick, V. A., Egeland, J. A., Eldridge, R. & Krusen, D. E. (1964). Dwarfism in the Amish: I. The Ellis van Creveld syndrome. *Bulletin of the Johns Hopkins Hospital,* **115,** 306.

Murdoch, J. L. & Walker, B. A. (1969). Ellis van Creveld syndrome. *Birth Defects Original Article Series 5,* Part 4, 279.

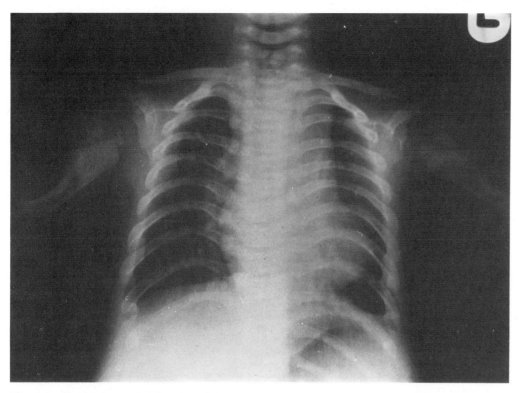

Fig. 8.1 Shortening and deformity of the humerus is seen and marked enlargement of the heart. (P.M.R.)

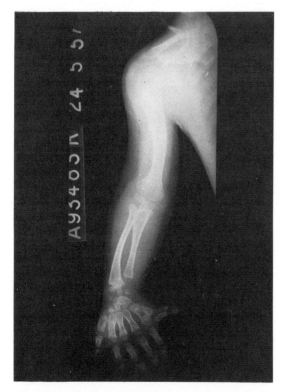

Fig. 8.2 The limb shortening is mainly of the distal segment. Post-axial polydactyly and the capitate and hamate bones are fused. (P.M.R.)

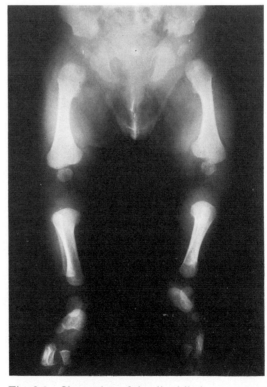

Fig. 8.3 Shortening of the distal limb segment and the bones are somewhat thickened. There is a hook-like projection of the ilium in the region of the triradiate cartilage. (P.M.R.)

9 The Metaphyseal Chondrodysplasias

The clinical types and classification of disorders affecting the metaphyses are in a considerable state of confusion. An increasing number of different varieties are being reported and both clinical and genetic delineation is frequently uncertain. There are many reports of single families with a 'new' type of disorder and these will not be described in detail here. The subject has been well reviewed by Sutcliffe and Stanley (1973).

METAPHYSEAL CHONDRODYSPLASIA— TYPE JANSEN (*Metaphyseal dysostosis*)

These patients are severely deformed with a short-limbed type of dwarfism, joint contractures of the hips and knees and expanded, cystic metaphyseal areas in all bones.

The first patient was described by Jansen (1934) and there have been only a few reported since then, including a follow-up of Jansen's original case by Haas, Boer and Griffioen (1969).

Inheritance. Most cases described have been sporadic but the condition may be of dominant inheritance since Lenz (1969) has referred to an affected mother and daughter.

Frequency. The condition is extremely rare, and is either apparent at birth or becomes so during infancy.

Clinical and radiographic features. This description of the clinical and radiographic features is taken mainly from Jansen's original case and from those described by Cameron, Young and Sissons (1954); Gram *et al* (1959) and Arroyo-Scotoliff (1973).

These children are severely dwarfed and may have widely spaced exophthalmic eyes, fronto-nasal hyperplasia and prominence of the superciliary arches. All limb bones are short but it is mainly the forearms and legs which are affected, these being curved. There are contractures of hip and knee joints.

The skull is not always severely affected but it may be brachycephalic with a short base and in one infant the calvarium was noted to have a peculiar reticular pattern. As the child grows the walls and base become thicker but the air sinuses remain small. The mandible may be hypoplastic. The vertebral column is normal, though scoliosis may develop.

The most striking feature is to be found in the metaphyses which are expanded, cystic and fragmented. In early infancy the changes are similar to those of rickets with cortical erosion, subperiosteal bone formation and wide cupping of the metaphyseal region (Holt, 1969). The epiphyses are normal though they may be delayed in appearance and widely separated from the metaphyses. The diaphysis is normal. The hands and feet are markedly affected and there may be clubfoot.

Pathology. Histology shows irregular masses of abnormal cartilage with hardly any enchondral ossification. The block in maturation appears to be at the level of vacuolated cartilage, and there are scanty, degenerate chondrocytes arranged in small clusters instead of rows.

Differential diagnosis. The fully developed case of metaphyseal chondrodysplasia type Jansen is very striking and unlikely to be confused with any other disorder except perhaps Ollier's dyschondroplasia, but in this latter condition there are no skull changes, the limb lesions are characteristically asymmetrical, and individuals are not severely dwarfed.

Progress and complications. Haas and colleagues in 1969, following up Jansen's original case, noted that there was a tendency to spontaneous improvement, although the individual was deaf. The radiographic appearance of the long bones was much improved, and the adult height about 125 cms (4′1″).

Clinical chemistry. In several patients hypercalcaemia has been reported, but this does not appear to produce any symptoms. A rise in alkaline phosphatase during growth has also been noted, but there are no other biochemical abnormalities.

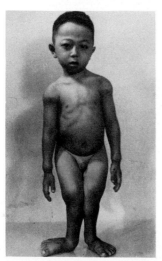

Fig. 9.1 (T.H.L. aged 7 years. Type Jansen.) Head and trunk are normal, deformities being only in the limbs. (Figs 9.1–9.5 by courtesy of Professor H. Sissons, London. Illustrations also in the HATF collection.)

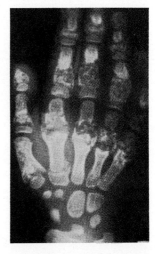

Fig. 9.2 (T.H.L.) Striking abnormality of the metaphyses which are expanded and fragmented.

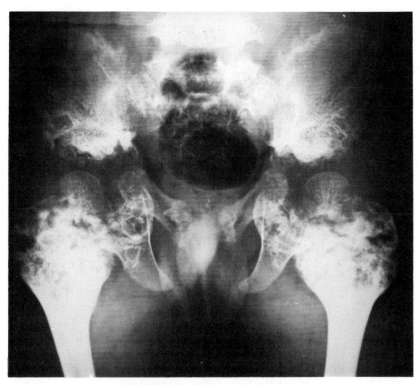

Fig. 9.3 (T.H.L.) The dysplasia affects principally the acetabular region of the pelvis and there is ballooning of the metaphyseal area of the femora. The capital femoral epiphyses are normal.

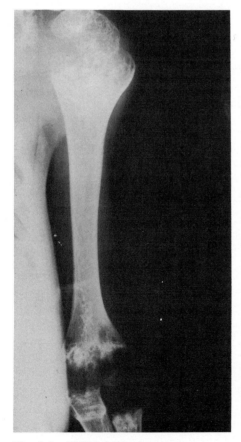

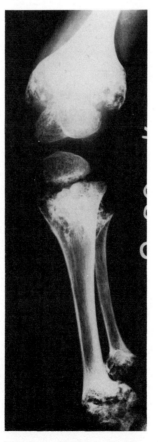

Fig. 9.4 (T.H.L.) The humeral metaphysis is ballooned in the same way as the femoral, the lower end of the humerus is ragged; epiphyses are normal.

Fig. 9.5 (T.H.L.) Similar enlarged, blotchy metaphyseal areas are seen around knee and ankle.

METAPHYSEAL CHONDRODYSPLASIA—TYPE SCHMID

This condition is considerably less severe than the Jansen type. There is some shortness of stature and the metaphyseal defect is chiefly in the lower limbs, usually affecting the hip to a greater extent than the knee, though bow legs are usual.

It was first described by Schmid (1949) subsequently by Maroteaux and Lamy (1958), and since then by many authors, though the severity of reported cases varies and the radiographic findings are not always identical. It is likely that more than one entity is currently being described under this name.

Inheritance. Type Schmid is probably of autosomal dominant inheritance, several families having been described with more than one generation affected (Stickler *et al*, 1962; Dent and Normand, 1964; Kozlowski, 1964; Rosenbloom and Smith, 1965). Kajii *et al* (1971) has described the condition in both of identical twins. Rosenbloom and Smith noted that the paternal age was raised in sporadic cases, indicating probably a spermatic mutation.

Frequency. The condition is a great deal more common than the Jansen type, though the population incidence is not known. It is not apparent at birth but usually becomes so during the second year of life.

Clinical and radiographic features. The first signs are some shortness of stature, lumbar lordosis and a waddling gait. As the child grows there is progressive shortening and genu varum develops.

Radiographically the skull is essentially normal in most cases although frontal bossing has been reported. The metaphyses of long bones are ragged, expanded and may be cupped, the picture being similar to that of healing rickets. The epiphyses are normal. Sutcliffe and Stanley (1973) noted a radiological feature not seen in rickets, namely fine spurs of sharply defined bone extending from the whole width of the metaphysis into the widened epiphyseal cartilage. The main deformity is at the hips where coxa vara develops.

Pathology. Dent and Normand (1964) noted that the histological changes in the cartilage were similar to rickets but the adjacent shaft was completely normal. Cooper and Ponseti (1973) carried out light and electromicroscopic studies of cartilage from the ulnar epiphyseal plate and iliac crest of a girl at 8 and then at 11 years of age. Clinically she appeared to have a condition more severe than type Schmid, but not so severe as the Jansen type. They noted that the cisternae of the chondrocytic endoplasmic reticulum was markedly dilated by a granular precipitate, and concluded that the specific defect resulted in storage of an undetermined substance in the rough surfaced endoplasmic reticulum.

Differential diagnosis. In the past this condition has usually been thought to be rickets, either vitamin-D resistant or some other type. However, the biochemistry is invariably normal. The main differential diagnosis is from metaphyseal chondrodysplasia type McKusick (formerly known as the cartilage-hair syndrome). In this condition the knees are more severely affected than the hips, many individuals have fine hair and in some cases there is an association with malabsorption, neutropenia and severe susceptibility to varicella.

Progress and complications. The final height of these individuals is between 130 and 160 cm (4′3″ and 5′3″) and apart from shortness of stature there are no particular symptoms. Since the epiphyses are not affected, degenerative osteoarthritis is not a feature. A case described by Kilburn (1973) was of normal stature.

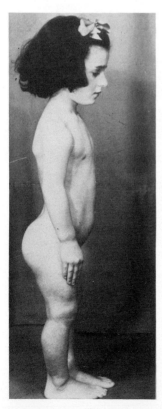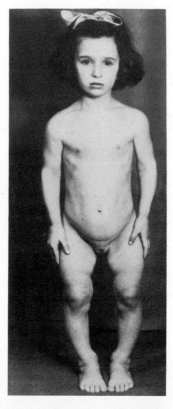

Fig. 9.6 (C.W. Type Schmid 7 year old girl) with shortness of stature, lumbar lordosis and genu varum. (H.A.T.F.)

THE METAPHYSEAL CHONDRODYSPLASIAS 35

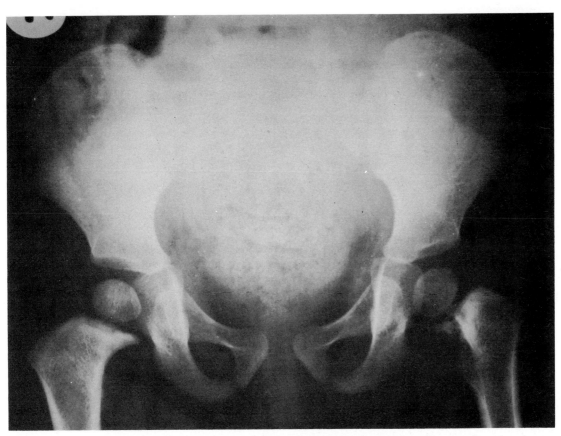

Fig. 9.7 (J.B. 2 year old female.) The pelvis is normal in shape at this age but the metaphyseal region of the femora, particularly the left, is abnormal and coxa vara is developing. (P.M.R.)

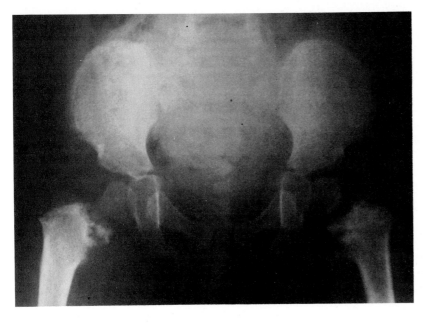

Fig. 9.8 (C.W. female aged 7 years.) The dysplastic changes in the neck of the femur are more severe than above. (H.A.T.F.)

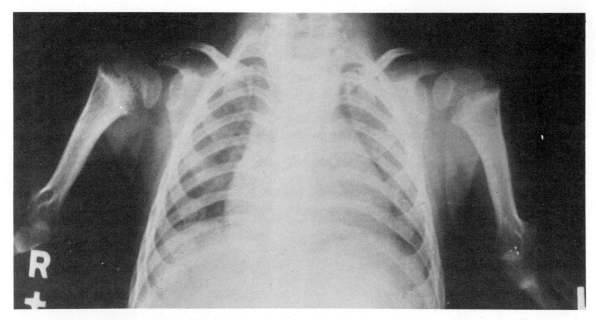

Fig. 9.9 (C.W.) Similar changes are seen in the metaphyseal region of the humerus. (H.A.T.F.)

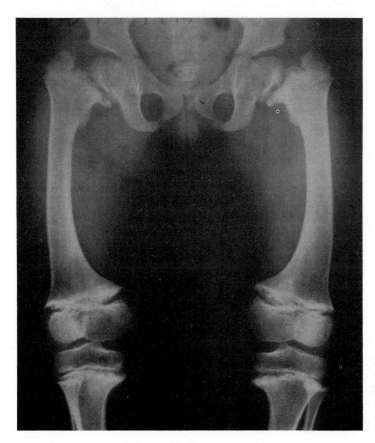

Fig. 9.10 (C.W.) The femora are shortened, bowed and the metaphyses particularly around the knee are flared and irregular. Coxa vara is well marked and the upper femoral metaphysis ragged. (H.A.T.F)

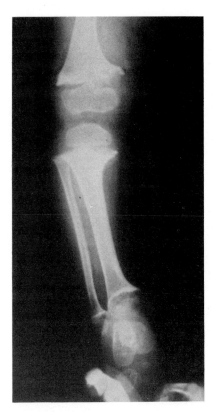

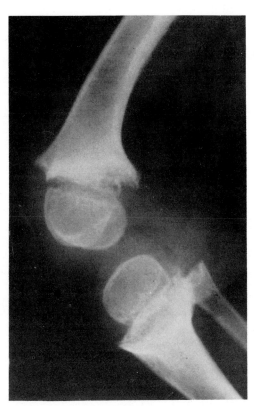

Fig. 9.11 (C.W.) The splayed and irregular metaphyses around the knee and ankle are shown, the latter being cupped. (H.A.T.F.)

Fig. 9.12 (C.W.) Lateral view of the knee emphasising the normal epiphysis in contrast with the ragged metaphysis. (H.A.T.F.)

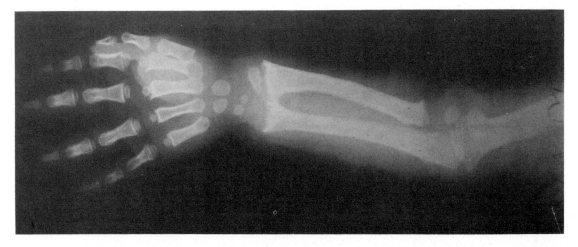

Fig. 9.13 (C.W.) The metaphyseal dysplasia affects the elbow and wrist region, though to a lesser extent than the lower limb. The hand is essentially normal. (H.A.T.F.)

METAPHYSEAL CHONDRODYSPLASIA—TYPE McKUSICK (*Cartilage Hair Hypoplasia*)

This disorder is characterised by shortness of limbs, fine sparse hair and abnormalities in the metaphyseal region. In some patients there is associated Hirschsprung disease and impaired cellular immunity. It was first described by McKusick (1964) and in more detail by McKusick et al (1965).

Inheritance. It is of autosomal recessive inheritance.

Frequency. It was noted to be the second most common form of dwarfism in the inbred Amish community of North America, reaching a level of 1 to 2 per 1,000 live births amongst them. Several cases have now been described elsewhere. The disorder is apparent at birth.

Clinical and radiographic features. These patients have fine, short and rather sparse fair hair, affecting the eyebrows and lashes as well as scalp hair. The short stature is usually of the short-limb type, sometimes there is generalised joint laxity, and the hands and feet are short and fat.

Radiographic features include involvement of the skull and spine, but these areas are less severely affected than the ribs and limb bones (Ray and Dorst, 1973). The skull has some tendency to brachycephaly and in infancy there may be defects in ossification of the calvarium, with an extension of the anterior fontanelle along the metopic suture, and a large sagittal fontanelle. Vertebrae tend to be small and there may be some reduction of the interpedicular distance in the lumbar region, though this is never as severe as in achondroplasia.

In the thorax the most striking feature is the cupping of the rib osteochondral junctions, associated with small cysts and the anterior portions of the ribs are wider than normal. There is premature fusion of the sternal sutures giving a pigeon breast deformity in the adult.

The limb bones show metaphyseal sclerosis and scalloping, sometimes with cyst-like areas; the proximal margin of the bony epiphysis partly conforms to the scalloped border of the adjacent metaphysis. Additional features in the upper limbs are dislocation or subluxation of the radial head and small hand bones.

The pelvic changes are not marked but the hip joints may be severely affected with coxa vara and an appearance of the femoral head like that seen in Perthes' disease (Beals, 1968). Metaphyseal changes are pronounced around the knee and ankle joints and a disproportionately long fibula at its lower end has been noted. There may be some bowing of the lower limbs but this is less severe than in the Schmid type of metaphyseal chondrodysplasia.

Pathology. The changes are non-specific, with a paucity of cartilage cells and failure to line up in columns. Ossification appears to proceed normally. Boothby and Bower (1973) noted that the hair in these individuals was one quarter of the normal diameter.

Differential diagnosis. This is from other metaphyseal chondrodysplasias, in particular type Schmid, where the hips tend to be more severely affected and the hands less so than in type McKusick. The metaphyseal lesions of rickets are similar, the disease being differentiated by the abnormal biochemistry. The metaphyseal chondrodysplasias associated with pancreatic insufficiency and neutropenia or thymolymphopenia tend to have less severe metaphyseal lesions than type McKusick and do not have abnormal hair.

Progress and complications. The adult height of these individuals is between 105 and 144 cm (3′5″ to 4′8″), though some are less severely affected and may reach 157 cm (5′2″). Apart from this shortness of stature they are not severely deformed.

Two disorders associated with this type of metaphyseal chondrodysplasia are of interest. First, intestinal malabsorption (a true Hirschsprung disease with congenital megacolon) may co-exist, and be the presenting feature of the disease. Secondly, Lux et al (1970) reported two children with metaphyseal chondrodysplasia type McKusick who developed a near-fatal varicella. They noted that chronic neutropenia and lymphopenia occurs in this disease as well as the abnormality in cellular immunity characterised by increased reaction to varicella. Smallpox vaccination has been fatal.

Treatment. This is directed to avoiding varicella and smallpox injections.

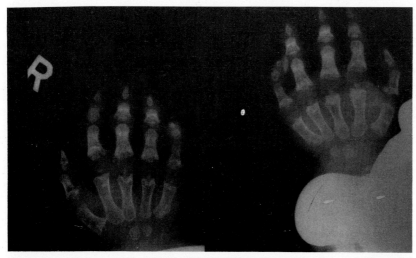

Fig. 9.14   (D.S. aged 15 months. Type McKusick.) In contrast with Type Schmid the hands are markedly affected with short wide phalanges and irregular metaphyseal areas. (H.A.T.F.)

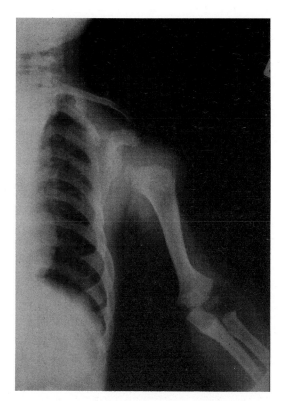

Fig. 9.15 (D.S.) There is a striking cupping of the ribs at the osteochondral junctions and metaphyseal irregularity and sclerosis particularly of the upper end of the humerus. (H.A.T.F.)

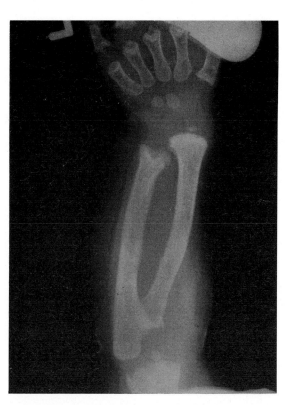

Fig. 9.16 (D.S.) The radius and ulna shafts are thickened and there is some sclerosis and irregularity of the metaphysis. (H.A.T.F.)

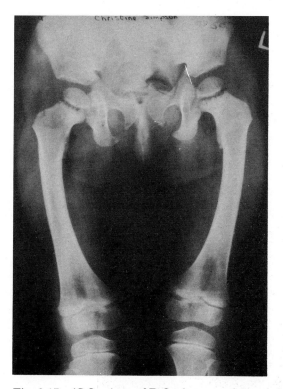

Fig. 9.17 (C.S., sister of D.S. above, aged 3 years.) There is some irregularity of the upper femoral metaphyseal area, but not so marked as in Type Schmid. Sclerosis of bone and flaring of the lower femoral metaphysis. Epiphyses are normal. (H.A.T.F.)

METAPHYSEAL CHONDRODYSPLASIA WITH CONGENITAL PANCREATIC INSUFFICIENCY AND NEUTROPENIA

Some years ago it was reported that pancreatic exocrine insufficiency can occur in children without any other features of cystic fibrosis of the pancreas (Bodian, Sheldon and Lightwood, 1964 and Shwachman et al, 1964). In 1967 Burke et al described associated bone lesions in this syndrome, and there have been more recent reports by Giedion et al (1968); Schmerling et al (1969), Taybi, Mitchell and Friedman (1969), and Stanley and Sutcliffe (1973).

Inheritance. The condition is likely to be of autosomal recessive inheritance, several affected sibs with normal parents having been reported.

Frequency. The population incidence is not known. The disorder becomes apparent during infancy.

Clinical and radiographic features. The symptoms relating to pancreatic insufficiency appear first, with infants failing to thrive and having diarrhoea with associated bulky offensive stools. Neutropenia is usually present at this stage, though it may be cyclic. Anaemia and thrombocytopenia also occur, but there is no immunoglobulin deficiency.

The bony changes affect chiefly the long bones, occasionally the vertebrae. There is sclerosis and irregularity of all metaphyses, the upper end of the femur particularly being affected, leading to coxa vara.

Differential diagnosis. This is from other metaphyseal chondrodysplasias, but the neutropenia and malabsorption symptoms differentiate this type.

Progress and complications. The natural history is related to the haematological and pancreatic disorders. There are frequent spontaneous remissions but without treatment death occurs within the first five years.

Schmerling and colleagues reported that diabetes developed in one of their patients, latent diabetes in his affected sister, and that there had been other cases of diabetes within the same family.

Clinical chemistry. Exocrine pancreatic function shows a very low concentration of both bicarbonate (ductulor) and enzyme (acinar) secretions, both before and after stimulation. There is a low chymotrypsin concentration in the stools in some cases. Cystic fibrosis of the pancreas is excluded by demonstration of normal sweat electrolytes. The neutropenia is either permanent or cyclic and frequently pancytopenia and a hypocellular bone marrow are present. The intestinal mucosa and immunoglobulins are normal.

Treatment. Schmerling and colleagues noted that treatment did not improve the neutropenia, dysostosis or growth, but large doses and prolonged use of pancreatic extract are indicated, together with antibiotics and vitamin supplements.

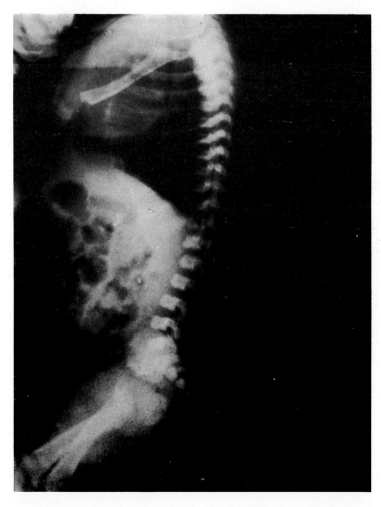

Fig. 9.18 Metaphyseal irregularity seen chiefly at the ends of the long bones and there is some vertebral irregularity. (G.O.S.)

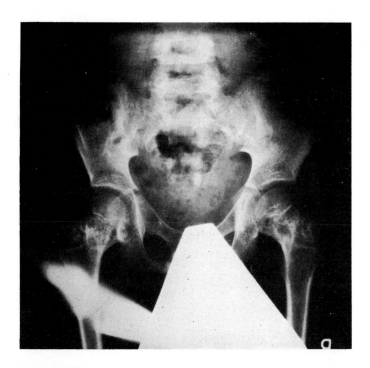

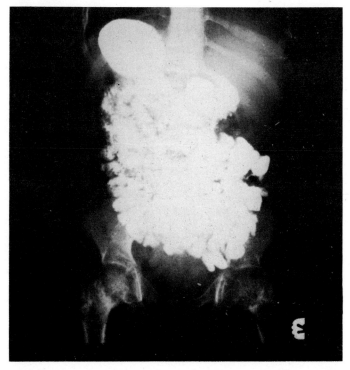

Figs 9.19 & 9.20 The characteristic metaphyseal defects at the upper end of the femora are seen. (G.O.S.)

METAPHYSEAL CHONDRODYSPLASIA WITH THYMOLYMPHOPENIA

Alexander and Dunbar (1968) first noted bone changes in thymic alymphoplasia, and Gatti et al (1969) reported the same condition in two affected sibs, as well as four sporadic cases of a lymphopenic agammaglobulinaemia associated with short stature and ectodermal dysplasia.

Inheritance. The disorder is likely to be of autosomal recessive inheritance.

Frequency. The population incidence is not known. The disease becomes apparent in early infancy.

Clinical and radiographic features. These children have sparse or absent hair, including the eyebrows, with ichthyosiform skin lesions, erythroderma and small dystrophic fingernails. The limbs are short, particularly the femur in relation to the tibia and fibula.

Radiographically the skull and vertebrae are normal, and the ribs somewhat short. The metaphyses of the long bones are wide and cupped particularly at the lower end of the ulna. The iliac part of the pelvis is shorter than normal and the superior acetabular surface almost horizontal.

Differential diagnosis. This is from other forms of metaphyseal chondrodysplasia, particularly the McKusick and Schmid types, but the low lymphocyte count and recurrent bacterial infections are characteristic.

Progress and complications. Hair may be present in infancy but falls out and fails to return. The lymphocyte count is initially normal but declines after the first few months of life. Bacterial infections are frequent and may lead to death from septicaemia.

Laboratory investigations. The main laboratory findings are lymphopenia, agammaglobulinaemia and thymic hypoplasia.

Treatment. This is related to the immunological deficiency and infection.

OTHER TYPES OF METAPHYSEAL CHONDRODYSPLASIA

It is among the metaphyseal disorders that individuals and families with minor differences from others in the group are perhaps most frequently reported. It is not yet known whether they will eventually prove to be specific entities, but until other examples are reported we do no more than list some of the more recently described.

Vaandrager type—ossification defects maximal in the metaphysis but extending some distance into the diaphysis. Autosomal dominant (Vaandrager, 1960).

Spahr type—clinically indistinguishable from type Schmid but of autosomal recessive inheritance (Spahr and Spahr-Hartmann, 1961).

Maroteaux type—similar to type Schmid but not all metaphyses affected, in particular the upper femur is normal (Maroteaux et al, 1963).

Kozlowski type—very mild disorder, with only very slight shortness of stature, otherwise similar to type Schmid (Kozlowski, 1964).

Peña type—all metaphyses affected with irregular ossification defects extending well into the diaphysis. Accompanied by dwarfing, scoliosis and defective ossification or platyspondyly of the cervical spine (Peña, 1965).

Wiedemann and Spranger type—congenital short-limbed dwarfism associated with metaphyseal changes similar to type Schmid. Normal hands and feet, and improvement with growth (Wiedemann and Spranger, 1970).

Metaphyseal chondrodysplasia calcificans—shortening of all long bones in infancy with expanded metaphyses and radiolucent defects extending into the shaft, similar to Ollier disease, but symmetrical. Later thick stripes of ossification and calcified spots extend from the metaphysis into the shaft (Van-Creveld et al, 1971).

Metaphyseal chondrodysplasia with peripheral location—conspicuous shortening of hands and feet, and to a lesser extent, other long bones. Cone-shaped epiphyses of the proximal and middle phalanges (Kozlowski and Rupprecht, 1972). There are likely to be others in this group.

REFERENCES

Alexander, W. J. & Dunbar, J. S. (1968). Unusual bone changes in thymic alymphoplasia. *Annals of Radiology*, **11**, 389.

Arroyo-Scotoliff, H. (1973). Metaphyseal dysostosis, Jansen type. *Journal of Bone & Joint Surgery*, **55A**, 623.

Beals, R. K. (1968). Cartilage-hair hypoplasia. *Journal of Bone & Joint Surgery*, **50A**, 1245.

Bodian, M., Sheldon, W. & Lightwood, R. (1964). Congenital hypoplasia of the exocrine pancreas. *Acta Paediatrics*, **53**, 282.

Boothby, C. B. & Bower, B. D. (1973). Cartilage-hair hypoplasia. *Archives of Diseases in Childhood*, **48**, 918.

Burke, V., Colebatch, J. H., Anderson, C. M. & Simons, M. J. (1967). Association of pancreatic insufficiency and chronic neutropenia in childhood. *Archives of Diseases in Childhood*, **42**, 147.

Cameron, J. A. P., Young, W. B. & Sissons, H. A. (1954). Metaphyseal dysostosis. *Journal of Bone & Joint Surgery*, **36B**, 622.

Cooper, R. R. & Ponseti, I. V. (1973). Metaphyseal dysostosis: description of an ultrastructural defect in the epiphyseal plate chondrocytes. *Journal of Bone & Joint Surgery*, **55A**, 485.

Creveld, S. van, Kozlowski, K., Pietron, K. & Valk, A van der (1971). Metaphyseal chondrodysplasia calcificans. A report on two cases. *British Journal of Radiology*, **44**, 773.

De Haas, W. H. D., De Boer, W. & Griffioen, F. (1969). Metaphysial dysostosis. *Journal of Bone & Joint Surgery*, **51B**, 290.

Dent, C. E. & Normand, I. C. S. (1964). Metaphyseal dysostosis, Type Schmid. *Archives of Diseases in Childhood*, **39**, 444.

Gatti, R., Platt, N., Pomerance, H. H., Hong, R., Langer, L. O., Kay, H. E. M. & Good, R. A. (1969). Hereditary lympho-penic agammaglobulinemia associated with a distinctive form of short-limbed dwarfism and ectodermal dysplasia. *Journal of Pediatrics*, **75**, 675.

Giedion, A., Prader, A. Hadorn, B., Schmerling, D. H. & Auricchio, S. (1968). Metaphysäre dysostose und angeborene Pankreasinsuffizienz. *Fortschritte auf dem Gebiete der Roentgenstrahlen und der Nuklearmedizin*, **108**, 51.

Gram, P. B., Fleming, J. L., Frame, B. & Fine, G. (1959). Metaphyseal chondrodysplasia of Jansen. *Journal of Bone & Joint Surgery*, **41A**, 951.

Holt, J. F. (1969). Discussion (on Jansen's disease). *Birth Defects Original Article Series 5*, **4**, 73.

Jansen, M. (1934). Über atypische Chondrodystrophie (Achondroplasie) und über ein noch nicht beschriebene angeborene Wachsumstörung des Knochensystems: Metaphysäre Dysostosis. *Zeitschrift für Orthopaedie Chirurgie*, **61**, 253.

Kajii, T., Ohsawa, T., Matsuda, I. & Sugai, M. (1971). Concordant metaphyseal dysostosis type Schmid in identical twins. *Human Genetics*, **13**, 151.

Kilburn, P. (1973). A metaphyseal abnormality. Report of a case with features of metaphyseal dysostosis. *Journal of Bone & Joint Surgery*, **55B**, 643.

Kozlowski, K. (1964). Metaphyseal dysostosis. Report of five familial and two sporadic cases of mild type. *American Journal of Roentgenology*, **91**, 602.

Kozlowski, K. & Rupprecht, E. (1972). Metaphyseal dysplasia with peripheral location. *Helvetica paediatrica acta*, **27**, 85.

Lenz, W. D. (1969). Discussion (on Jansen's disease). *Birth Defects Original Article Series 5*, **4**, 71.

Lux, S. E., Johnston, R. B., August, C. S., Say, B., Penchaszadek, V. B., Rosen, F. S. & McKusick, V. A. (1970). Chronic neutropenia and abnormal cellular immunity in cartilage-hair hypoplasia. *New England Journal of Medicine*, **282**, 231.

Maroteaux, P. & Lamy, M. (1958). La dysostose métaphysaire. *Semaine des Hôpitaux, Paris*, **34**, 1729.

Maroteaux, P., Savart, P., Lefebvre, J. & Royer, P. (1963). Les formes partielles de la dystose métaphysaire. *Presse Médicale*, **71**, 1523.

McKusick, V. A. (1964). Metaphyseal dysostosis and thin hair; a 'new' recessively inherited syndrome. *Lancet*, **1**, 832.

McKusick, V. A., Eldridge, R., Hostetler, J. A., Ruangwit, U. & Egeland, J. A. (1965). Dwarfism in the Amish: II. Cartilage-hair hypoplasia. *Bulletin of the Johns Hopkins Hospital*, **116**, 285.

Peña, J. (1965). Disostosis metafisaria. Una revision. Con aportacion de una observacion familiar. Una forma mieva de la enfermedael. *Radiología*, **47**, 3.

Ray, H. C. & Dorst, J. P. (1973). Cartilage-hair hypoplasia. In *Progress in Pediatric Radiology*, ed. Kaufmann, H. J., vol. 4, p. 270. Karger, Basel.

Rosenbloom, A. L. & Smith, D. W. (1965). The natural history of metaphyseal dysostosis. *Journal of Pediatrics*, **66**, 857.

Schmerling, D. H., Prader, A., Hitzig, W. H., Giedion, A., Hadorn, B. & Kühni, M. (1969). The syndrome of exocrine pancreatic insufficiency, neutropenia, metaphyseal dysostosis and dwarfism. *Helvetica Paediatrica Acta*, **24**, 547.

Schmid, F. (1949). Beitrag zur Dysostosis enchondralis metaphysaria. *Monatsschrift für Kinderheilkunde*, **97**, 393.

Shwachman, H., Diamond, L. K., Oski, F. & Kon-T Khaw. (1964). The syndrome of pancreatic insufficiency and bone marrow dysfunction. *Journal of Pediatrics*, **65**, 645.

Spahr, A. & Spahr-Hartmann, I. (1961). Dysostose métaphysaire familiale. Étude de 4 cas dans une famille. *Helvetica paediatrica acta*, **16**, 836.

Stanley, P. & Sutcliffe, J. (1973). Metaphyseal chondroplasia with dwarfism, pancreatic insufficiency and neutropenia. *Pediatric Radiology*, **1**, 119.

Stickler, G. B., Maher, F. T., Hunt, J. C., Burke, E. C. & Rosevear, J. W. (1962). Familial bone disease resembling rickets (hereditary metaphyseal dysostosis). *Pediatrics*, **29**, 996.

Sutcliffe, J. & Stanley, P. (1973). Metaphyseal chondrodysplasias. In *Progress in Pediatric Radiology*, ed. Kaufmann, H. J., vol. 4, p. 250. Karger, Basel.

Taybi, H., Mitchell, A. D. & Friedman, G. D. (1969). Metaphyseal dysostosis and the associated syndrome of pancreatic insufficiency and blood disorders. *Radiology*, **93**, 563.

Vaandrager, G. J. (1960). Metafysaire dysostosis. *Nederlands tijdschrift voor geneeskunde*, **104**, 547.

Wiedemann, H. R. & Spranger, J. (1970). Chondrodysplasia metaphysaria (dysostosis metaphysaria)—ein neuer Type. *Zeitschrift für Kinderheilkunde*, **108**, 171.

10   The Hypophosphatasias

The hypophosphatasias are inherited disorders some-what similar to rickets but characterised by a low serum alkaline phosphatase. There is first a severe congenital form in which the child is stillborn or dies during the first year of life, secondly a less severe (tarda) form presenting around 6 months of age, and thirdly, a mild disorder presenting only in adult life as osteomalacia. The infantile types are of autosomal recessive inheritance, and it is likely that both the severe congenital and the milder, tarda varieties are of the same aetiology since both have been reported in the same family. The variant which presents in adult life is probably a distinct aetiological entity since several cases of autosomal dominant inheritance have been reported (Bethung and Dent, 1960; Silverman, 1962).

INFANTILE HYPOPHOSPHATASIA

The best known of the hypophosphatasias is the very severe congenital form described by Rathbun (1948), in which there is absent ossification of large areas of the skeleton, in particular the skull, facial bones and the long bones of the hands and feet. Death usually occurs within the first few days of life.

A rather less severe form of infantile hypophos-phatasia develops around 6 months of age. It presents with failure to thrive and signs of rickets. The onset is gradual and these patients may have few problems apart from frequent fractures.

Inheritance. Both the congenital lethal form and the tarda form are of autosomal recessive inheritance, many affected sibs with normal parents having been reported (Currarino et al, 1957; Fraser, 1957). The disorder is particularly common amongst inbred communities (MacPherson, Kroeker and Houston, 1972; Mehes et al, 1972).

Clinical and radiographic features. In the more severe form the infant suffers from prenatal fractures and at birth has marked deformities of the limbs, with a soft globular head and soft skeleton. If not stillborn, then death from respiratory failure occurs usually within the first few days of life, or, more rarely, at a few months of age.

In the most extreme form, there is practically no mineralisation at all of the skeleton seen on radio-graphy. More usually there are wide suture lines in the skull, or perhaps absent ossification of major portions of the calvaria. The ribs are thin and the ends unossified. The neural arches may be invisible and the pectoral and pelvic girdles small. The long bones are characteristic with large jagged metaphyseal defects extending far into the diaphysis.

The tarda form has a slower onset, later in infancy, and is likely to be confused with rickets. These infants have general symptoms of failure to thrive with anorexia, vomiting, convulsions and muscular hypo-tonia. Fractures are common and there is premature loss of deciduous teeth. In infancy the cranial sutures are wide apart but as the child grows there may be premature fusion with craniostenosis and signs of raised intracranial pressure. Shortness of stature and rachitic deformities develop as the child grows (Jacobsen and McClain, 1967).

Pathology. The pathological changes in bone resemble those of rickets. Although the resting cartilage is normal, large parts of the skeleton consist of unmineralised osteoid.

Differential diagnosis. The severe lethal form of hypophosphatasia must be differentiated from osteo-genesis imperfecta and from lethal forms of short-limbed dwarfism such as achondrogenesis and thana-tophoric dwarfism. In none of these conditions is large areas of the skull unossified and neither is a low alkaline phosphatase a feature.

The less severe tarda form must be distinguished from rickets (nutritional, associated with renal tubular disease or with uraemic osteodystrophy). Again a low alkaline phosphatase is not a feature of these disorders and the jagged, punched-out metaphyseal defects are quite characteristic of hypophosphatasia.

Progress and complications. Infants with the severe lethal form usually die of respiratory insufficiency in the first few days or months of life. This is likely to be caused by infection developing due to the soft thoracic cage. Those few children who survive the neo-natal period are severely affected by rickets with stunt-ing, limb deformities, and a general failure to thrive.

In the tarda form, premature fusion of the cranial sutures gives rise to craniostenosis, a raised intra-cranial pressure and mental retardation in some cases. However, if the infant survives the first year of life there is likely to be spontaneous improvement.

Laboratory investigations. The main feature is the very low alkaline phosphatase, although the level does not correlate with the severity of the clinical disease (Paterson, 1974). A further chemical finding is the presence of large amounts of phosphoethanolamine in the urine. In some severely affected infants there may be hypercalcaemia and nephrocalcinosis.

It is possible to detect heterozygotes (that is, the clinically unaffected parents) since they usually have a rather low serum alkaline phosphatase and may also excrete phosphoethanolamine in the urine.

Treatment. There is no specific treatment which will influence the calcification defects.

MILD (ADULT) HYPOPHOSPHATASIA

This form of the disease presents in adults with signs of osteomalacia. Alternatively, there may be a history of persistent rickets since childhood, the disease perhaps having undergone exacerbations and remissions (Jardon, Burney and Fink, 1970).

Clinical and radiographic features. The presenting sign is usually a fracture, and on radiography, long-standing rachitic changes may be seen. In mild cases there may be little in the way of radiographic signs.

It is likely that this form of hypophosphatasia is of autosomal dominant inheritance and therefore of different aetiology from the severe hypophosphatasias of infancy.

REFERENCES

Bethune, J. E. & Dent, C. E. (1960). Hypophosphatasia in the adult. *American Journal of Medicine*, **28,** 615.

Currarino, G., Neuhauser, E. B. D., Reyersbach, G. C. & Sobel, E. H. (1957). Hypophosphatasia. *American Journal of Roentgenology*, **78,** 392.

Fraser, D. (1957). Hypophosphatasia. *American Journal of Medicine*, **22,** 730.

Jacobson, D. P. & McClain, E. J. (1967). Hypophosphatasia in monozygotic twins. *Journal of Bone & Joint Surgery*, **49A,** 377.

Jardon, O. M., Burney, D. W. & Fink, R. L. (1970). Hypophosphatasia in an adult. *Journal of Bone & Joint Surgery*, **52A,** 1477.

Mehes, K., Klujber, L., Lassu, G. & Kajtar, P. (1972). Hypophosphatasia: screening and family investigations in an endogamous Hungarian village. *Clinical Genetics*, **3,** 60.

MacPherson, R. I., Krocker, M. & Houston, C. S. (1972). Hypophosphatasia. *Journal de l'association Canadienne des Radiologistes*, **23,** 16.

Paterson, C. R. (ed.) (1974). Hypophosphatasia. *Metabolic Disorders of Bone*. Chapter 16, p. 266. Oxford: Blackwell Scientific Publications.

Rathbun, J. C. (1948). 'Hypophosphatasia'. A new developmental anomaly. *American Journal of Diseases of Children*, **75,** 822.

Silverman, J. L. (1962). Apparent dominant inheritance of hypophosphatasia. *Archives of Internal Medicine*, **110,** 191.

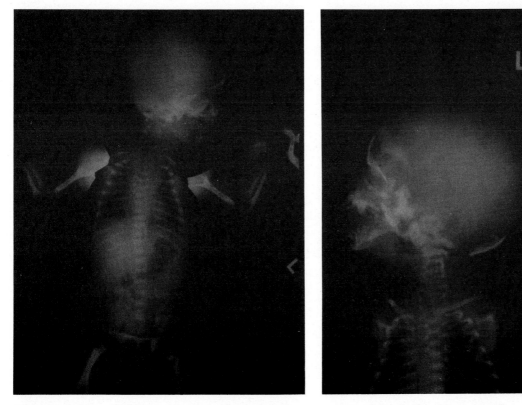

Figs 10.1 & 10.2   (Baby C.) Absent ossification of the greater part of the skull and large jagged metaphyseal defects in all long bones. Ribs are thin. (H.A.T.F.)

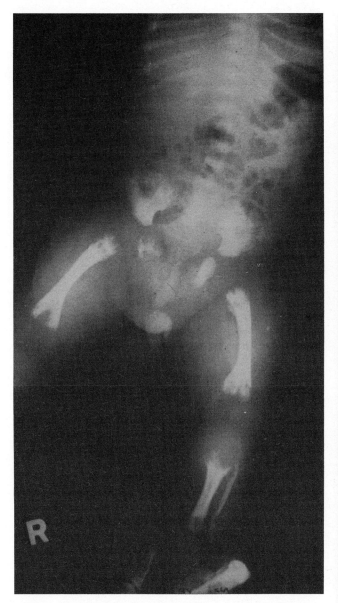

Fig. 10.3   (Baby C.) The pelvis is poorly ossified and the metaphyseal defects extend far into the diaphyses. (H.A.T.F.)

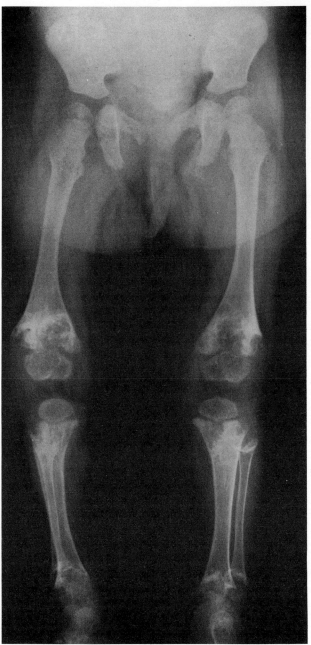

Fig. 10.4   (M.M.) The tarda form of infantile hypophosphatasia with wide rachitic-like deformities of the lower limb metaphyses. (H.A.T.F.)

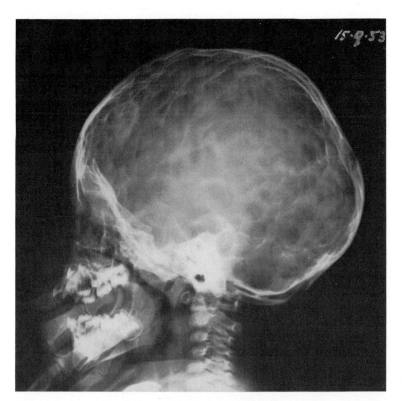

Fig. 10.5 (M.M.) Premature fusion of cranial sutures with signs of raised intracranial pressure. (H.A.T.F.)

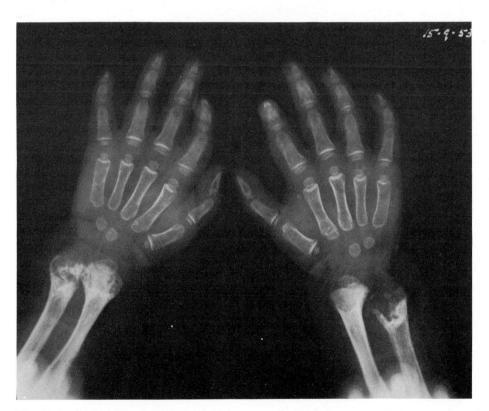

Fig. 10.6 (M.M.) The jagged punched-out metaphyseal lesions are well shown at the wrist. (H.A.T.F.)

11 Brachyolmia

In this condition the only defect is that the vertebral bodies are flattened. It was described by Maroteaux *et al* (1968).

The disorder appears to be of little clinical importance other than that of differentiation from the spondyloepiphyseal dysplasias and other vertebral disorders.

Inheritance. Cases of affected sibs have been described and so it is probably of autosomal recessive inheritance. Maroteaux (1974) suggests there is also a dominant variety.

REFERENCES

Maroteaux, P., Wiedemann, R., Spranger, J., Kozlowski, K. & Lenzi, L. (1968). *Essai de classification des dysplasies spondylo-éphysaires,* Simep editions, Lyon.

Maroteaux, P. (1974). *Maladies Osseuses De L'Enfant.* Flammarion Médecine-Sciences, Paris.

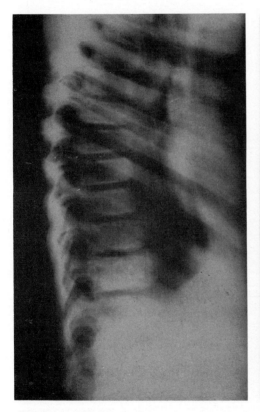

Fig. 11.1 (J.S. female aged 8 years.) Vertebral flattening and no other defect. (H.A.T.F.)

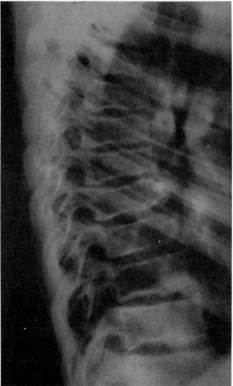

Fig. 11.2 (J.S. aged 12 years.) Platyspondyly and some irregularity of epiphyseal plates. (H.A.T.F.)

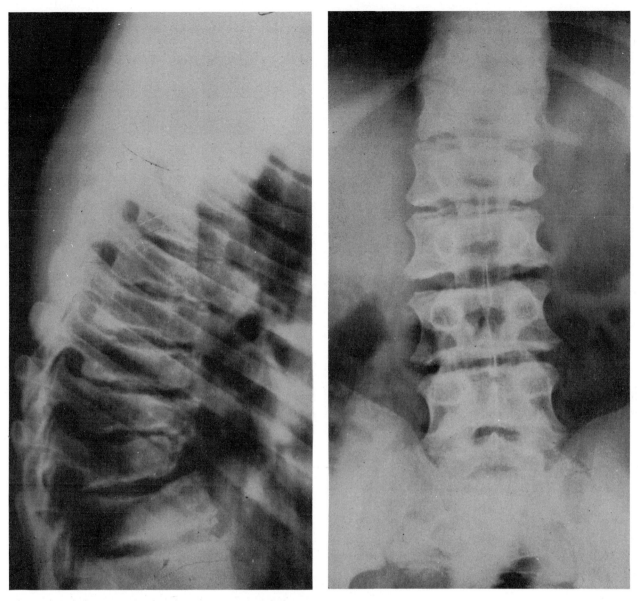

Figs 11.3 & 11.4   (E.S. brother of J.S. above, aged 16 years.) He has the same vertebral flattening and irregularity of the epiphyseal end plates. (H.A.T.F.)

12   The Spondyloepiphyseal Dysplasias

This group of diseases is characterised by disordered epiphyseal growth and flattened vertebrae with irregular surfaces and narrowed disc spaces. There are two clear-cut varieties in which the inheritance, clinical and radiographic features are distinctive. First, X-linked spondyloepiphyseal dysplasia tarda (described in this chapter) and secondly, spondyloepiphyseal dysplasia congenita (Chapter 15). This latter form (of dominant inheritance) is of great severity and since the metaphyses are also involved it is included amongst the spondylo-epi-metaphyseal disorders.

There are likely to be other varieties of spondyloepiphyseal dysplasia, since both dominant and recessive inheritance has been reported where there are vertebral and principally large proximal joint changes (Hoback, 1961; Carter and Sutcliffe, 1970; Diamond, 1970). Precise delineation of these conditions has not yet been made.

SPONDYLOEPIPHYSEAL DYSPLASIA TARDA (X-LINKED)

This is a relatively benign form of spondyloepiphyseal dysplasia, of late onset, affecting mainly the spine and giving a short trunk type of dwarfism with only mild dysplastic changes in the hips and shoulders.

Early reports in the literature confused the disorder with Morquio disease (Jacobsen, 1939). The first clear description was given by Maroteaux, Lamy and Bernard (1957), who described three families with 20 affected males in four generations.

Inheritance. Many subsequent surveys have established that the disorder is of X-linked recessive inheritance, being apparent only in males and transmitted by carrier females. Bannerman, Ingell and Mohn (1971) investigated 7 males between the age of 26 and 67 years, and commented that the heterozygous females in these families showed no consistent changes, neither could they find any close linkage with the Xg blood groups or with colour blindness.

Frequency. The population incidence is not known. Males only are affected and the diagnosis is not usually made until between 5 and 10 years of age.

Clinical and radiographic features. The presenting signs are usually of short stature, due to impaired growth of the spine, and back pain. There may be protrusion of the sternum.

Radiographically the appearance of the vertebrae is quite distinctive, being somewhat flat but humped in the posterior part, both superiorly and inferiorly. These humps are sclerosed, the disc spaces are narrow, and there may be disc calcification. The platyspondyly extends from the second cervical vertebra downwards (Langer, 1964). The absence of ossification at the anterior margins of the lumbar vertebral bodies is reminiscent of lumbar osteochondritis, but even in the lower thoracic spine little, if any, kyphosis develops. The thorax has an increased anteroposterior diameter, and because of the platyspondyly the lower ribs are close to the iliac crests.

There are mild dysplastic changes in all the large joints but particularly the shoulder and hip. The pelvis appears to be small, often markedly so, and the discrepancy between this and the rib cage is striking. The acetabulae are deep and the femoral necks short. The distal limb epiphyses are not affected.

The condition is a fairly benign one and therefore it is important to distinguish it from other more serious disorders (Harper, Jenkins and Laurence, 1973).

Differential diagnosis. Multiple epiphyseal dysplasia is somewhat similar but there is no 'hump' of the vertebrae, and frequently no vertebral changes at all. Also, the distal epiphyses of the limbs in multiple epiphyseal dysplasia are severely involved. Spondyloepiphyseal dysplasia congenita is differentiated by reason of being a far more severe disorder and apparent at birth. It has a characteristic configuration of the upper femur with a greatly enlarged trochanteric region, absence of the capital femoral epiphyses and high-riding trochanters. Morquio disease is characterised by a more severe degree of platyspondyly, without the characteristic vertebral hump; the disorder is apparent at an earlier age than X-linked spondyloepiphyseal dysplasia and abnormal excretion of mucopolysaccharide is present in the urine.

Progress and complications. The adult height of patients with X-linked spondyloepiphyseal dysplasia is between 130 and 150 cm (4′3″ to 4′11″). Limitation of movement and pain in the back and large proximal joints appear usually during adolescence, and there is early spondylosis. Bannerman (1969) studied Jacobsen's original case, and found the patient had marked secondary arthritis in his 30's, and Weinfeld, Ross and Sarasohn (1967) also reported premature osteoarthritis.

Treatment. This is related to the secondary osteoarthritis.

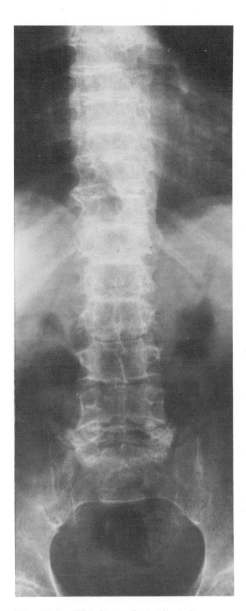

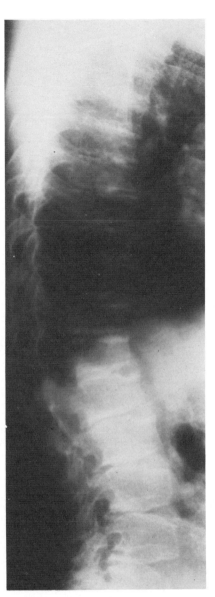

Fig. 12.1 (K.) Some flattening of vertebral bodies and narrowing of disc spaces. (Courtesy of Professor J. I. P. James, Edinburgh.)

Fig. 12.2 (K.) Characteristic defects of X-linked S.E.D. in anterior part of vertebral bodies, with sclerosis particularly of posterior part. (Courtesy of Professor, J. I. P. James, Edinburgh.)

REFERENCES

Bannerman, R. M. (1969). X-linked spondyloepiphyseal dysplasia tarda (SDT). *Birth Defects Original Article Series 5,* Part 4, 48.

Bannerman, R. M., Ingall, G. B. & Mohn, J. F. (1971). X-linked spondyloepiphyseal dysplasia tarda: clinical and linkage data. *Journal of Medical Genetics,* **8,** 291.

Carter, C. & Sutcliffe, J. (1970). Genetic varieties of spondyloepiphyseal dysplasia. In *Symposium Ossium,* Livingstone, Edinburgh.

Diamond, L. S. (1970). A family study of spondyloepiphyseal dysplasia. *Journal of Bone & Joint Surgery,* **52A,** 1587.

Harper, P. S., Jenkins, P. & Laurence, K. M. (1973). Spondyloepiphyseal dysplasia tarda: a report of four cases in two families. *British Journal of Radiology,* **46,** 676.

Hobaek, A. (1961). *Problems of Hereditary Chondrodysplasias,* Oslo University Press, Oslo.

Jacobsen, A. W. (1939). Hereditary osteochondrodystrophia deformans. *Journal of American Medical Association,* **113,** 121.

Langer, L. O. (1964). Spondyloepiphyseal dysplasia tarda. *Radiology,* **82,** 833.

Maroteaux, P., Lamy, M. & Bernard, J. (1957). La dysplasie spondylo-épiphysaire tardive; description clinique et radiologique. *La Presse Médicale,* **65,** 1205.

Weinfeld, A., Ross, M. W. & Sarasohn, S. H. (1967). Spondyloepiphyseal dysplasia tarda, a cause of premature osteoarthritis. *American Journal of Roentgenology,* **101,** 851.

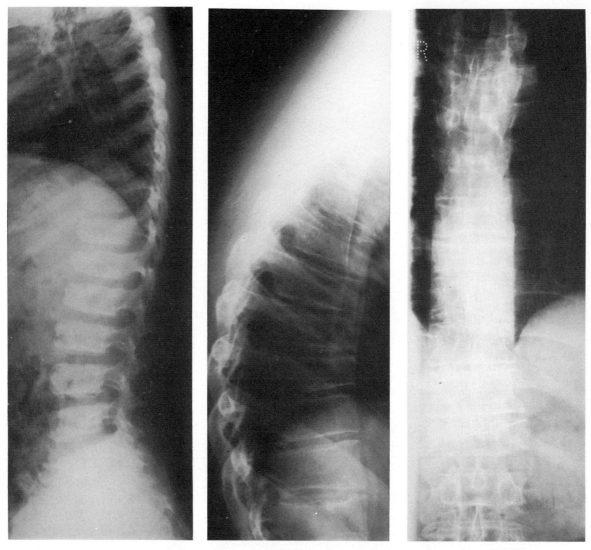

Figs 12.3, 12.4 & 12.5   (K. & J.H. Father and son.) Autosomal dominant form of spondyloepiphyseal dysplasia tarda. Platyspondyly with irregularity of epiphyseal plates. (A.H.)

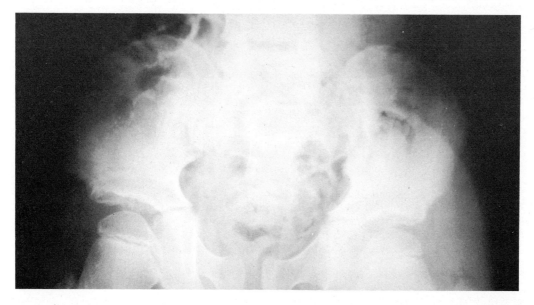

Fig. 12.6   (J.H.) Small pelvis with mild dysplastic changes in the hips. (A.H.)

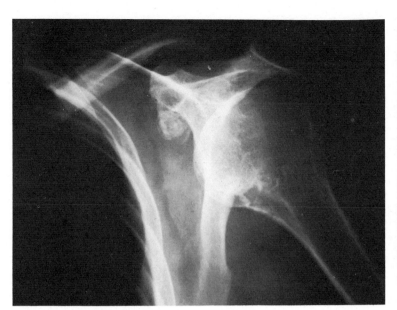

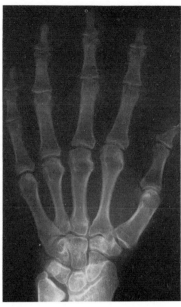

Fig. 12.7 (K.H.) Mild dysplastic changes at the shoulder joint. (A.H.)

Fig. 12.8 (J.R.) Some changes at the wrist but the hand is unaffected. (G.O.S.)

13 Spondylometaphyseal Dysplasia—Kozlowski Type

In this disorder there is a short trunk type of dwarfism with platyspondyly accompanied by defective metaphyseal ossification. The epiphyses are only minimally affected. It was first described by Kozlowski, Maroteaux and Spranger in 1967.

Inheritance. The disorder appears to be of autosomal dominant inheritance. Riggs and Summitt (1971) have described an affected mother and son.

Frequency. This disorder is not apparent until after the second year of life.

Clinical and radiographic features. The disorder is not very severe and individuals are of normal intelligence. The presenting sign is usually shortness of stature due to the short trunk and scoliosis may develop in later childhood.

Radiographically the vertebrae are markedly flattened and there is irregular metaphyseal ossification of the long bones, most marked in the proximal femur. The pelvis has short iliac wings with a narrowed outlet. The acetabulum is irregular and in children the upper part more horizontal than normal. Coxa vara is a feature and genu valgum has been present in some cases. The only other feature of note is the late appearance of rather small carpal bones.

Differential diagnosis. Metatropic dwarfism in older children has a similarly affected vertebral column but the disorder, including the scoliosis, is more severe, and is accompanied by epiphyseal changes.

Progress and complications. There is a normal expectation of life and the adult height is about 140 cm (4'7").

REFERENCES

Kozlowski, K., Maroteaux, P. & Spranger, J. (1967). La dysostose spondylo-metaphysaire. *La Presse Médicale*, **75**, 2769.
Riggs, W. & Summitt, R. L. (1971). Spondylometaphyseal dysplasia (Kozlowski). *Radiology*, **101**, 375.

14 Pseudoachondroplasia

This is a form of short-limbed dwarfism in which the vertebral column and both metaphyses and epiphyses are affected. It was first clearly described by Maroteaux and Lamy (1959). In 1961 Ford, Silverman and Kozlowski described three patients and noted the differences between this form of short-limbed dwarfism and classical achondroplasia, as well as differentiating it from other types of spondyloepiphyseal dysplasia. Since then there has been a number of reports (Hall and Dorst, 1969; Wadia, 1969; Fisher, 1974).

Inheritance. Most cases appear to be of dominant inheritance but 'pseudoachondroplasia' may well be a hereogeneous group as some (more severe) cases appear to be of autosomal recessive inheritance.

Frequency. The population incidence is not known, many cases in the past having been confused with true achondroplasia. The disorder is not apparent at birth, diagnosis usually being made during the second year of life or even later.

Clinical features. The head is normal, and it is shortness of stature (which may be very severe) that is the presenting feature. The trunk is shortened by reason of platyspondyly and there is a lumbar lordosis similar to that of classical achondroplasia. Scoliosis may develop as the child grows. The hands are short and stubby and there is frequently genu valgum or varum.

Radiographically the skull is normal. The vertebrae are characteristically shaped, being flat with a distinctive anterior tongue-like protrusion of the central part of the bodies. There is no narrowing of the interpedicular distance in the lumbar region.

The long bones are all severely affected, the metaphyses being markedly flared and irregular and the epiphyses small and very irregular. It is only *articular* cartilage which is affected, not that at the base of the skull, or associated with the pelvis, ribs or spinal pedicles.

Apart from some irregularity of the acetabulum the pelvis is normal, not showing the slit-like sciatic notch present in classical achondroplasia.

Pathology. Cooper, Ponseti and Maynard (1973) carried out electronmicroscope studies of the iliac crest and fibula epiphyseal plates in pseudoachondroplasia and noted a specific defect—a swelling of the endoplasmic reticulum cisternae due to an accumulating synthesis of products. They suggested that the material was an abnormal lipoprotein or glycoprotein.

Differential diagnosis. This is from classical achondroplasia, which is differentiated by an abnormal skull, interpedicular narrowing in the lumbar region and the fact that the epiphyses are unaffected. Also, the configuration of the pelvis is different with its narrowed sciatic notch. True achondroplasia can be diagnosed at birth, unlike pseudoachondroplasia which only becomes apparent at about 2 years of age.

Multiple epiphyseal dysplasia, if severe, is rather similar to pseudoachondroplasia but here the vertebral changes are absent or only minimal and the metaphyses are unaffected. However, by the time the child reaches adolescence and in adult life, differentiation between the two may be very difficult, particularly as the vertebral column in pseudoachondroplasia tends to become more normal in appearance with growth.

Progress and complications. The adult height of these individuals is between 82 and 130 cm (2'8" to 4'3"). Life expentancy is normal, the chief problems arising from premature osteoarthritis, particularly of the hip and knee.

REFERENCES

Cooper, R. R., Ponseti, I. V. & Maynard, J. A. (1973). Pseudoachondroplastic dwarfism: A rough surfaced endoplasmic reticulum storage disorder. *Journal of Bone & Joint Surgery*, **55A,** 475.

Fisher, R. L. (1974). Unusual spondyloepiphyseal and spondylometaphyseal dysplasias of childhood. *Clinical Orthopaedics and Related Research*, **100,** 78.

Ford, N., Silverman, F. N. & Kozlowski, K. (1961). Spondylo-epiphyseal dysplasia (Pseudoachondroplastic type). *American Journal of Roentgenology*, **86,** 462.

Hall, J. G. & Dorst, J. P. (1969). Pseudoachondroplastic SED, recessive Maroteaux–Lamy type. *Birth Defects Original Article Series 5*, Part 4, 254.

Maroteaux, P. & Lamy, M. (1959). Les formes pseudo-achondroplastiques des dysplasies spondylo-epiphysaires. *La Presse Médicale*, **10,** 383.

Wadia, R. (1969). Pseudoachondroplastic spondyloepiphyseal dysplasia: dominant Maroteaux–Lamy type in three generations of whom three affected persons are described here. *Birth Defects Original Article Series 5*, Part 4, 250.

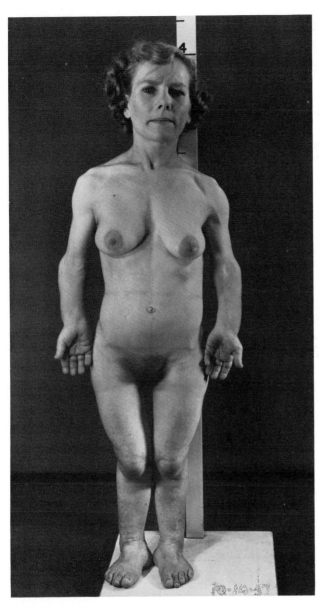

Fig. 14.1 (P.H.) Aged 28 years, height 125·7 cm (4'1½"). Normal skull, and limbs disproportionately short compared with the trunk. (H.A.T.F.)

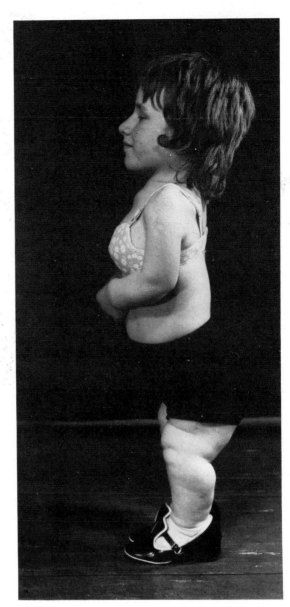

Fig. 14.2 (F.G.) Aged 14½ years. Height 88 cm (2'10½"). (Courtesy of Professor J. I. P. James, Edinburgh.)

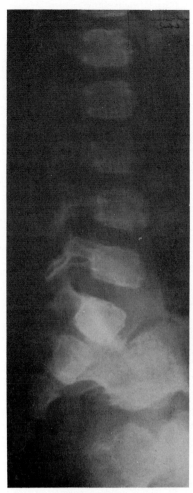

Fig. 14.3 (C.D.) Female aged 6 years. (H.A.T.F.)

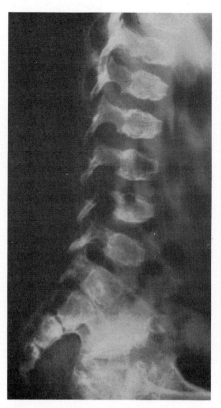

Fig. 14.4 (A.M.) Male aged 11 years. The anterior tongue-like process is well shown at this age. (H.A.T.F.)

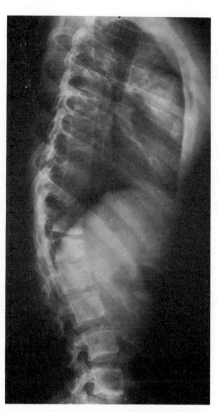

Fig. 14.5 (P.H.) Female aged 28 years. The vertebral column is almost normal by this age, just showing slight deformities still in the lower thoracic and upper lumbar region. (H.A.T.F.)

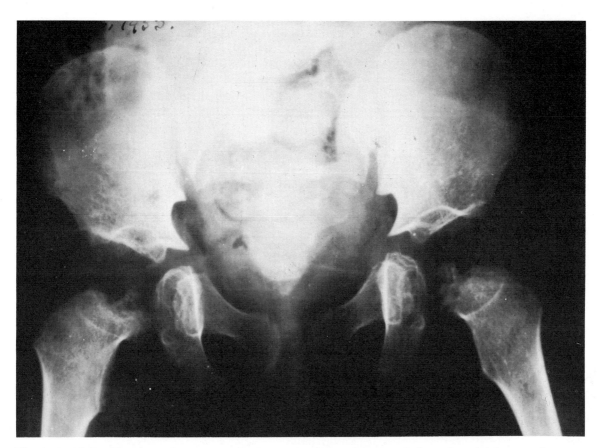

Fig. 14.6 (C.D.) Female aged 6 years. Apart from irregularity of the acetabulum, the pelvis is normal. There is no interpedicular narrowing in the lower lumbar spine. The capital femoral epiphyses are small and very irregular and there is metaphyseal irregularity. (H.A.T.F.)

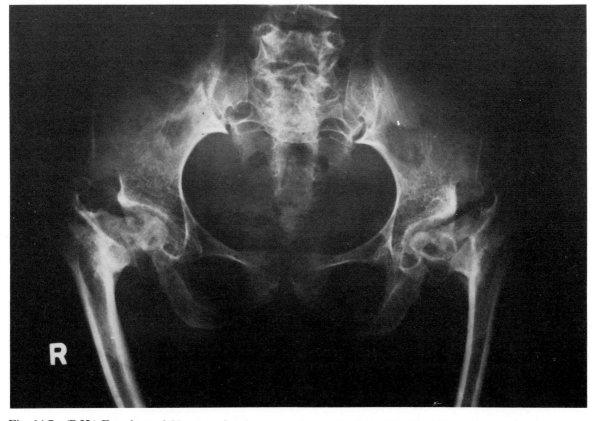

Fig. 14.7 (P.H.) Female aged 28 years, showing gross disorganisation of the hip joint and upper femur. The pelvic ring is well formed. (H.A.T.F.)

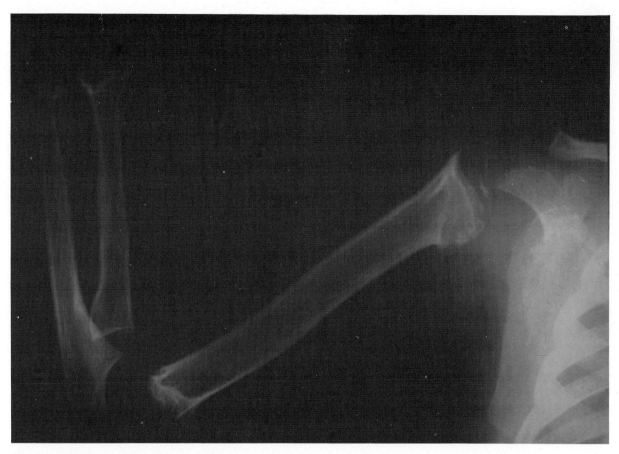

Fig. 14.8 (C.D.) Female aged 6 years. The metaphyses are widened and epiphyses irregular and late in appearing. (H.A.T.F.)

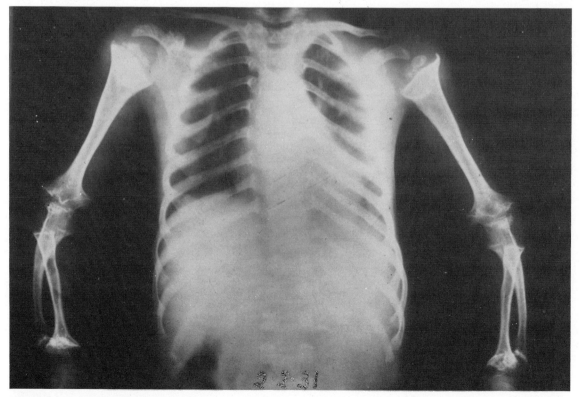

Fig. 14.9 (P.H.) Female aged 8 years. The metaphyseal flaring is more obvious, and epiphyses are still small or absent. (H.A.T.F.)

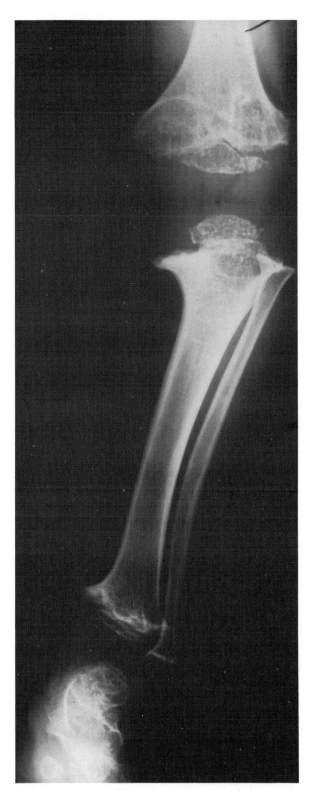

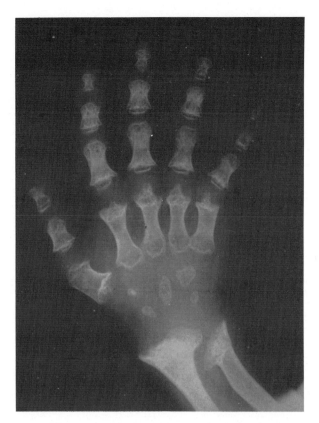

Fig. 14.11 (A.M.) Male aged 11 years. The hands are short and stubby with late appearance of the carpal epiphyses and widening of all metaphyses in the metacarpals and phalanges. (H.A.T.F.)

Fig. 14.10 (C.D.) Female aged 6 years. The metaphyseal flaring and late, irregular epiphyses are seen at both knee and ankle joints. (H.A.T.F.)

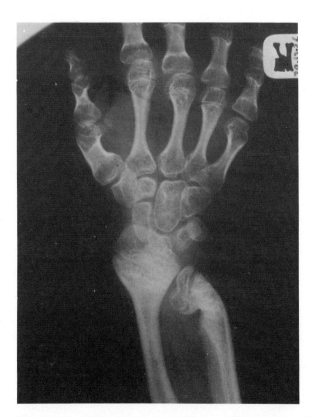

Fig. 14.12 (P.H.) Female aged 13 years. The metacarpals remain short with broad metaphyses, and the lower end of the radius and ulna are severely deformed. (H.A.T.F.)

15 Spondyloepiphyseal Dysplasia Congenita

This is a rare, very severe disorder characterised by a short trunk type of dwarfism with irregular platy-spondyly, and gross disorganisation of the upper femur.

Spranger and Wiedemann (1966) reported on 6 of their own patients and 14 from the previous literature, and Spranger and Langer (1970) reviewed 29 patients. The disorder has previously been confused with Morquio disease and other ill-defined spondylo-epiphyseal dysplasias.

Inheritance. Most cases are sporadic but it is likely the condition is of dominant inheritance.

Frequency. The condition is rare and the sexes are equally affected. It is present at birth and can be diagnosed radiographically then, but clinically, is not usually noticed until the infant is a few months old.

Clinical and radiographic features. The face is typically flat, the thorax increased in its antero-posterior diameter, kyphosis develops early and lordosis is present. Cleft palate and clubfoot are occasional features. Bach *et al* (1967) and Fraser *et al* (1969) have described a similar condition in which there is also a high degree of myopia, primary cataracts, buphthalmos and deafness.

On radiography the skull is normal apart from a steep floor to the anterior fossa. Vertebrae are flattened with an oval or pear-shaped appearance on the lateral view. There is hypoplasia and delayed ossification of the odontoid process, giving instability in this region.

The most striking feature of the disorder is the upper femoral region. Ossification is grossly retarded (Spranger and Langer noted a boy of 14 years still without a capital femoral epiphysis) and there is a gross degree of coxa vara with high-riding trochanters. Ossification of the pelvis is also retarded. In other bones there are minor epiphyseal and perhaps meta-physeal changes, with some delay of ossification around the knee joint. The hands and feet are only slightly involved, if at all.

Differential diagnosis. The main disorder likely to cause confusion is Morquio disease, but this is mani-fest at a later age, the pelvis has a distinctive configura-tion, coxa valga is present and the hands are charac-terised by shortened phalanges and metacarpals, with some failure of modelling and a pointed base of the second to fifth metacarpals. The feet are also involved in Morquio disease, but to a lesser degree. Corneal opacities are usually present and there is keratan sulphate in the urine.

There are probably other varieties of spondylo-epiphyseal dysplasia as yet to be delineated which will need to be differentiated from this type.

Progress and complications. Children are not usually mentally retarded. Adult height ranges from 85 to 130 cm (2′9″ to 4′3″). Problems arise from the very severely affected hip joints, from developing scoliosis, atlanto-axial instability, and from the eye problems in which the myopia is associated with retinal detachment and glaucoma. Treatment is related to these complications.

REFERENCES

Bach, C., Maroteaux, P., Schaeffer, P., Bitan, A. & Crumiere, C. (1967). Dysplasie spondyloépiphysaire congenitale avec anomalies multiples. *Archives Françaises de Pédiatrie*, **24**, 23.

Fraser, G. R., Friedmann, A. I., Maroteaux, P., Glen-Bott, A. M. & Mittwoch, U. (1969). Dysplasia spondyloepiphysaria congenita and related generalised skeletal dysplasias among children with severe visual handicaps. *Archives of Diseases in Childhood*, **44**, 490.

Spranger, J. W. & Wiedemann, H. R. (1966). Dysplasia spondyloepiphysaria congenita. *Helvetica Paediatrica Acta*, **21**, 598.

Spranger, J. W. & Langer, L. O. (1970). Spondyloepiphyseal dysplasia congenita. *Radiology*, **94**, 313.

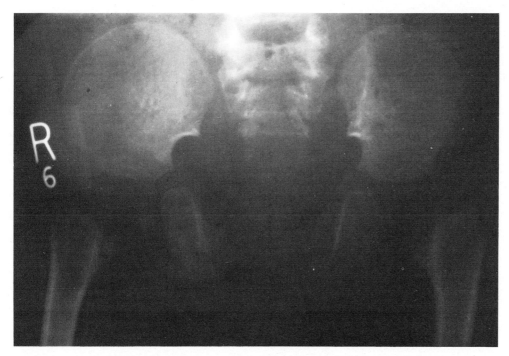

Fig. 15.1 (D.H.) Retarded ossification of pelvis and head of femur. (G.O.S.)

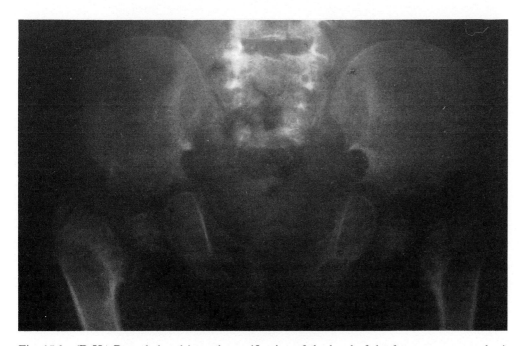

Fig. 15.2 (D.H.) Retarded and irregular ossification of the head of the femur; coxa vara; horizontal acetabular roofs. (G.O.S.)

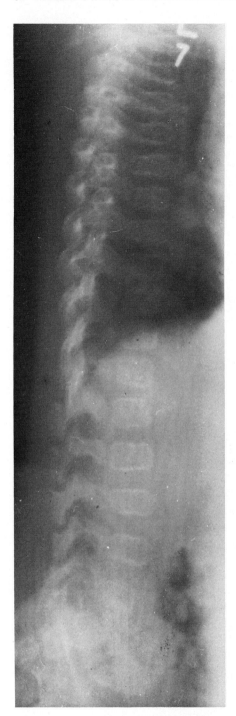

Fig. 15.3 (D.H.) Flattened vertebrae with *posterior* wedging, seen particularly in the thoracic region. (G.O.S.)

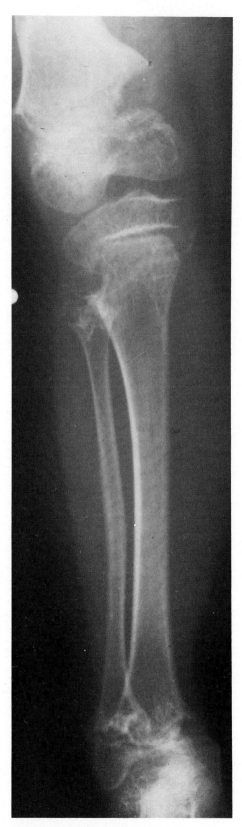

Figs 15.4 & 15.5 (D.H.) Metaphyseal and epiphyseal disorders. (G.O.S.)

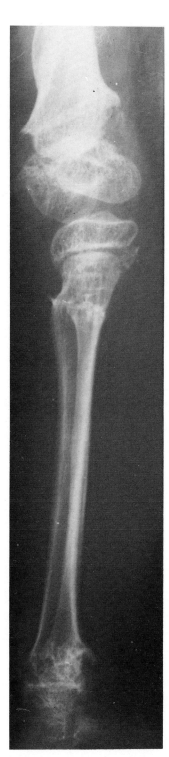

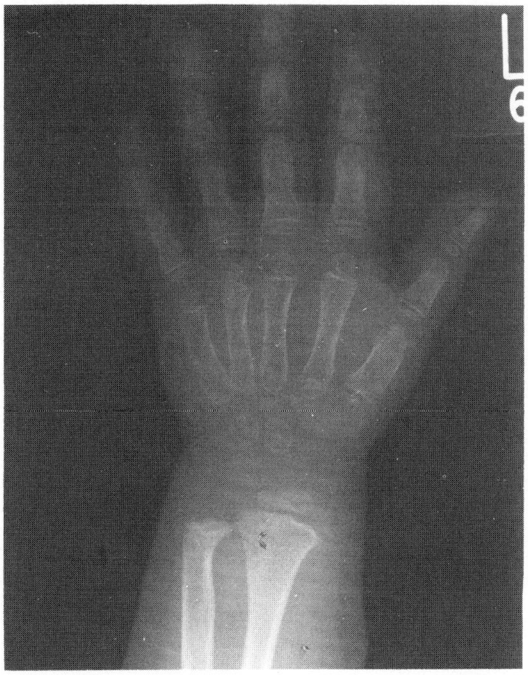

Fig. 15.6 (D.H.) Apart from delayed appearance of carpal ossification centres, the hand is relatively normal. (G.O.S.)

Fig. 15.5

16 Metatropic Dwarfism

In this form of dwarfism the infant is at first disproportionately short limbed, but subsequently the vertebral anomalies and developing scoliosis lead to a short trunk type of dwarfism.

It was first clearly delineated by Maroteaux, Spranger and Wiedemann in 1966, previous reports in the literature having described the condition as a type of Morquio disease (Michail *et al*, 1956). A more recent report in the English literature was by Jenkins, Smith and McKinnell (1970).

Inheritance. Some cases are likely to be of autosomal recessive inheritance, since more than one affected sib has been reported, but the disorder may well be a heterogeneous group as there have also been cases of apparent autosomal dominance.

Frequency. The population incidence is not known but the condition is very rare. It is immediately apparent at birth.

Clinical and radiographic features. At birth these infants have short extremities with a long trunk and narrow chest. Frequently there is a small tail-like appendage overlying the sacrum. Scoliosis is probably present at birth and as the child grows the defective ossification of vertebral bodies leads to flattening and a short trunk type of dwarfism, accentuated by the progressive scoliosis.

Radiographically the skull is normal and the thoracic cage resembles infants with asphyxiating thoracic dystrophy (Jeune disease), but there is not always respiratory deficiency in metatropic dwarfism.

The long bones are characteristic, being short with very wide flaring and irregularity of the metaphyses (dumb-bell shaped). The epiphyses are late in appearing and dysplastic.

In the infant the vertebrae are small and flat or diamond shaped in the lateral view, with wide intervertebral disc spaces. In later life there is platyspondyly with anterior wedging of the vertebrae.

The pelvis has short iliac wings and a horizontal acetabular roof. The capital femoral epiphysis is late appearing and there is considerable hyperplasia in the trochanteric region, though not as marked as in Kniest disease.

Pathology. There is an almost complete absence of enchondral ossification.

Differential diagnosis. This is from Morquio disease, which is characterised by a pigeon-breast type of deformity; the limbs are not shortened, and radiographic changes in the hands with the pointed base of the metacarpals is characteristic. There is an excess of keratan sulphate in the urine.

Kniest disease is somewhat similar but these patients do not have the characteristic narrow thorax, and the huge expansion of the trochanteric region of the femur is distinctive.

In later childhood the Kozlowski type of spondylometaphyseal dysplasia is similar so far as the vertebral changes are concerned, but does not have the characteristic dumb-bell shaped long bones, nor such a severe degree of dwarfing.

Progress and complications. The infant mortality in metatropic dwarfism is increased due to the reduced thoracic volume, and as growth progresses the kyphoscoliosis leads to further respiratory and cardiac problems. The final height of these patients is between 110 and 120 cm (3'7" to 3'11").

REFERENCES

Jenkins, P., Smith, M. B. & McKinnell, J. S. (1970). Metatropic dwarfism. *British Journal of Radiology*, **43**, 561.

Maroteaux, P., Spranger, J. & Wiedemann, H. R. (1966). Der metatropische Zwergwuchs. *Archiv für Kinderheilkunde*, **173**, 211.

Michail, J., Matsoukas, J., Theodorou, S. & Houliaras, K. (1956). Maladie de Morquio (ostéochondrodystrophie polyépiphysaire déformante) chez deux frères. *Helvetica Paediatrica Acta*, **11**, 403.

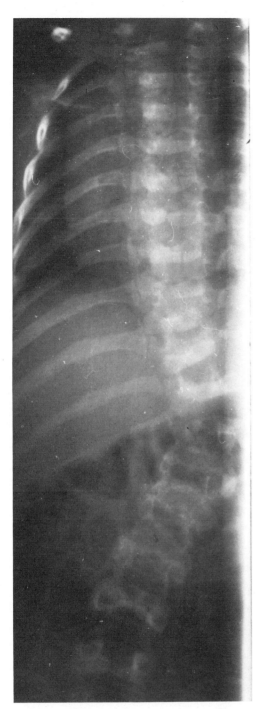

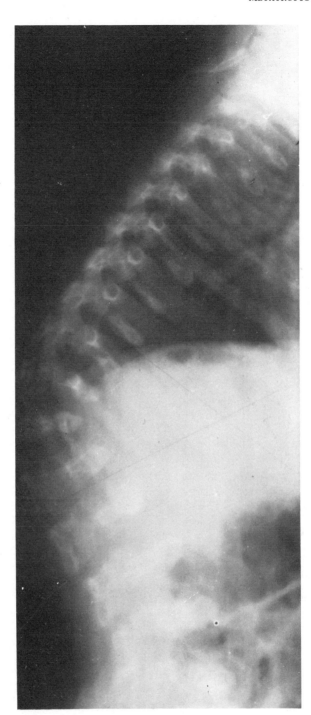

Fig. 16.1 (S.R.) Flattened vertebrae with wide intervertebral spaces and scoliosis. (G.O.S.)

Fig. 16.2 (S.R.) Vertebrae small, flattened or diamond shaped, with kyphosis. (G.O.S.)

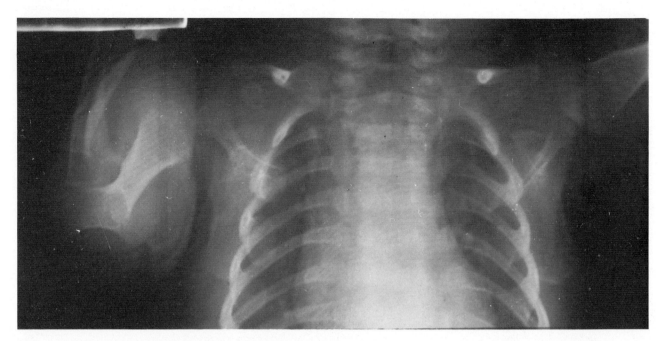

Fig. 16.3 (S.R.) Narrow thorax in infant. (G.O.S.)

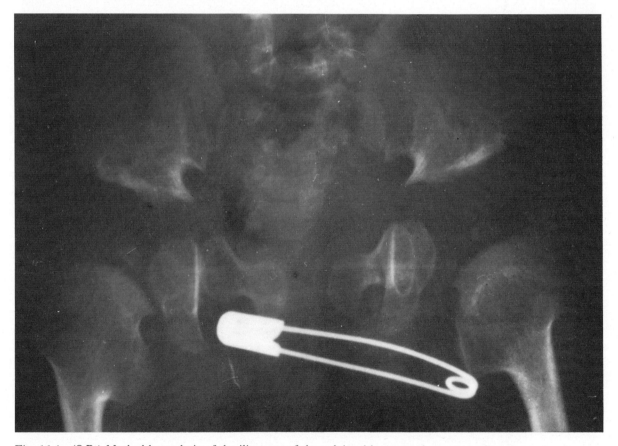

Fig. 16.4 (S.R.) Marked hypoplasia of the iliac part of the pelvis with great enlargement of trochanteric region. (G.O.S.)

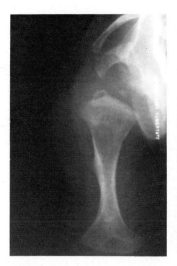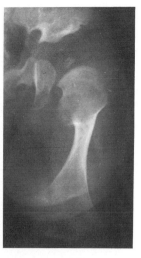

Figs 16.5 & 16.6 (S.R.) The humerus and femur show the typical dumb-bell shape, with dysplastic changes in both the metaphyses and epiphyses. (G.O.S.)

17 Kniest Disease

This is a recently delineated type of dwarfism with a short trunk, rather short curved limbs, a short broad thorax and a characteristic face with hypertelorism and a depressed nasal bridge.

The disorder was fully described and named 'Kniest disease' by Maroteaux and Spranger (1973), quoting the first likely case in the literature reported by Kniest (1952). The diagnosis has previously been confused with metatropic dwarfism, but the two conditions appear to be quite distinct.

Inheritance. It is of dominant inheritance, there being as yet insufficient evidence to state whether it is autosomal or X-linked.

Frequency. It is extremely rare, and is clinically apparent either at birth or within the first few months of life.

Clinical and radiographic features. The presenting sign is either shortness of stature, or enlargement of joints, particularly the knees. The face is characteristic, with hypertelorism, a flat mid-face and depressed nasal bridge. Cleft palate is present in about half the patients and there may be both conductive and neural hearing loss. Myopia is often a feature. The trunk is short and kyphosis may develop. The thorax is broad with sternal protrusion somewhat like Morquio disease. There may be joint contractures and sometimes clubfoot.

Radiographically there is platyspondyly with some anterior wedging of the first lumbar vertebra, and the epiphyseal surfaces of the vertebrae are very irregular. The long bones have broad metaphyses and disorganised epiphyses. Some of the most characteristic features are in the lower limbs, where the capital femoral epiphysis is very small and late in appearing but the trochanteric region is enormously enlarged. The epiphyses around the knee are large and irregular and together with the metaphyseal splaying are responsible for the clinical enlargement of this joint. The ilia are broad and hypoplastic in their basilar portions. The hands may show extra ossification centres at the distal end of the middle phalanges.

Differential diagnosis. This is from metatropic dwarfism, where the thorax is narrow and the vertebrae are diamond or oval-shaped rather than flat. Spondyloepiphyseal dysplasia congenita has similar features in the pelvis and spine but the characteristic upper end of the femur in Kniest disease is diagnostic.

Progress and complications. The final height of these individuals is between 106 and 145 cm (3′6″ to 4′9″). Patients suffer from restricted joint mobility and premature osteoarthritis. Complications arise from chronic otitis and deafness, and the myopia may lead to retinal detachment. The four cases described by Roaf, Longmore and Forrester (1967) were thus affected and are likely to be examples of Kniest disease.

REFERENCES

Kniest, W. (1952). Zur Abgrenzung der Dysostosis enchondralis von der Chondrodystrophie. *Zeitschrift für Kinderheilkunde,* **70,** 633.

Maroteaux, P. & Spranger, J. (1973). La maladie de Kniest. *Archives Françaises de Pédiatrie,* **30,** 735.

Roaf, R., Longmore, J. B. & Forrester, R. M. (1967). A childhood syndrome of bone dysplasia, retinal detachment and deafness. *Developmental Medicine and Child Neurology,* **9,** 464.

18   Diastrophic Dwarfism

This is a form of short-limbed dwarfism associated with a severe intractable scoliosis, talipes equino-varus and contractures of most joints.

It was first named by Lamy and Maroteaux in 1960, though patients had been reported before this, described as 'atypical achondroplasia'. The first report in the English literature was by Taybi (1963) and Walker et al (1972) reviewed 51 patients.

Inheritance. The condition is of autosomal recessive inheritance, as many affected sibs with normal parents have been described.

Frequency. The population incidence is not known, though it appears to be less common than classical achondroplasia. The sexes are affected equally and the condition is apparent at birth.

Clinical and radiographic features. Apart from the short limbs, a striking feature present at birth, or developing within the first few days of life, is a cystic swelling of the ear present in three-quarters or more of these patients. The swelling subsequently calcifies, then ossifies giving a 'cauliflower ear' appearance in the adult. Apart from this defect the head appears normal, though cleft palate is present in between one quarter and one half of cases.

Scoliosis develops as the child grows, and may become very severe.

There are multiple joint contractures (of shoulders, elbows, hands, hips and knees) though some joints unaffected by contractures may be abnormally lax and dislocations are frequent. The hands and feet are short and broad and there is a particularly resistant talipes equino-varus. A curious feature is a short first metacarpal, resulting in the thumb being apparently placed too far proximally (Stober, Hayes and Holt, 1963; Wilson, Chrispin and Carter, 1969).

Radiographically the skull is normal, the vertebrae may have disorders of segmentation, and there may be hypoplasia of the odontoid process and instability in this region. It is usually only the cervical vertebrae that are abnormal, the remainder of the vertebral column is structurally unremarkable apart from some slight narrowing of the interpedicular distance in the lumbar vertebrae, not so severe as in classical achondroplasia.

The epiphyses of the long bones are delayed in appearing and flat and distorted when they do. The metaphyses are flared. The hip joints are severely affected, with wide, irregular acetabulae, short wide femoral necks and deformed femoral heads. The radiographic appearances around the knee are characteristic in that the lower femoral and upper tibial epiphyses are flattened and apparently shifted medially.

There is disproportionate shortening of the ulna and fibula. Langer (1965) noted that the carpal bones, in contradistinction to other areas, showed accelerated maturation. The metacarpals, metatarsals and phalanges have delayed appearance of secondary ossification centres and occasionally symphalangism. The first metacarpal and metatarsal are characteristically oval or triangular in shape and disproportionately short.

Pathology. The histology has been studied by Caplan et al (1961) and Salle et al (1966). They found a reduction in the number of chondrocytes in the resting, proliferative and columnar zones and the thickness of the proliferative and columnisation zones was only half the normal. The cells were flattened and atrophic and there were cystic areas scattered throughout the matrix.

Differential diagnosis. Diastrophic dwarfism was for many years confused with classical achondroplasia but this is clearly differentiated by its abnormal skull and pelvis and the lack of scoliosis and clubfoot. Confusion has also arisen with arthrogryposis multiplex congenita, but these children do not have a short-limbed type of dwarfism and the tubular shape of their limbs is quite characteristic.

Progress and complications. There is a considerable infant mortality in diastrophic dwarfism, probably due to respiratory difficulties, but if they survive this period then life expectancy appears to be normal.

Scoliosis (which is never present at birth) develops during the early years of life and is, like the clubfoot, particularly intractable. Cervical vertebral anomalies and the hypoplastic odontoid in particular may lead to compression of the cord in the atlanto-axial region and tetraplegia. The final height of these individuals is between 80 and 140 cm (2'7" to 4'7").

Treatment. Treatment is directed toward the scoliosis, joint contractures and clubfeet, and it is necessary to be watchful of the cervical cord area.

REFERENCES

Kaplan, M., Sauvegrain, J., Hayem, F., Drapeau, P., Maughey, F. & Boulle, J. (1961). Etude d'un nouveau cas de nanisme diastrophique. *Archives Françaises de Pédiatrie*, **18**, 981.

Lamy, M. & Maroteaux, P. (1960). La nanisme diastrophique. *La Presse Médicale*, **68**, 1977.

Langer, L. O. (1965). Diastrophic dwarfism in early infancy. *American Journal of Roentgenology*, **93**, 399.

Salle, B., Picot, C., Vauzelle, J. L., Deffrenne, P., Monnet, P., Francois, R. & Robert, J. M. (1966). Le nanisme diastrophique —à propos de trois observations chez le nouveau-né. *Pédiatrie*, **21**, 311.

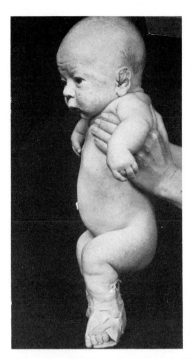

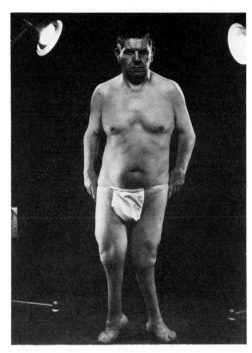

Fig. 18.1 (S.H. aged 6 weeks.) Short upper limbs particularly, feet under treatment for talipes equino varus. The cystic ear lesion is visible. (Courtesy of Mr G. C. Lloyd-Roberts, London.)

Fig. 18.2 (R.B. 55 year old male.) Marked shortening of the upper limbs particularly. End result of severe intractable talipes equino varus. (Courtesy of Mr G. P. Mitchell, Edinburgh.)

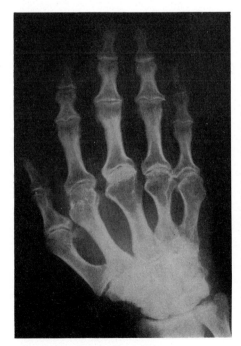

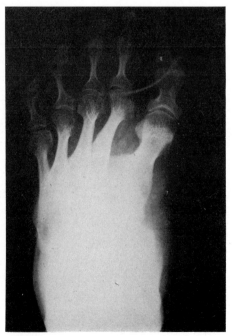

Fig. 18.3 (R.B.) The hands, particularly the metacarpals, are short and stubby but he does not show the characteristic shortening of the first metacarpal. (Courtesy of Mr G. P. Mitchell, Edinburgh.)

Fig. 18.4 (R.B.) The feet also are short and stubby and the first metatarsal shorter than the others. (Courtesy of Mr G. P. Mitchell, Edinburgh.)

Stover, C. N., Hayes, J. T. & Holt, J. F. (1963). Diastrophic dwarfism. *American Journal of Roentgenology*, **89**, 914.
Taybi, H. (1963). Diastrophic dwarfism. *Radiology*, **80**, 1.
Walker, B. A., Scott, C. I., Hall, J. G., Murdoch, J. L. & McKusick, V. A. (1972). Diastrophic dwarfism. *Medicine*, **51**, 41.
Wilson, D. W., Chrispin, A. R. & Carter, C. O. (1969). Diastrophic dwarfism. *Archives of Diseases in Childhood*, **44**, 48.

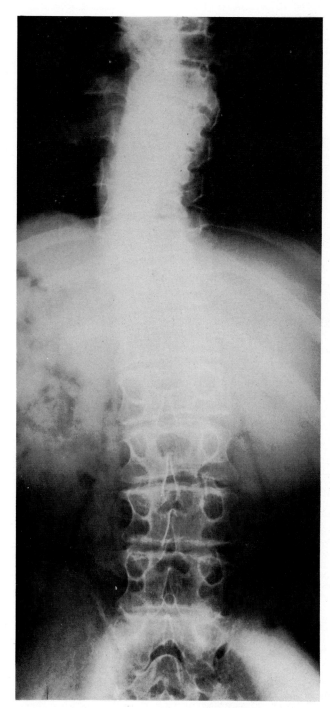

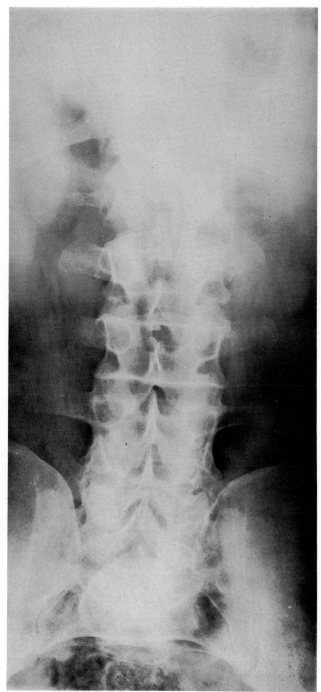

Fig. 18.5 (S.H. aged 15 years.) Thoraco-lumbar scoliosis. The interpedicular distance of the first and last lumbar vertebrae are approximately equal, as in hypochondroplasia. Normally the distance widens from first to last vertebra. (Courtesy of Mr G. C. Lloyd-Roberts, London.)

Fig. 18.6 (R.B.) The lumbar vertebrae show the same defect as patient S.H. (Courtesy of Mr G. P. Mitchell, Edinburgh.)

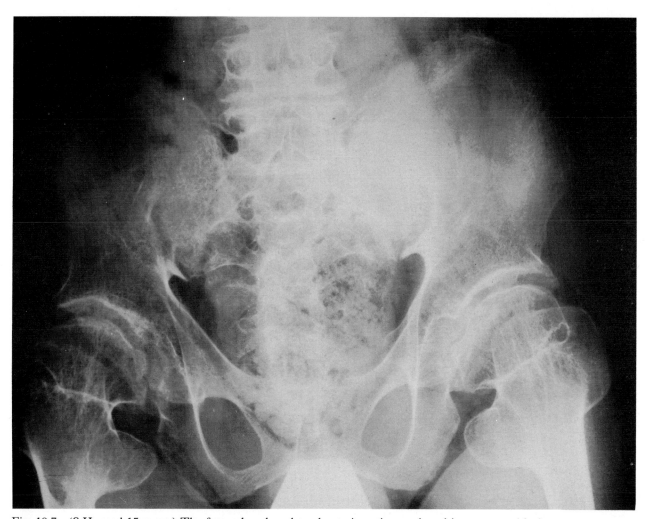

Fig. 18.7 (S.H. aged 15 years.) The femoral neck and trochanteric region are broad in contrast with the rather narrow femoral shaft but the pelvis is not markedly abnormal. (Courtesy of Mr G. C. Lloyd-Roberts, London.)

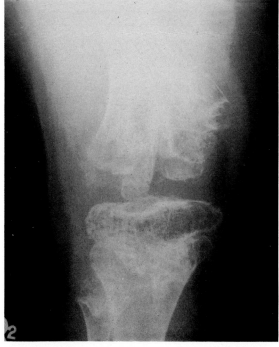

Fig. 18.8 (S.H. aged 10 years.) There is epiphyseal and metaphyseal dysplasia with a cone-shaped deformity at the lower end of the femur. (Courtesy of Mr G. C. Lloyd-Roberts, London.)

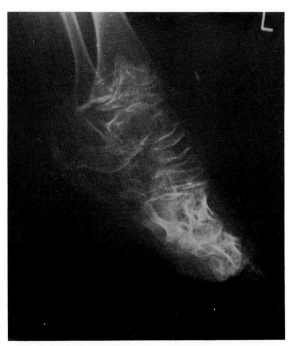

Fig. 18.9 (S.H. aged 9 years.) Osteoporotic, equinus foot. (Courtesy of Mr G. C. Lloyd-Roberts, London.)

19 Parastremmatic Dwarfism

This is an extremely rare, severe form of dwarfism with bizarre, asymmetrical lower limb deformities in which it appears that the bones have twisted around their long axes.

It was described by Langer, Petersen and Spranger (1970), who suggested the name, but there are probably earlier cases in the literature; Langer and colleagues suggest that the patients described by Apert, Liege and Denet (1934) and by Rask (1963) suffered from parastremmatic dwarfism.

Inheritance. Very few cases have been described but there is one instance of father to daughter inheritance, the rest have been sporadic. It is likely therefore that the disorder is of dominant inheritance, either autosomal or X-linked.

Frequency. The disorder is extremely rare; it is not apparent at birth, but becomes so during the first year of life.

Clinical and radiographic features. The presenting sign is a bending deformity, mainly of the lower limbs, similar to rickets. Walking is delayed and the gait abnormal from infancy. Dwarfism is severe and scoliosis present as well as joint contractures.

Radiographically the skull is normal but the vertebrae are flat with irregularly ossified end plates. The long bones are shortened and distorted with very deformed epiphyses and metaphyses. The latter are characterised by irregular stippling and streaks giving a distinctive flocculated appearance.

At a certain stage of development the pelvis shows a remarkable lace-like appearance of the developing iliac crests. The capital femoral epiphyses are small and late in ossifying (Horan & Beighton, 1976).

Pathology. Langer and colleagues reported that biopsy material from the proximal femur showed enchondral bone formation decreased and irregular with a diminished number of osteoblasts and osteoclasts. There was complete lack of columnisation of cartilage cells.

Differential diagnosis. This is from those conditions characterised by platyspondyly and scoliosis together with metaphyseal and epiphyseal changes, (the spondyloepiphyseal dysplasias, metatropic dwarfism, Kniest disease and pseudoachondroplasia.) However in none of these does the bone have a flocculated appearance, nor is there asymmetrical bending of the long bones of the lower limb.

Progress and complications. These children have delayed motor development probably due to the stiff joints and twisted limbs present from infancy. Although the skeletal deformities are so severe these individuals can survive to adulthood, the final height being between 90 and 110 cm (3′ to 3′7″).

REFERENCES

Apert, M. M., Liege, R. & Denet, J. (1934). Dystrophie ostéo-articulaire grave chez une fille de 12 ans. *Bulletin de la Société de Pédiatrie de Paris*, **32**, 577.

Horan, F. & Beighton, P. (1976). Parastremmatic dwarfism. *Journal of Bone & Joint Surgery*, **58A** (in press).

Langer, L. O., Petersen, D. & Spranger, J. (1970). An unusual bone dysplasia: parastremmatic dwarfism. *American Journal of Roentgenology*, **110**, 550.

Rask, M. R. (1963). Morquio–Brailsford osteochondrodystrophy and osteogenesis imperfecta: Report of a patient with both conditions. *Journal of Bone & Joint Surgery*, **45A**, 561.

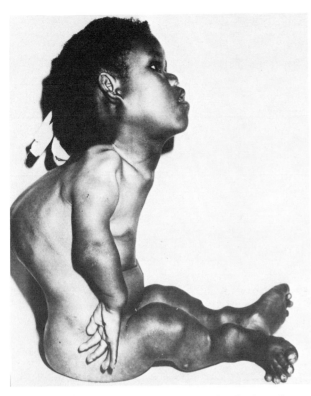

Fig. 19.1   (S.V.B.) Aged 5 years, gross kyphosis and bending deformation of limbs. (Courtesy of Professor P. Beighton, Cape Town.)

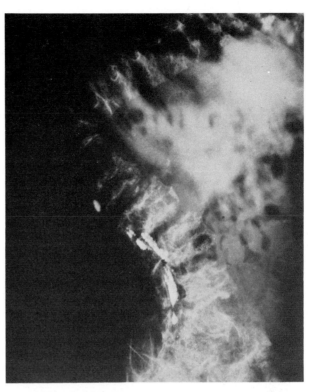

Fig. 19.2   (S.V.B.) Aged 9 years. Somewhat flattened vertebrae with irregularly ossified end plates. (Courtesy of Professor P. Beighton, Cape Town.)

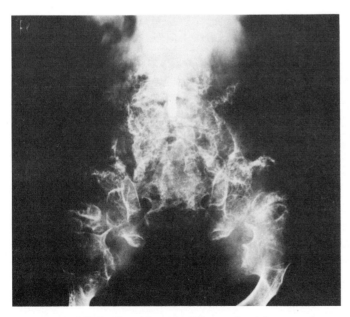

Fig. 19.3   (S.V.B.) Aged 9 years. Distorted epiphyses and metaphyses with gross disorganisation of the hip joint. (Courtesy of Professor P. Beighton, Cape Town.)

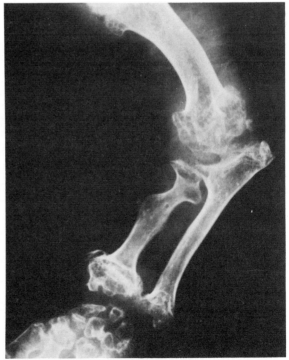

Fig. 19.4   (S.V.B.) Shortening of long bones, widened and distorted metaphyses with irregular streaks and blotches. (Courtesy of Professor P. Beighton, Cape Town.)

20 Dyggve–Melchior–Clausen Disease

This is a form of short trunk dwarfism formerly confused with Morquio disease, but the children are usually mentally retarded and there is no mucopolysaccharide in the urine.

The disorder was first described by Dyggve, Melchior and Clausen in 1962, in three severely mentally retarded sibs whose parents were consanguineous.

Inheritance. It is of autosomal recessive inheritance.

Clinical and radiographic features. The disorder is extremely rare, though it is possible that some cases which have been described as non-keratan sulphate excreting Morquio disease belong to this group (Linker, Evans and Langer, 1970). The disorder becomes apparent during infancy or early childhood, by reason of a short trunk type of dwarfism and mental retardation.

Radiographically the vertebral bodies are flat and have a characteristic notch on the superior and inferior surfaces. The long bones are somewhat short with irregular epiphyseal and metaphyseal ossification.

The hands may show cone-shaped epiphyses of the phalanges.

The pelvis is short and broad with disordered ossification of the iliac crest. The capital femoral epiphysis is late in appearing and there is a characteristic spur on the medial aspect of the neck.

Pathology. Affifi *et al* (1974) have described five sibs thought to have this syndrome with unique membranous inclusions within the muscle fibres of one of them. They noted a banding pattern characteristically in subsarcolemmal sites.

Differential diagnosis. This is from Morquio disease which is characterised by normal intelligence, sometimes corneal clouding, no disorder of ossification of the iliac crest, and a pointed base to the metacarpals. Keratan sulphate appears in the urine.

Progress and complications. Children with the Dyggve–Melchior–Clausen syndrome are likely to be mentally retarded. The height of the only two adults known was 119 and 128 cm (3′11″ and 4′2″).

REFERENCES

Affifi, A. K., der Kaloustian, V. M., Bahuth, N. B. & Mire-Salman, J. (1974). Concentrically laminated membranous inclusions in myofibres of Dyggve–Melchior–Clausen syndrome. *Journal of the Neurological Sciences*, **21**, 335.

Dyggve, H. V., Melchior, J. C. & Clausen, J. (1962). Morquio–Ullrich's disease: an inborn error of metabolism? *Archives of Diseases in Childhood*, **37**, 525.

Linker, A., Evans, L. R. & Langer, L. O. (1970). Morquio's disease and mucopolysaccharide excretion. *Journal of Pediatrics*, **77**, 1039.

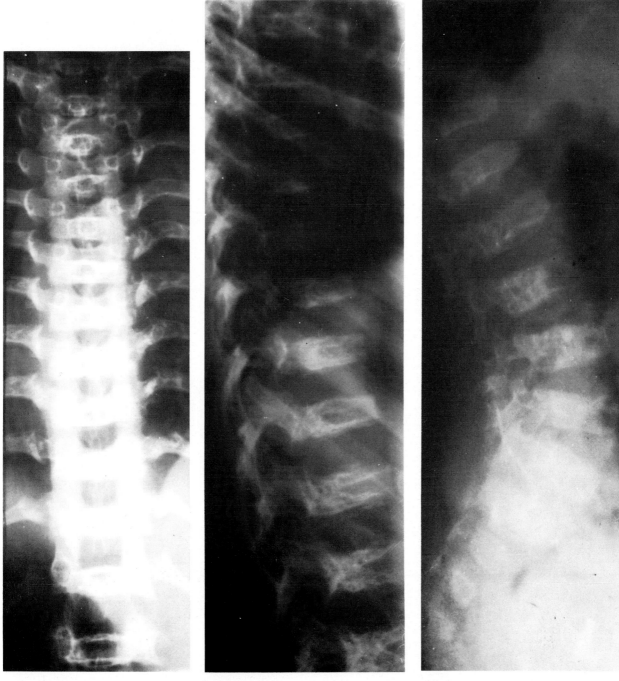

Figs 20.1 & 20.2 (S.F.) AP and lateral of spine show platyspondyly with rather wide intervertebral spaces. (G.O.S.)

Fig. 20.3 (S.F.) Irregular flattening of vertebral bodies. (G.O.S.)

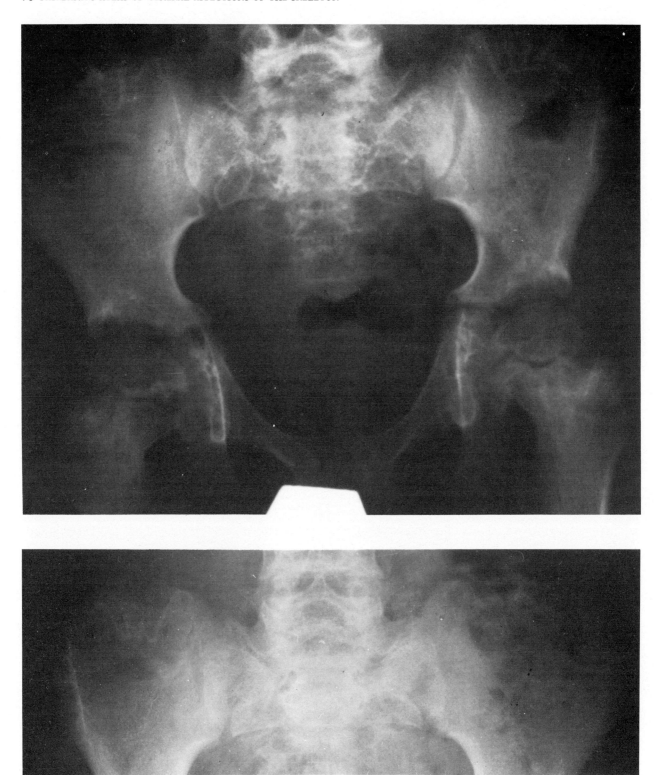

Figs 20.4 & 20.5   (S.F.) Male at 9 and 14 years showing lace-like ossification in the region of the iliac crest and irregular ossification of the femoral epiphyses and metaphyses. (G.O.S.)

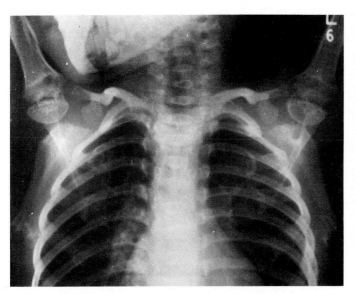

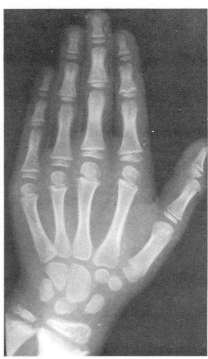

Fig. 20.6   (S.F.) Metaphyseal and epiphyseal irregularity at the upper end of the humerus and a defect in ossification at the lower end of the scapula. (G.O.S.)

Fig. 20.7   (S.F.) The hand is relatively normal but there are marked metaphyseal changes at the lower end of the radius and ulna. (G.O.S.)

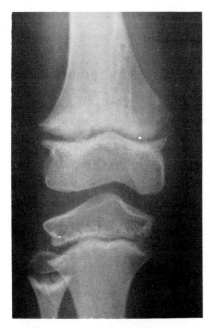

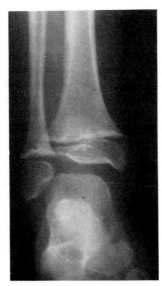

Fig. 20.8   (S.F.) Metaphyseal and epiphyseal irregularities at the knee. (G.O.S.)

Fig. 20.9   (S.F.) Metaphyseal and epiphyseal irregularities at the ankle. (G.O.S.)

Osteogenesis Imperfecta
Fragilitas Ossium

This disorder, characterised by fragility of bone and blue sclerae, has been known for centuries. It is often accompanied by other disorders of connective tissue such as generalised joint laxity, undue ease of bruising, poor scar formation and by the onset of deafness in the second or third decade. The first major report in the English literature was by Bell (1928).

For some time argument has centred around whether the condition is essentially one or more diseases, one extreme of the condition being the mild tarda form, starting usually during infancy or childhood with only occasional fractures, blue sclerotics, little or no bone deformity and a strong family history of autosomal dominant inheritance. At the other extreme there is the severe congenital form which is clearly of prenatal onset in that children may be born with multiple fractures. It is accompanied by severe dwarfing and the prognosis is poor. These are nearly always sporadic cases. Current evidence suggests that whereas osteogenesis imperfecta tarda is clinically and genetically a clear cut entity, the congenita type is likely to be heterogeneous. With this in mind, the two extremes of severity are here discussed.

SEVERE CONGENITAL FORM OF OSTEOGENESIS IMPERFECTA

These infants have multiple fractures pre- and postnatally, dwarfing and progressive deformity due to malunion of fractures and bending of the soft bones.
Inheritance. The great majority of cases are sporadic, indicating either that this entity is a new mutation of a dominant gene, or non-genetic in origin. However, there has been an occasional report of more than one affected sib with normal parents (Goldfarb and Ford, 1954; McKusick, 1972), indicating that at least in some instances the condition can be of autosomal recessive inheritance. There is also an occasional report of a patient with the severe congenital type born to a mother with the milder, tarda form, indicating that the congenita and tarda forms can have the same aetiology (Seedorf, 1949), though this does not usually appear to be the case. The genetics of the severe congenital form of osteogenesis imperfecta are not yet fully established and it may well be a heterogeneous group. No relationship with parental age or birth rank has been reported (Smårs, 1961).
Frequency. The population incidence is around 1 in 50,000 births, the sexes being equally affected. The condition is immediately apparent at birth.
Clinical and radiographic features. In addition to the severe dwarfing, multiple fractures and limb deformities, the limbs are disproportionately short at birth. The head is large, and the face small and triangular. The bones of the vault are membranous in character and soft to the touch. The teeth may be abnormal with defective dentine giving them a somewhat transparent and brownish appearance. The sclerae are blue at birth—as indeed are those of all newborn children, but in the congenita form they often become white as the child grows, as do those of a normal child (Bauze, Smith and Francis, 1975). Other clinical characteristics are generalised joint laxity in about 45 per cent of cases, sometimes a tendency to easy bruising, poor wound healing and congenital herniae. Scoliosis develops in a high proportion of patients—King and Bobechko (1971) reported its occurrence in 50 per cent, and Hoek (1975) in 70 per cent of patients.

Radiographic appearances are very variable, though always striking. The large vault of the skull with a temporal bulge and small face beneath is well known. Wormian bones are present in the suture lines. The bones of the vertebral column are normal in shape initially, but they are soft and later develop platyspondyly or the biconcave deformity of osteoporosis. The appendicular skeleton is very variably affected—which is part of the reason for regarding the congenita form as a heterogeneous group. Fairbank (1951) described three types: thick bone; slender, fragile bone, and cystic bone. Certainly all these have been reported since then in severe congenital osteogenesis imperfecta, though it is likely that one form may progress to another. Bauze and colleagues (1975) noted in some instances that buttressing developed on the concave side of a long bone deformity, though other cases were apparently unable to do this. In the thick-boned type there is telescoping of fractures and the major long bones are shortened. In the thin-bone type the shafts are extremely narrow with a very thin cortex and marked osteoporosis. The marrow cavity may be completely obliterated. Another difference between patients is that in some cases the bones bend (perhaps related to multiple micro-fractures?), whereas in others they break and angulate.

The epiphyses are essentially normal and in severely affected cases the metaphyses appear relatively expanded by comparison with the narrowed diaphyses.
Differential diagnosis. The diagnosis is not usually in doubt, the only rather similar condition to severe osteogenesis imperfecta present at birth being congenital hypophosphatasia, a lethal condition characterised by a low serum alkaline phosphatase and large areas of absent ossification in the skull and other bones.
Progress and complications. These infants are often stillborn with multiple fractures and intracranial haemorrhage associated with cranial damage. If they survive the perinatal period, they suffer from

considerable deformity from the softening of bone and continuing tendency to fracture, and further osteoporosis results from the necessity to immobilise them. Little growth takes place and children living to their teens or even later may still be less than 90 cm (2′11″) in height. Neurological complications related to platybasia have been described.

The fractures are very variable in number and are commoner in the lower limbs, but they tend to diminish with age and usually heal normally. Hyperplastic callus does develop in a few cases with much swelling, heat, throbbing pain and tenderness, and has been reported by many writers (Baker, 1946; Fairbank and Baker, 1948; Vandermark and Page, 1948; Apley, 1951; Strach, 1953; Banta, Schreiber and Kulikwj, 1971). Bauze et al (1975) reported two sets of parent and child with hyperplastic callus and noted that in these cases the bone did not remodel with time, indicating a persistent abnormality in the fracture healing process. All authors stress the difficulty and importance of distinguishing hyperplastic callus from acute osteomyelitis and from neoplasm. Klenerman, Ockenden and Townsend (1967) reported two cases in which there was a genuine osteosarcoma present but they questioned whether this could be considered more common in osteogenesis imperfecta than in the general population—both conditions being extremely rare.

The otosclerosis and deafness that develops in osteogenesis imperfecta tarda may or may not be a feature in the congenital type of disease: most of these infants die before the second or third decade when this feature usually presents.

MILDER TARDA FORM OF OSTEOGENESIS IMPERFECTA

Many features of this slightly later developing disease are similar to the congenita form of osteogenesis imperfecta, but fractures are less frequent as well as being of later onset.

Inheritance. Nearly all reported cases are of autosomal dominant inheritance.

Frequency. This is probably around 1 in 20,000 live births, the sexes being equally affected. The condition may occasionally be apparent soon after birth, but the usual age of onset is during infancy or childhood, the greatest number of fractures being reported around the ages of 2 or 3 years, and then at 6 or 7 years (Smårs, 1961).

Clinical and radiographic features. There is the same broadening of the skull and temporal region, with a small triangular face as in the congenita form. Blue sclerotics are nearly always present throughout life, and other features are ligamentous laxity, thin skin with increased width of scars and sometimes undue ease of bruising due to increased capillary fragility. Pectus excavatum and scoliosis are common, as is platyspondyly and biconcave vertebrae. Most cases of the 'tarda' form are of the thin-bone type, with thin cortices and decreased bone density.

In about one-quarter of cases otosclerosis and deafness develop during the second or third decade

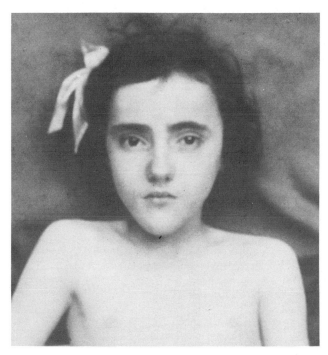

Fig. 21.1 (L.) Elfin-shaped face with broad forehead and pointed chin. (H.A.T.F.)

of life. This disorder is associated with enlargement of the foot plate of the stapes, and may respond to stapedectomy.

Differential diagnosis. Mild cases of osteogenesis imperfecta with onset in infancy may be difficult to distinguish from the 'battered baby', though in the latter the typical shape of the skull, blue sclerotics, teeth abnormalities and vertebral changes are not present. There may also be difficulties in diagnosing other conditions which cause osteoporosis in childhood, such as the early stages of leukaemia, before the typical blood picture is apparent, and in later childhood idiopathic juvenile osteoporosis. This latter does not develop until a year or so before puberty and is a self limiting disorder.

PATHOGENESIS

Osteogenesis imperfecta, whether congenita or tarda, results from defective collagen formation. Whether this defect is of the collagen itself or of the cells which produce it is not known, though histological studies have shown cellular abnormalities (Follis, 1953; Falvo and Bullough, 1973). Doty and Mathews (1970) found on osteoblast anomaly in their electronmicroscope and histochemical studies of osteogenesis imperfecta, and suggested that this probably led directly to immaturity of the collagen fibres. Riley and Jowsey (1973) found the ultrastructure of osteocytes and scleral collagen was normal but that corneal collagen fibres were half the normal diameter.

Laboratory investigation has not always been precisely related to the clinical picture in these patients and it may well be that various contradictory findings are descriptions of essentially different disorders.

Bauze, Smith and Francis (1975) divided patients into mild, moderate and severe groups according to the degree of deformity of the long bones, and found that in the severe group polymeric collagen from skin was unstable, though normal in amount. In the mild group, however, the reverse was found—the polymeric skin collagen was stable but reduced in amount. Since the overall metabolism of collagen is similar in all tissues, they considered that their findings in skin collagen reflected those in bone, and implied a collagen cross-linkage defect in severe osteogenesis imperfecta (Francis, Smith and Macmillan, 1973). Further clarification must await progress in collagen chemistry and an accurate link-up with clinical, radiological and genetic types of the disease.

Solomons and Miller (1973) refer to a hypermetabolic state in osteogenesis imperfecta with increased risk of malignant hyperthermia induced by anaesthetic agents. They suggest a prolonged immaturity state in a variety of tissues, including bone. Cropp and Myers (1972) also refer to a defect in energy metabolism, similar to hyperthyroidism.

TREATMENT

This is mainly directed to the care of fractures, immobilising the patient as little as possible in order to avoid further osteoporosis and further risk of fracturing. Fragmentation and rodding, particularly of the lower limb bones, has been practised for many years (Sofield and Millar, 1959; Williams, 1965; Tiley and Albright, 1973), and allows correction of deformity with early mobilisation of the patient. This enables many patients to walk, with or without the aid of protective calipers, whereas in the past they would have been confined to a spinal carriage or wheelchair.

A wide range of chemical treatments has been advocated in osteogenesis imperfecta, but there is no evidence that any of them has an effect on the fracture rate. Calcium and vitamin D are not without their dangers; fluoride may give some improvement of the teeth but has no other benefit (Albright and Grunt, 1971). Anabolic steroids have no effect on the fracture

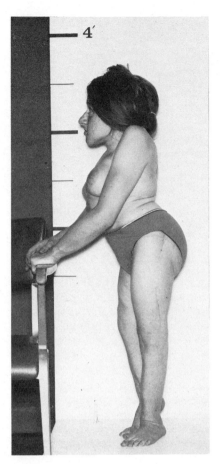

Fig. 21.2 Fully grown female with shortness of stature and deformities. (A.H.)

rate and many adverse side-effects (Cattell and Clayton, 1968). Magnesium oxide has also been found to be of no value (Dietrich and Stryker, 1975). More recently, ascorbic acid has been used (Winterfeldt, Eyring and Vivian, 1970) and calcitonin (Castells et al, 1972; Goldfield et al, 1972), but more clinical trials are needed before their value can be established.

REFERENCES

Albright, J. A. & Grunt, J. A. (1971). Studies of patients with osteogenesis imperfecta. *Journal of Bone & Joint Surgery,* **53A,** 1415.

Apley, A. G. (1951). Hyperplastic callus in osteogenesis imperfecta. *Journal of Bone & Joint Surgery,* **33B,** 591.

Baker, S. L. (1946). Hyperplastic callus simulating sarcoma in two cases of fragilitas ossium. *Journal of Pathology & Bacteriology,* **58,** 609.

Banta, J. V., Schreiber, R. R. & Kulik, W. J. (1971). Hyperplastic callus formation in osteogenesis imperfecta simulating osteosarcoma. *Journal of Bone & Joint Surgery,* **53A,** 115.

Bauze, R. J., Smith, R. & Francis, M. J. O. (1975). A new look at osteogenesis imperfecta. *Journal of Bone & Joint Surgery,* **57B,** 2.

Bell, J. (1928). Blue sclerotics and fragility of bone. *Treasury of Human Inheritance,* **2,** Part 3.

Castells, S., Inamdar, S., Baker, R. K. & Wallach, S. (1972). Effects of porcine calcitonin in osteogenesis imperfecta tarda. *Journal of Pediatrics,* **80,** 757.

Cattell, H. S. & Clayton, B. (1968). Failure of anabolic steroids in the therapy of osteogenesis imperfecta. *Journal of Bone & Joint Surgery,* **50A,** 123.

Cropp, G. J. A. & Myers, D. N. (1972). Physiological evidence of hypermetabolism in osteogenesis imperfecta. *Pediatrics,* **49,** 375.

Dietrich, S. L. & Stryker, W. S. (1975). Magnesium oxide in the treatment of osteogenesis imperfecta. *Journal of Bone & Joint Surgery*, **57A,** 136.

Doty, S. B. & Mathews, R. S. (1970). Electron microscopy and histochemical studies in osteogenesis imperfecta. *Journal of Bone & Joint Surgery*, **52A,** 601.

Fairbank, H. A. T. & Baker, S. L. (1948). Hyperplastic callus formation with or without evidence of a fracture in osteogenesis. *British Journal of Surgery*, **36,** 1.

Fairbank, T. (1951). *An Atlas of General Affections of the Skeleton*, 1st edition. Edinburgh & London: E. & S. Livingstone.

Falvo, K. A. & Bullough, P. G. (1973). Osteogenesis imperfecta: A histometric analysis. *Journal of Bone & Joint Surgery*, **55A,** 275.

Follis, R. H. Jun. (1953). Histochemical studies on cartilage and bone. III. Osteogenesis imperfecta. *Bulletin of the Johns Hopkins Hospital*, **93,** 386.

Francis, M. J. O., Smith, R. & Macmillan, D. C. (1973). Polymeric collagen from biopsies of human skin. *Clinical Science*, **44,** 429.

Goldfarb, A. A. & Ford, D. (1954). Osteogenesis imperfecta congenita in consecutive siblings. *Journal of Pediatrics*, **44,** 264.

Goldfield, E. B., Braiker, B. M., Prendergast, J. J. & Kolb, F. O. (1972). Synthetic salmon calcitonin: treatment of Paget's disease and osteogenesis imperfecta. *Journal of the American Medical Association*, **221,** 1127.

Hoek, K. J. (1975). Scoliosis in osteogenesis imperfecta. *Journal of Bone & Joint Surgery*, **57A,** 136.

King, J. D. & Bobechko, W. P. (1971). Osteogenesis imperfecta. An orthopaedic description and surgical review. *Journal of Bone & Joint Surgery*, **53B,** 72.

Klenerman, L., Ockenden, B. G. & Townsend, A. C. (1967). Osteosarcoma occurring in osteogenesis imperfecta. *Journal of Bone & Joint Surgery*, **49B,** 314.

McKusick, V. (1972). *Heritable Disorders of Connective Tissue*, 4th edition, Mosby, St. Louis.

Riley, F. C. & Jowsey, J. (1973). Osteogenesis imperfecta: morphologic and biochemical studies of connective tissue. *Pediatric Research*, **9,** 757.

Seedorf, K. S. (1949). *Osteogenesis Imperfecta*, Monksgaard, Copenhagen.

Småirs, G. (1961). *Osteogenesis imperfecta in Sweden.* Scandinavian University Books, Stockholm.

Sofield, H. A. & Millar, E. A. (1959). Fragmentation, realignment and intramedullary rod fixation of deformities of the long bones in children. *Journal of Bone & Joint Surgery*, **41A,** 1371.

Solomons, C. C. & Millar, E. A. (1973). Osteogenesis imperfecta—new perspectives. *Clinical Orthopaedics & Related Research*, **96,** 299.

Strach, E. H. (1953). Hyperplastic callus formation in osteogenesis imperfecta. *Journal of Bone & Joint Surgery*, **35B,** 417.

Tiley, F. & Albright, J. A. (1973). Osteogenesis imperfecta: treatment by multiple osteotomy and intramedullary rod insertion. *Journal of Bone & Joint Surgery*, **55A,** 701.

Vandemark, W. E. & Page, M. A. (1948). Massive hyperplasia of bone following fractures of osteogenesis imperfecta. *Journal of Bone & Joint Surgery*, **30B,** 1015.

Williams, P. F. (1965). Fragmentation and rodding in osteogenesis imperfecta. *Journal of Bone & Joint Surgery*, **47B,** 23.

Winterfeldt, E. A., Eyring, E. J. & Vivian, V. M. (1970). Ascorbic-acid treatment for osteogenesis imperfecta. *Lancet*, **1,** 1347.

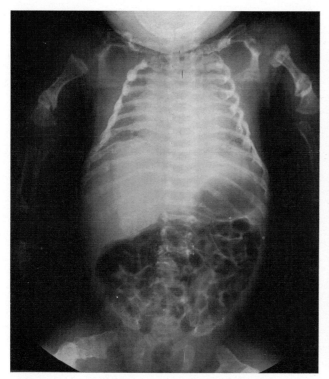

Fig. 21.3 (J.B.) Newborn infant with severe disease and multiple fractures, including clavicles and ribs. (H.A.T.F.)

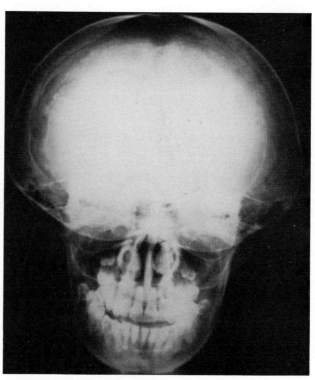

Fig. 21.4 (S.C.) Characteristic skull with much enlarged vault, temporal bulge and small face beneath. (A.H.)

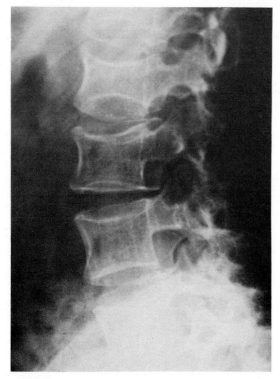

Fig. 21.5 (E.H.) Aged 23 years with osteoporosis and biconcave vertebrae. (H.A.T.F.)

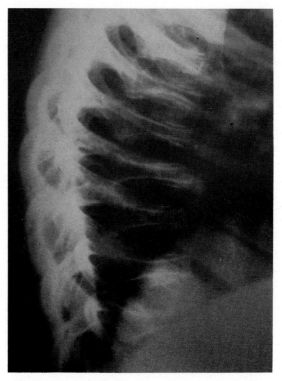

Fig. 21.6 (H.S.) Again osteoporosis but here the vertebrae are more flattened. (H.A.T.F.)

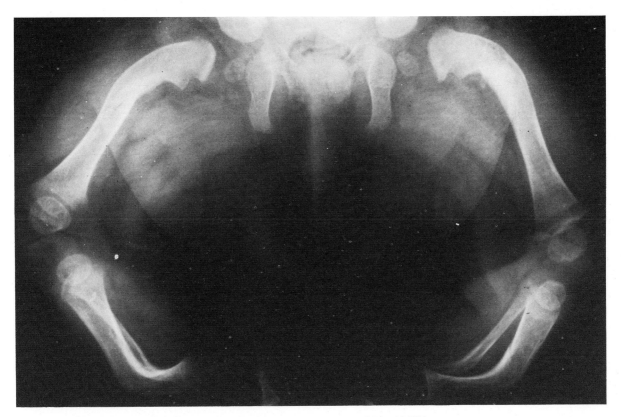

Fig. 21.7 Infant with severe disease with bending of femora and tibiae. (A.H.)

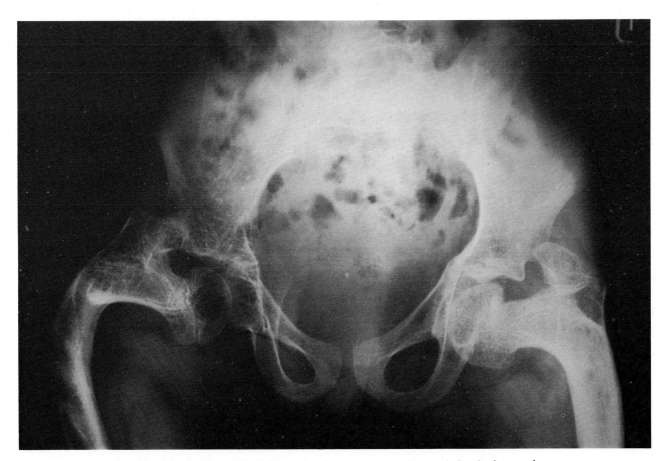

Fig. 21.8 (S.C.) Considerable bending of both femora and the greater trochanter is impinging on the ilium. The pelvic ring is distorted. (A.H.)

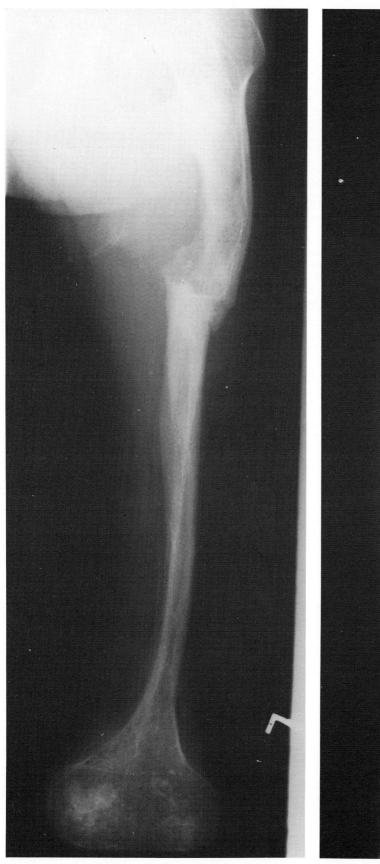

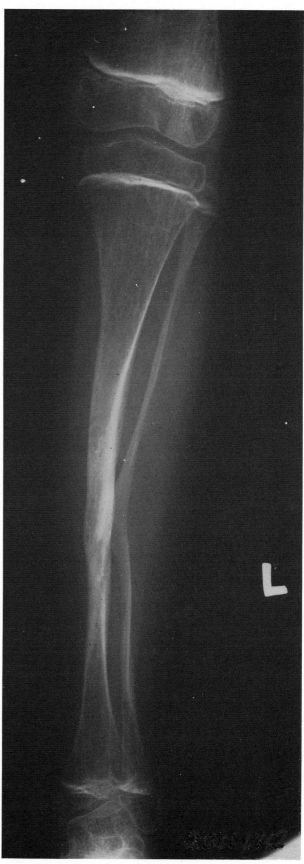

Fig. 21.9 (J.C.) Osteoporosis and a healing fracture are obvious, this patient has developed the thin bone type of disease. (A.H.)

Fig. 21.10 (P.W. male aged 4 years.) Considerable thinning of the tibia and fibula with thin cortices. (H.A.T.F.)

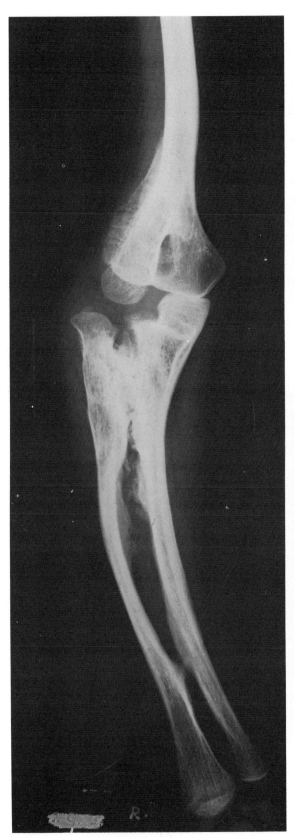

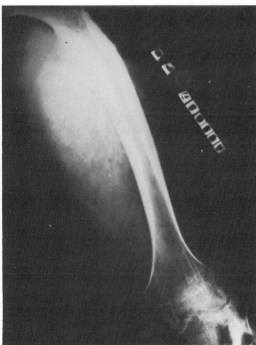

Figs 21.12 & 21.13   A fracture of the upper femoral shaft showing hyperplastic callus. (H.A.T.F.)

Fig. 21.11   (P.W.) Bowing of both humerus and forearm bones, probably synostosis of radius and ulna following fracture. (H.A.T.F.)

22 Idiopathic Juvenile Osteoporosis

Idiopathic osteoporosis may develop with acute onset in childhood, a year or so before puberty. It is of variable severity, and spontaneous remission occurs in two to five years. It was described by Dent and Friedman (1965), but they referred to Schippers (1938), who probably described the first case. Transient childhood osteoporosis is similar but develops at a slightly earlier age (Dent, 1976). Jackson (1958) reported osteoporosis of unknown cause in 'younger people', but the youngest man was 23 and the woman 21 and most were much older. This does not appear to be the same disorder, though he noted a slow symptomatic improvement in them.

Aetiology. The cause of idiopathic juvenile osteoporosis is not yet known. The cases so far described have been sporadic. These children appear to have inability to absorb dietary calcium.

Frequency. The disorder is extremely rare. The age of onset is about 2 years before puberty, thus girls are affected usually at a rather earlier age than boys.

Clinical and radiographic features. Up to the acute onset of this disorder childhood is apparently normal. There are variable degrees of severity in the disease, but the presenting feature is usually back pain due to compression fractures of vertebrae, or pathological fracture of other bones.

The skull is normal. The vertebrae are predominantly affected by multiple compression fractures, anterior wedging, and development of the biconcave vertebrae more usually seen in senile osteoporosis.

There may, however, be Schmorl nodes or local depressions. There is accompanying loss of vertebral height and thus the sitting height of these children is reduced.

The bone shows disappearance of the normal trabecular pattern and there is an extremely thin cortex. Fractures of ribs and long bones are common, particularly of the femora and around the hip and knee joints. In severe cases there may be gross rarefaction of the metaphyseal area (Dent, 1969).

Differential diagnosis. Osteoporosis in children is extremely rare, but the following need to be excluded:

Osteogenesis imperfecta tarda is characterised by a family history of the condition (autosomal dominant inheritance) and these patients usually have blue sclerae; the vertebral column is normal, the limbs being the more affected part of the skeleton. Osteoporosis which is secondary to liver disease, Cushing disease or steroid therapy is excluded by the appropriate investigations. The early stages of acute leukaemia may present in a similar way to idiopathic juvenile osteoporosis, a problem which may only be resolved when the typical blood and marrow picture of leukaemia develops.

Progress and complications. The disorder characteristically lasts from 2 to 5 years and then spontaneously remits. During this time fractures heal well and complications related to secondary deformity of bone only occur if these are inadequately treated.

Clinical chemistry. During the acute phase of the disease there is a negative calcium balance, and following immobilisation there is some hypercalcaemia, but apart from this there are no specific findings.

Treatment. During the acute phase the problem is to protect the child from fractures and to treat those that do occur.

Treatment with sex hormones is probably harmful in that premature fusion of epiphyses will occur, and it is preferable to wait for the spontaneous remission of the disease.

REFERENCES

Dent, C. E. (1976). Personal communication.
Dent, C. E. & Friedman, M. (1965). Idiopathic juvenile osteoporosis. *Quarterly Journal of Medicine,* **34,** 177.
Dent, C. E. (1969). Idiopathic juvenile osteoporosis (IJO). *Birth Defects Original Article Series 5,* Part 4, 134.
Jackson, W. P. U. (1958). Osteoporosis of unknown cause in younger people. *Journal of Bone & Joint Surgery,* **40B,** 420.
Schippers, J. C. (1938). A case of 'spontaneous' generalised osteoporosis in girl 10 years old. *Maandschrift voor Kindergeneeskunde,* **8,** 109.

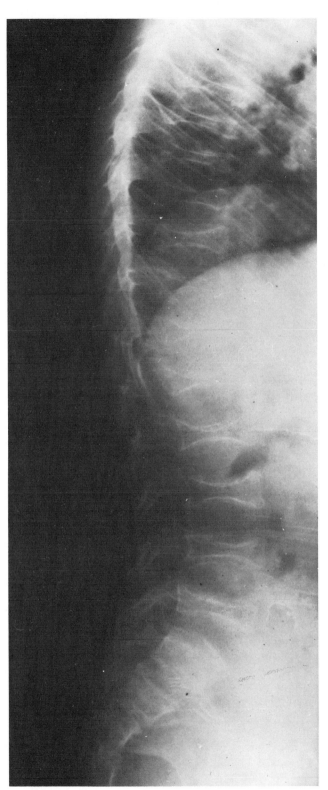

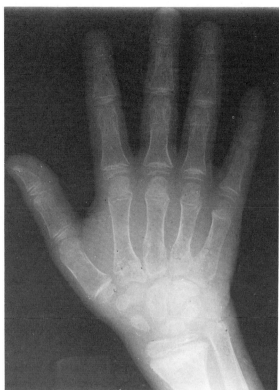

Figs 22.1 & 22.2 (A.H.) Marked osteoporosis shown in the spine and hand of a pre-pubertal male. (Courtesy Professor C. Dent, London.)

23   The Osteolyses

Cases of osteolysis or 'disappearing bones' present a striking clinical and radiological picture. The classification and aetiology is somewhat confused, many different varieties with a rather similar appearance occurring. There are at least three groups of these disorders likely to have a separate aetiology:

1. Osteolysis of the hands and feet, often hereditary. There may be several entities in this group.
2. Massive osteolysis associated with a preexisting congenital vascular defect such as a haemangioma.
3. Massive osteolysis not associated with any congenital lesion, presenting as a slowly progressive and destructive lesion more akin to a tumour than the previous groups.

OSTEOLYSES AFFECTING PRINCIPALLY THE HANDS AND FEET

Familial. There have been several reports of carpal and tarsal osteolysis of autosomal dominant inheritance. Cheney (1965) reported a mother and four of her six children affected, Gluck and Miller (1972) have described three generations of one family affected and Kohler (1973) reported a family in which a father and three children were affected. Earlier reports of disappearing bones in the carpus and tarsus were by Omer and Mossman (1958) and Normand and Smellie (1962). In this latter case there was also erosion of the proximal ends of the metacarpals and some osteolysis at the elbows and knees.

The onset of the disease is usually during childhood when there are rheumatoid arthritis-like episodes with pain, swelling and increased sensibility to touch and temperature. This apparent acute arthritis of the wrists and ankles may be followed by a quiescent phase and subsequently, during adolescence, osteolysis and collapse of the carpal and tarsal bones occur, perhaps with extrusion of involved bones into the adjacent joints. However, the course of the disease is not always the same and in some cases there is a slow onset during childhood perhaps associated with mild trauma or a mild specific illness. The carpus and tarsus may grow but the bones have a bizarre shape. The disease may 'burn itself out', but perhaps leaving contractures and deformities.

Whether the cases of osteolysis described as 'multicentric' are the same or a different entity is uncertain. Sometimes additional features have been noted: Cheney's family for example were of short stature and the family described by Kohler and colleagues were of Marfan-like appearance and had frontal bossing, micrognathia and pes cavus. Another feature in this latter family was a hyperinflammatory response; for example when the daughter had a wrist operation there was inflammation followed by fusion of the elbow on the same side.

Osteolysis of the phalanges was reported by Lamy and Maroteaux (1961) affecting a mother and son, and this would appear to be a separate entity. Torg et al (1969) described three sibs with osteolysis of the carpal and tarsal bones together with a more generalised osteoporosis, cortical thinning and increase in calibre of the long bones. The parents were related and in this instance the disorder is likely to have been of recessive inheritance.

Hollister et al (1974) investigated a patient with progressive lysis of the carpal and tarsal bones and found replacement of bone by dense fibrous tissue containing abnormal blood vessels. There were scanty trabeculae in cortical bone but normal resting cartilage and growth plates. There was hypervascularity apparently associated with osteolysis at large joints and widespread proliferation of ultrastructurally abnormal fibroblasts. Clinically the skin was thick and leathery with contractures and some hyperpigmentation and hypertrichosis. There was also dwarfism.

Association with nephropathy. Symmetrical osteolysis of the hands and feet associated with hypertension and renal failure has been reported by Torg and Steel (1968) and Macpherson, Walker and Kowall (1973). The onset is in early childhood and cases do not appear to be familial. Histology has shown chronic glomerulonephritis. On biopsy Shurtleff et al (1964) noted there was an absence of inflammatory tissue but that arteriolar thickening was present.

MASSIVE OSTEOLYSIS

In this condition there is unifocal extensive disappearance of pre-existing bone. Gorham and Stout (1955) summarised 24 cases, noting that the disease usually occurred in childhood with slow, progressive absorption over several years. Bone was replaced by fibrous tissue and there was marked proliferation of vascular spaces somewhat resembling haemangioendothelioma. They noted no regeneration of bone. Johnson and McClure (1958), found that the destruction of bone did eventually undergo arrest. Kery and Wouters (1970) reported a patient in whom the lytic process began in the opposite tibia 12 years after the first side. They noted that the lesion did not resemble an ordinary haemangioma of bone but was more like the proliferation of capillaries associated with an arteriovenous fistula.

Sage and Allen (1974) examined an amputation specimen from a woman of 36 years and found that the metatarsals and cuneiform bones had been replaced by spongy tissue which had eroded the surrounding muscles. They found no communication with any major blood vessels and the abnormal vessels were not obviously malignant. Fornasier (1970) reported a patient who had had skin haemangiomata all his life and presented with a pathological fracture in a lytic area.

The massive osteolyses, whether associated with congenital vascular lesions or not, are not familial in nature.

REFERENCES

Cheney, W. D. (1965). Acro-osteolysis. *American Journal of Roentgenology*, **94,** 595.

Fornasier, V. L. (1970). Haemangiomatosis with massive osteolysis. *Journal of Bone & Joint Surgery*, **52B,** 444.

Gluck, J. & Miller, J. J. (1972). Familial osteolysis of the carpal and tarsal bones. *Journal of Pediatrics*, **81,** 506.

Gorham, L. W. & Stout, A. P. (1955). Massive osteolysis. *Journal of Bone & Joint Surgery*, **37A,** 985.

Hollister, D. W., Rimoin, D. L., Lachman, R. S., Cohen, A. H., Reed, W. B. & Westin, G. W. (1974). The Winchester Syndrome: a nonlysosomal connective tissue disease. *Journal of Pediatrics*, **84,** 701.

Johnson, P. M. & McClure, J. G. (1958). Observations in massive osteolysis. *Radiology*, **71,** 28.

Kery, L. & Wouters, H. W. (1970). Massive osteolysis. *Journal of Bone & Joint Surgery*, **52B,** 452.

Kohler, E., Babbitt, D., Huizenga, B. & Good, T. A. (1973). Hereditary osteolysis. *Radiology*, **108,** 99.

Lamy, M. & Maroteaux, P. (1961). Acroostéolyse dominante. *Archives Françaises de Pédiatrie*, **18,** 693.

Macpherson, R. I., Walker, R. D. & Kowall, M. H. (1973). Essential osteolysis with nephropathy. *The Journal of the Canadian Association of Radiologists*, **24,** 98.

Normand, I. C. S. & Smellie, J. M. (1962). Disappearing carpal bones. *Proceedings of the Royal Society of Medicine*, **55,** 978.

Omer, G. E. & Mossman, D. L. (1958). Bone agenesis. A case involving the carpus and tarsus. *Journal of Bone & Joint Surgery*, **40A,** 917.

Sage, M. R. & Allen, P. W. (1974). Massive osteolysis. *Journal of Bone & Joint Surgery*, **56B,** 130.

Shurtleff, D. B., Sparkes, R. S., Clawson, K., Guntheroth, W. G. & Mottet, N. K. (1964). Hereditary osteolysis with hypertension and nephropathy. *Journal of American Medical Association*, **188,** 363.

Torg, J. S. & Steel, H. H. (1968). Essential osteolysis with nephropathy. *Journal of Bone & Joint Surgery*, **50A,** 1629.

Torg, J. S., De George, A. M., Kirkpatrick, J. A. & Trujillo, M. M. (1969). Hereditary multicentric osteolysis with recessive transmission: A new syndrome. *Journal of Pediatrics*, **75,** 243.

24   Osteopetrosis

In this condition there is generalised osteosclerosis and bone fragility. There are two quite distinct forms of the disease: the first, presenting at birth or in early infancy, is of great severity and death from pancytopenia due to the obliteration of marrow cavities occurs usually in the first decade of life. The second type is of milder degree, variable in its age of onset and severity, and may only be discovered incidentally during adult life.

OSTEOPETROSIS CONGENITA

This severe congenital form of the disease was first described by Sick (1914).

Inheritance. It is of autosomal recessive inheritance, there being several reports of affected sibs with unaffected consanguinous parents (Ennell and Pehrson, 1958; Tips and Lynch, 1962).

Frequency. The population incidence is not known, but the sexes are equally affected, and the disorder is apparent at birth or in very early infancy.

Clinical and radiographic features. In severely affected cases the foetus is stillborn: those that survive are of small stature and fail to thrive. The bone is fragile and pathological fractures are common. As the sclerotic bone encroaches on and replaces the marrow spaces, there is compensatory enlargement of the liver and spleen.

Additional problems arise from the sclerotic bone of the skull, where narrowed foramina in the base result in cranial nerve palsies, particularly of the 2nd, 7th and 8th nerves. Hydrocephalus may occur, probably in association with the narrowed foramen magnum. Dentition is delayed and the teeth are small.

The radiographic picture of the congenital form of osteopetrosis is quite characteristic with the thickened and sclerotic bone affecting both the base and vault of the skull, with an absence of air cells and sinuses. The vertebrae may be uniformly dense or have a 'sandwich' appearance in which there are segments of increased density above and below separated by a band of more translucent bone. All other bones in the body are dense and sclerotic with no distinction between cortical and cancellous bone.

The metaphyses of the long bones are expanded or 'club shaped', the enlargement usually ending abruptly at the diaphysis. Although the epiphyses are sclerotic they are of normal shape. In cases which are of less severity there appears to be fluctuating activity of the disease with transverse bands of greater and lesser density in the long bones, and the epiphyses may show a dense centre surrounded by a halo of less dense bone. Metacarpals and phalanges may show a 'bone within a bone' appearance, and occasionally the ilium may have arcuate bands.

Pathology. Engfeldt et al (1960) found the cartilage was normal in osteopetrosis as was calcification and penetration by vessels. However, the calcified matrix persisted in a greater degree than normal and rows of vesicular cartilage cells were seen far down the metaphysis, many surrounded by calcified substance. Instead of the normal marrow cavity there were columns of calcified cartilage and enchondral bone. The failure of resorption of calcified tissue may have occasional spontaneous remissions, during which time there may be resorption and reconstruction of bone. It would appear that such remissions are general rather than local, that is all bones are affected at the same time.

Differential diagnosis. The severe recessive form of osteopetrosis congenita is unlikely to be confused with any other disease. It differs from the tarda form by reason of its recessive inheritance, degree of severity and age of onset.

Progress and complications. The usual outcome is death in childhood from progressive anaemia and pancytopenia, associated with recurrent respiratory and other infections. Osteomyelitis of the mandible and maxilla may occur, as well as complications relating to cranial nerve palsies and possibly hydrocephalus.

Laboratory investigations. The blood picture in osteopetrosis is of anaemia with erythroblastosis, a moderate leucocytosis with a myeloid reaction, and late thrombocytopenia. The plasma calcium and phosphate are usually normal or inconsistently altered.

Treatment. The fluctuating activity of the osteosclerotic process in older patients prompted Dent, Smellie and Watson (1965) to attempt treatment of these children. They noted the anaemia could be controlled by corticosteroids but only at dosages that slowed growth. They found that most of the active red cell formation was in the liver and spleen, and most red cell destruction in the spleen—and indeed splenectomy improved the anaemia. This point had been studied by Sjolin (1959) who had suggested there was some degree of hypersplenism in osteopetrosis since the degree of anaemia did not always fit the radiographic appearances. Thus, the anaemia is in part a haemolytic one, which can be corrected by splenectomy (Besselman, 1966).

Dent and colleagues attempted to deplete the body of calcium by dietary means but found this only partially controlled bone density. They commented that excessive calcium absorption seemed to be an important feature of the disease.

Yu et al (1971) reported some success in the treatment of a child on low calcium intake, cellulose phosphate and steroids.

Other aspects of treatment relate to dental care and possibly decompression of cranial nerves.

OSTEOPETROSIS TARDA

This milder form of osteopetrosis was described by Albers Schönberg (1904). It appears to be a distinct form of the disease, being of later onset, milder in degree and of autosomal dominant inheritance, but it is not certain that all 'tarda' cases have the same aetiology (Spranger, Langer and Wiedemann, 1974).

Inheritance. Certainly the main form is of autosomal dominant inheritance, with much variation in severity and sometimes with skipped generations (Johnston *et al*, 1968).

Frequency. The population incidence is not known. The sexes are equally affected and the age of onset is variable, often during childhood but on occasions the disease is not found until adult life. Hinkel and Beiler (1955), reported several adults only diagnosed between 55 and 66 years of age.

Clinical and radiographic features. The appearances are similar though less severe than the congenita form, with dense sclerotic bone, pathological fractures, transverse striations and club-shaped expanded metaphyses. Signs of fluctuating activity with translucent bands in the long bones, 'sandwich' vertebrae, and the 'bone-within-a-bone' appearance of the small bones of the hand and foot are rather more common than in the congenita type.

In some cases there may be anaemia and there are occasional reports of cranial nerve paralysis and osteomyelitis of the mandible, as in osteopetrosis congenita, but all complications are less common in this milder form of the disease.

Differential diagnosis. There is a large number of disorders in which increased density of bone is a feature, but many of these will be apparent on ordinary clinical and laboratory investigations—such as congenital syphilis, fluoride and heavy metal poisoning, myelofibrosis and neoplasms.

The craniometaphyseal and craniodiaphyseal disorders are somewhat similar but the vertebrae are unaffected. In pycnodysostosis the bone is dense but the skull is quite characteristic with its open fontanelles, and the ragged appearance of the terminal phalanges distinguishes this condition from osteopetrosis. In dysosteosclerosis there is more extreme widening of the metaphyses with a clear area between the metaphysis and diaphysis, and platyspondyly is also a feature. Paget's disease is usually asymmetrical and the alkaline phosphatase is high.

Treatment. This is directed in the main to care of the teeth, of the fractures and, as in the congital type of osteopetrosis attempts to control the anaemia by corticosteroids or splenectomy have been made.

REFERENCES

Albers-Schönberg, H. (1904). Röntgenbilder einer seltenen Knochenerkrankung. *Munchener Medizinische Wochenschrift*, **51**, 365.

Besselman, D. M. (1966). Splenectomy in the management of the anemia and thrombocytopenia of osteopetrosis. *Journal of Pediatrics*, **69**, 455.

Dent, C. E., Smellie, J. M. & Watson, L. (1965). Studies in osteopetrosis. *Archives of Diseases in Childhood*, **40**, 7.

Enell, H. & Pehrson, M. (1958). Studies in osteopetrosis. I. Clinical report of three cases with genetic considerations. *Acta Paediatrica*, **47**, 279.

Engfeldt, B., Fajers, C. M., Lodin, H. & Pehrson, M. (1960). Studies in osteopetrosis. III. Roentgenological and pathologic-anatomical investigations on some of the bone changes. *Acta Paediatrica*, **49**, 391.

Hinkel, C. L. & Beiler, D. D. (1955). Osteopetrosis in adults. *American Journal of Roentgenology*, **74**, 46.

Johnston, C. C., Lavy, N., Lord, T., Vellios, F., Merritt, A. D. & Deiss, W. P. (1968). Osteopetrosis. A clinical, genetic, metabolic and morphologic study of the dominantly inherited benign form. *Medicine*, 47, 149.

Sick, P. (1914). Über drei Fälle einer seltenen Skeletterkrankung. (Marmorknochen nach Albers-Schönberg.) Festschr. z. Feier. d. 5 Jahr. Bestehens des Eppendorfer Krankenhauses.

Sjolin, S. (1959). Studies in osteopetrosis. II. Investigations concerning the nature of the anaemia. *Acta Paediatrica*, **48**, 529.

Spranger, J. W., Langer, L. O. & Wiedemann, H. R. (1974). *Bone Dysplasias: An Atlas of Constitutional Disorders of Skeletal Development*. W. B. Saunders Company, Philadelphia.

Tips, R. C. & Lynch, H. T. (1962). Malignant congenital osteopetrosis resulting from a consanguinous marriage. *Acta Paediatrica*, **51**, 585.

Yu, J. S., Oates, R. K., Walsh, H. & Stuckey, S. J. (1971). Osteopetrosis. *Archives of Diseases in Childhood*, **46**, 257.

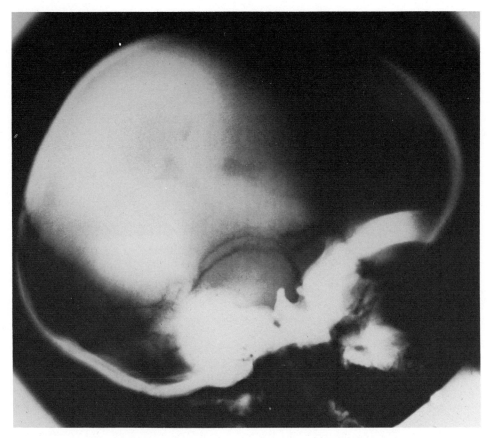

Fig. 24.1 (P.) The thickened sclerotic bone affects both the base and vault of the skull and there is absence of air cells and sinuses. (Courtesy of Mr A. G. Apley, Pyrford.)

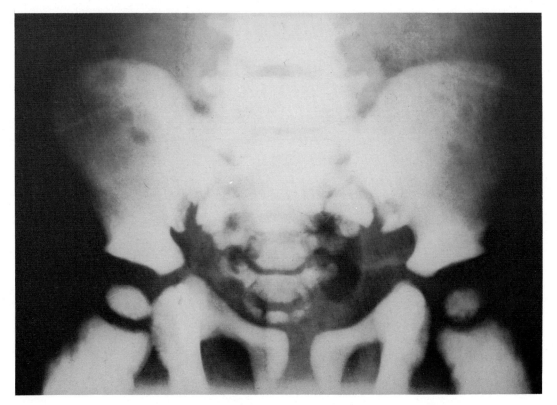

Fig. 24.2 The pelvis and upper femora of this child are uniformly sclerotic. (Courtesy of Mr A. G. Apley, Pyrford.)

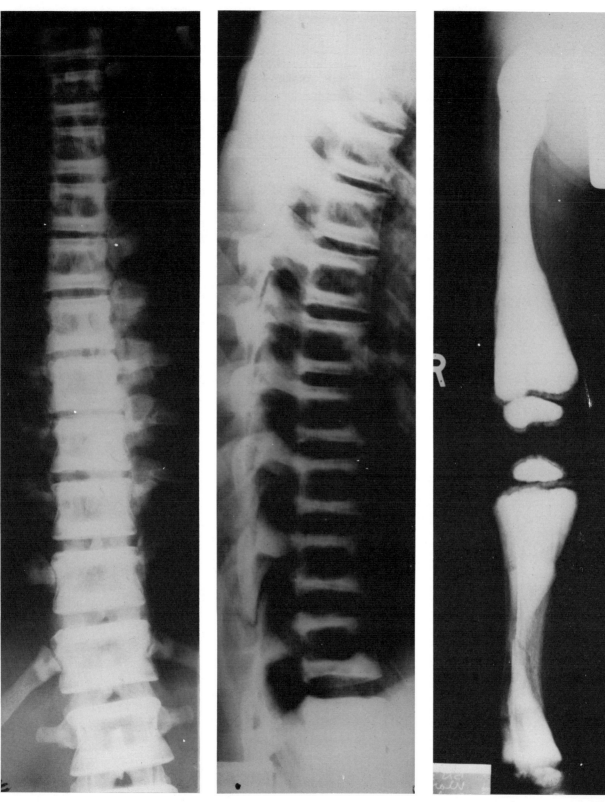

Figs 24.3 and 24.4 (L.H.) Typical 'sandwich' or 'rugger jersey' appearance, with segments of increased density separated by a band of translucent bone. (A.H.)

Fig. 24.5 (P.) No distinction between cortical and cancellous bone, the metaphyses are club-shaped, with the expansion extending well into the diaphysis. Pathological fracture of tibia and fibula. Epiphyses are essentially normal but show a halo of less dense bone. (Courtesy of Mr A. G. Apley, Pyrford.)

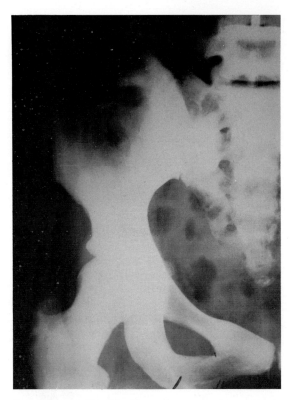

Fig. 24.6 (L.H.) The ilium shows an arcuate band, seen rather more rarely than bone of uniform density. (A.H.)

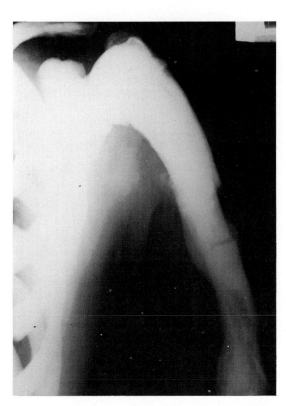

Fig. 24.7 (A.S.) Adult with severe involvement showing thick sclerotic ribs, scapula and humerus, the latter with a healing pathological fracture. (Courtesy of Mr A. G. Apley, Pyrford.)

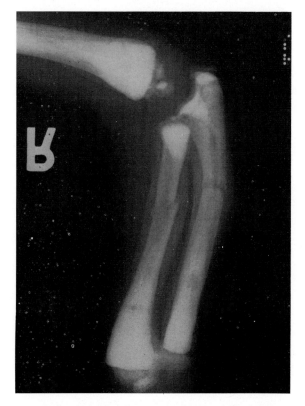

Fig. 24.8 (P.) The forearm bones show the typical deformity with epiphyses having a halo of less dense bone. (Courtesy of Mr A. G. Apley, Pyrford.)

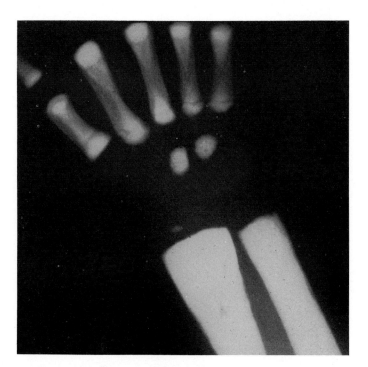

Fig. 24.9 (P.) Under-modelled metaphyses of the radius and ulna. The metacarpals show the bone-within-a-bone appearance. (Courtesy of Mr A. G. Apley, Pyrford.)

25 Dysosteosclerosis

In this condition there is osteosclerosis with short stature and platyspondyly, together with increased bone fragility.

It was named by Spranger et al (1968) who distinguished it from osteopetrosis tarda. The condition described by Roy et al also in 1968 is likely to be the same. Earlier reports in the literature referred to an atypical form of Albers-Schönberg disease (Ellis, 1937; Field, 1938).

Inheritance. The condition is probably of autosomal recessive inheritance, as in the few cases described there have been affected sibs and consanguinous parents.

Frequency. The disorder is extremely rare. The age of onset is during early childhood.

Clinical and radiographic features. The findings are very similar to osteopetrosis with dense, fragile bone and short stature. There are dental anomalies with poorly calcified enamel and failure of the second dentition to erupt. Spranger and colleagues reported occasional macular atrophy of the skin and flattened fingernails. Cranial nerve palsies and bulbar paralysis can occur with upper motor neuron involvement.

On radiography both the calvarium and base of the skull are thick with frontal and parietal bossing. The air cells are absent or decreased in size. Vertebrae are flat, dense and deformed in shape sometimes with dorsal wedging. The ribs, scapula and clavicle are sclerotic. In the long bones, the diaphyses are short, thick and curved and the metaphyses expanded, like those in osteopetrosis, but there is a characteristic radiolucent area of non-sclerotic bone between the metaphysis and diaphysis.

Differential diagnosis. This is chiefly from osteopetrosis tarda, but in this disorder there is no platyspondyly or a metaphyseal translucent area, and it is characterised by marrow and haematological problems. In pycnodysostosis the vertebrae are normal and the skull is typical of the disease, with delayed closure of fontanelles and Wormian bones in the suture lines. Also, the hypoplasia of the terminal phalanges is quite characteristic.

Progress and complications. The complications of dysosteosclerosis relate to the abnormal fragility of bone and, sometimes, due to the skull changes, there is optic atrophy, progressive mental retardation and progressive upper motor neuron signs. Blood and marrow problems do not arise.

REFERENCES

Ellis, R. W. B. (1937). Osteopetrosis. *Proceedings of the Royal Society of Medicine*, **27**, 1563.

Field, C. E. (1938). Albers-Schönberg disease. An atypical case. *Proceedings of the Royal Society of Medicine*, **32**, 320.

Roy, C., Maroteaux, P., Kremp, L., Courtrecuise, V. & Alagille, D. (1968). Un nouveau syndrome osseux avec anomalies cutaneés et troubles neurologiques. *Archives Francaises de Pédiatrie*, **25**, 983.

Spranger, J., Albrecht, C., Rohwedder, H. J. & Wiedemann, H. R. (1968). Die dysosteosklerose—eine sonderform der generalisierten osteosklerose. *Fortschritte auf dem Gebiete der Roentgenstrahlen und der Nuklearmedezin*, **109**, 504.

26 Pycnodysostosis

This is characterised by some shortness of stature due to short limbs, persistent open fontanelles, increased density and fragility of bone and dysplastic terminal phalanges.

It was described and named by Maroteaux and Lamy (1962), though they referred to Montanari as having described the first series of cases in 1923, under the title of 'osteopetrosis and cranio-cleido dysostosis'. It is likely that the case described by Fairbank (1948) as atypical osteopetrosis is in fact pycnodysostosis. By 1968, Sedano, Gorlin and Anderson were able to review 73 cases.

Inheritance. The condition is clearly of autosomal recessive inheritance and consanguinity of parents has been reported in about 25 per cent of cases.

Frequency. The disorder is rare: the sexes are equally affected. It is usually diagnosed during infancy, not at birth, though some mild cases are only discovered incidentally late in adult life.

Clinical and radiographic features. There is a short-limb type of dwarfism and the head is markedly abnormal and quite characteristic of this disease. There is bulging both of the frontal and occipital regions and the anterior fontanelle remains open even in adults. The face is small and the chin receding. There may be dental anomalies with premature or delayed eruption of teeth. The hands are characteristic, being short and square with very short terminal phalanges. An occasional feature is kyphosis or scoliosis, and possibly other deformities relating to the pathological fractures to which these children are liable.

On radiography the increased bone density of the whole skeleton is most noticeable, though the fragility varies greatly from one patient to another. Radiography confirms the anomalies of the skull with widened suture lines, persistence of fontanelles, and the presence of Wormian bones. There is hypoplasia of the facial bones and the angle of the mandible is more obtuse than normal.

The vertebral column may show lack of segmentation at the level of the atlas and axis, and sometimes in the lower lumbar vertebrae, and several cases of spondylolisthesis have been reported. The vertebral bodies have concave anterior and posterior borders, but the alternating bands of greater and lesser density seen in osteopetrosis do not occur (Maroteaux and Fauré, 1973).

The appendicular skeleton, in addition to the overall increase in density, shows moderate metaphyseal undermodelling. The clavicles are thin, often with hypoplasia of the lateral end. Apart from these findings the main abnormality is of the hands and feet, where characteristically the terminal phalanges are absent or represented only by small bony fragments. The metacarpals, metatarsals and other phalanges are dense and slender but are not usually otherwise affected.

Pathology. Lacey, Eyring and Shaffer (1970) noted that the pathogenesis of this disorder differs from osteopetrosis in that there is simultaneous reduction of formation and resorption of bone. Elmore (1967) found that a medullary canal was always present even though small and imperfect, and there was always microscopic evidence of haemopoiesis.

Differential diagnosis. This is from the two disorders with which the disease was first confused, namely cranio-cleido-dysostosis and osteopetrosis. The increased bone density, characteristic terminal phalanges, and the absence of marrow and cranial nerve complications differentiate it.

Progress and complications. The frequency of pathological fractures is variable, some individuals having only one or two. A history of fractured mandible during tooth extraction is not uncommon (Elmore, 1967) but apart from this it is usually the lower limbs that are affected. Fracture healing appears to be normal. Unlike osteopetrosis and other conditions in which there is sclerosis of the skull base, the cranial nerves are not affected in this condition.

The adult height of these individuals varies from 130 to 150 cm (4'3" to 4'11"). Life expectation is probably normal and there are few complications, though Maroteaux and Fauré (1973) noted a case in which there had been dyspnoeic spells due to recurrent obstruction of the airway resulting from the retrognathia and small size of the mandible. As in osteopetrosis, osteomyelitis of the mandible has been reported.

REFERENCES

Elmore, S. M. (1967). Pycnodysostosis: A review. *Journal of Bone & Joint Surgery*, **49A**, 153.

Fairbank, H. A. T. (1948). Osteopetrosis. *Journal of Bone & Joint Surgery*, **30B**, 339.

Lacey, S. H., Eyring, E. J. & Shaffer, T. E. (1970). Pycnodysostosis: A case report of a child with associated trisomy X. *Journal of Pediatrics*, **77**, 1033.

Maroteaux, P. & Lamy, M. (1962). La Pycnodysostose. *La Presse Médicale*, **20**, 999.

Maroteaux, P. & Fauré, C. (1973). Pycnodysostosis. In *Progress in Paediatric Radiology*, Volume 4. Intrinsic Diseases of Bones, p. 403. Ed. by Karger, Basel.

Sedano, H. D., Gorlin, R. J. & Anderson, V. E. (1968). Pycnodysostosis. Clinical and genetic considerations. *American Journal of Diseases in Childhood*, **116**, 70.

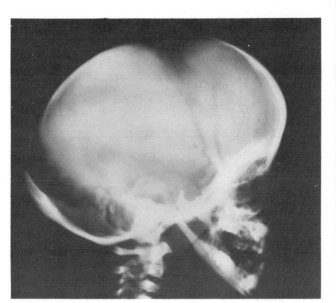
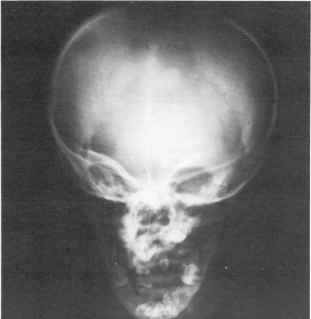

Figs 26.1 and 26.2 (I.D.) The skull shows increased density, Wormian bones and delayed closure of suture lines. The mandibular angle is almost non-existent. (G.O.S.)

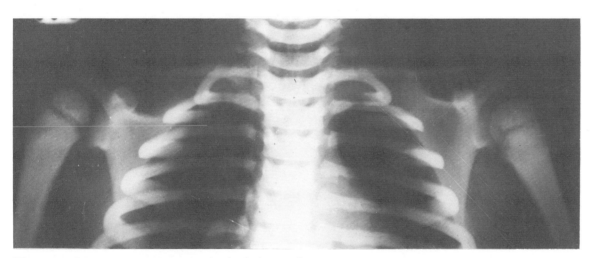

Fig. 26.3 (I.D.) Increased bone density is obvious and the clavicles are thin and underdeveloped. (G.O.S.)

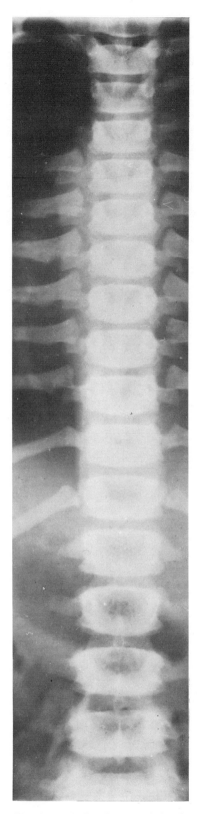

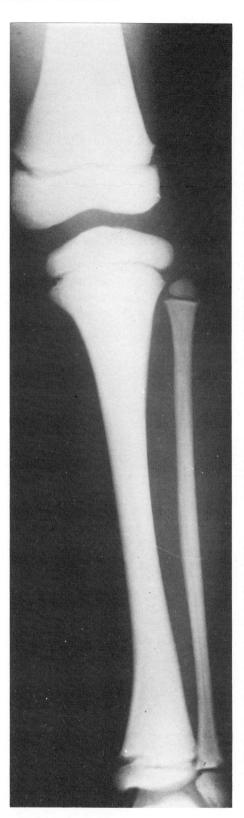

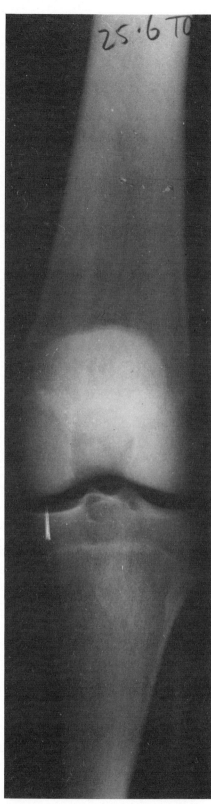

Fig. 26.4 (I.D.) Increased density of the vertebral bodies but not the alternating bands seen in osteopetrosis. (G.O.S.)

Fig. 26.5 (I.D.) Increased density of the femur, tibia and fibula and some lack of metaphyseal modelling. (G.O.S.)

Fig. 26.6 (J.D.) Adult patient with similar under-modelling of the metaphyseal region. (G.O.S.)

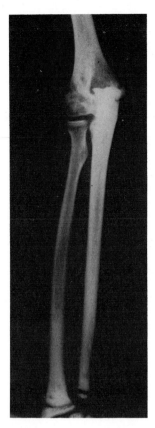

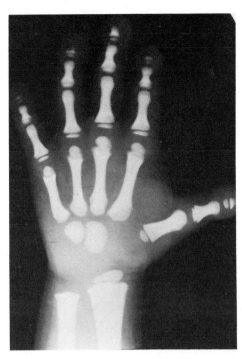

Fig. 26.7 (D.B. aged 12 years.) There is some irregular increase of density of the forearm and some under-modelling. (H.A.T.F.)

Fig. 26.8 (I.D.) Increased density of all hand bones is seen together with dysplastic terminal phalanges. (G.O.S.)

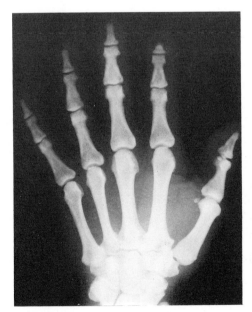

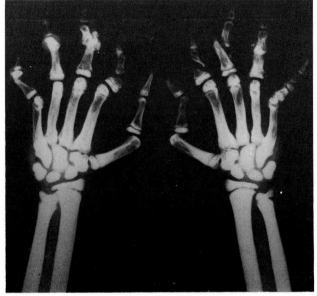

Fig. 26.9 (J.D.) This patient is less severely affected, only the terminal phalanx of the index finger being abnormal. (G.O.S.)

Fig. 26.10 (D.B. aged 12 years.) This patient had other features of pycnodysostosis, although unusually the phalangeal dysplasia primarily affects the proximal bones. (H.A.T.F.)

27 Sclerosteosis

This is a familial generalised osteosclerosis chiefly involving the skull and accompanied by syndactyly and other digital anomalies.

It was named by Hausen (1967) but 'osteopetrosis with syndactyly' had been noted earlier in the literature, for example by Falconer and Ryrie (1937) and by Truswell (1958).

Inheritance. It is of autosomal recessive inheritance, affected sibs and parental consanguinity having been reported in many instances.

Frequency. The population incidence is not known. The disease becomes apparent in early childhood.

Clinical and radiographic features. The head and face are characteristic with a high forehead, hypertelorism, a broad flat nasal bridge and prognathism with a broad square mandible. The head is enlarged.

The hands are characteristic, with cutaneous syndactyly usually only extending as far as the proximal interphalangeal joint. Syndactyly of the toes may be present. Sujiura and Yasuhara (1975) noted dysplasia of the nails of the index and middle fingers and of the second and third toes. The mother of their patient lacked a nail of the right index finger and so possibly in this instance the condition may have been of dominant inheritance.

On radiography the skull is greatly thickened, and the outer and inner tables of the calvarium cannot be distinguished. Gorlin, Spranger and Koszalka (1969) noted that the vertebrae, ribs, clavicles and pelvis were uniformly sclerotic. The long bones were straight 'like canes', with increased density and lack of diaphyseal modelling. Radiographs of the hands may show complete absence of the middle phalanx or only a small triangular bone at this site.

Differential diagnosis. This is from hyperphosphatasia tarda and from craniodiaphyseal dysplasia but in neither of these conditions are the hands involved.

Progress and complications. Patients with sclerosteosis are of normal stature. Complications arise from bony encroachment on the foramina in the base of the skull and cranial nerve palsies, particularly of the second, fifth, seventh and eighth may occur.

REFERENCES

Beighton, P. (1975). Robert Jones Prize Essay, British Orthopaedic Association, London.

Falconer, A. W. & Ryrie, B. J. (1937). Report on a familial type of generalised osteosclerosis. *Medical Press,* **195,** 12.

Gorlin, R. J., Spranger, J. & Koszalka, M. F. (1969). Genetic craniotubular bone dysplasias and hyperostoses. A critical analysis. *Birth Defects Original Article Series 5,* Part 4, p. 79.

Hausen, H. G. (1967). Sklerosteose, in *Handbuch der Kinderheilkunde,* ed. Opitz, H. & Schmid, F., Springer, Berlin.

Sugiura, Y. & Yasuhara, T. (1975). Sclerosteosis. *Journal of Bone & Joint Surgery,* **57A,** 273.

Truswell, A. S. (1958). Osteopetrosis with syndactyly. A morphological variant of Albers-Schönberg's disease. *Journal of Bone & Joint Surgery,* **40B,** 208.

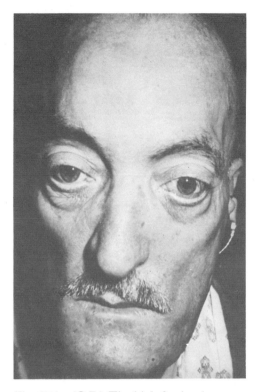

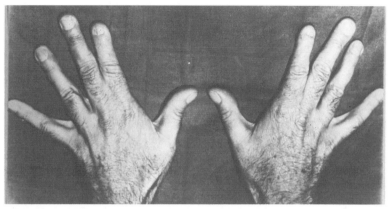

Fig. 27.1 (G.B.) The high forehead, hypertelorism and flattened nasal bridge are characteristic. (Courtesy of Professor P. Beighton, Capetown.)

Fig. 27.2 (G.B.) Characteristic hands with cutaneous syndactyly extending nearly as far as the proximal inter-phalangeal joints of index and middle fingers. The nails of the index fingers are dysplastic. (Courtesy of Professor P. Beighton, Capetown.)

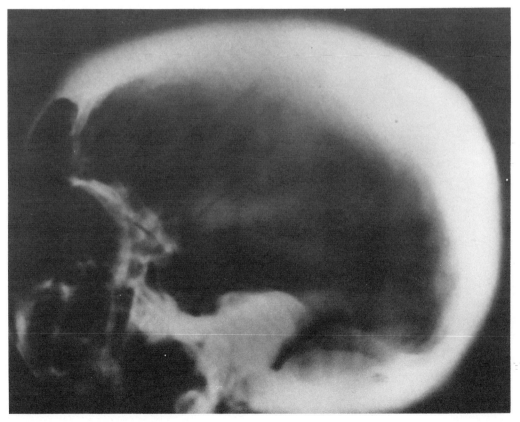

Fig. 27.3 The skull is greatly thickened and the outer and inner tables cannot be distinguished. (Courtesy of Professor P. Beighton, Capetown.)

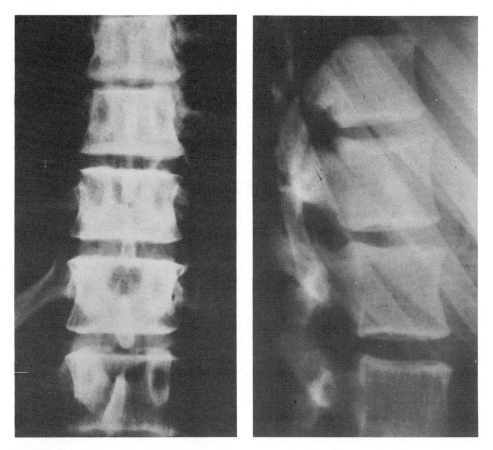

Figs 27.4 and 27.5 The vertebrae are normal in shape with generalised sclerosis. (Courtesy of Professor P. Beighton, Capetown.)

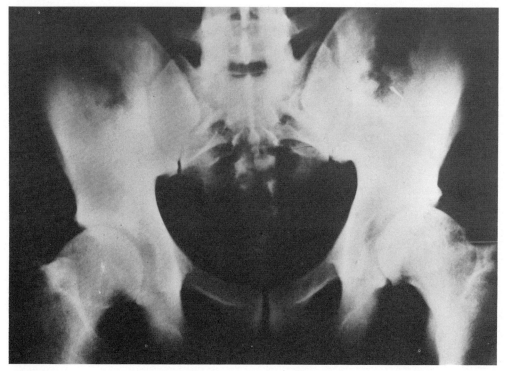

Fig. 27.6 Uniform sclerosis of the pelvis and upper femora. (Courtesy of Professor P. Beighton, Capetown.)

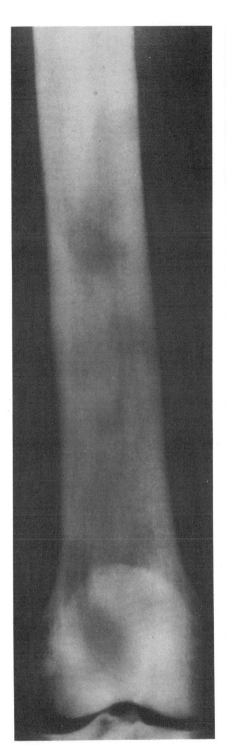
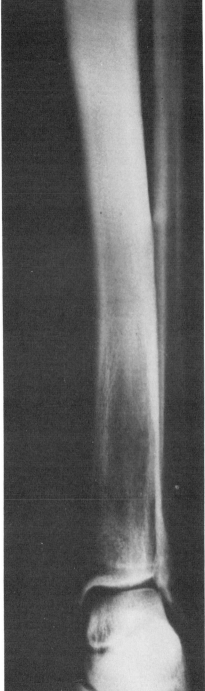

Figs 27.7 and 27.8   The long bones show increased
density and almost total lack of diaphyseal modelling.
(Courtesy of Professor P. Beighton, Capetown.)

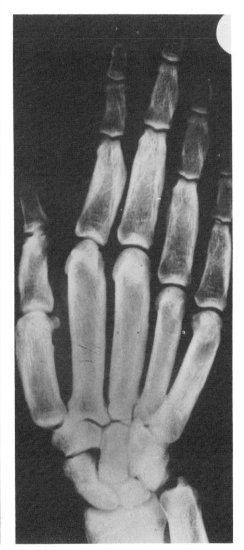

Fig. 27.9   Patchy sclerosis of
metacarpals and phalanges with
almost complete lack of modelling
in the more proximal bones.
(Courtesy of Professor P. Beighton,
Capetown.)

28 Craniometaphyseal Dysplasia

This disorder was first clearly defined by Jackson *et al* (1954) who differentiated it from other disorders of bone modelling with increased density affecting the skull, and particularly from familial metaphyseal dysplasia (Pyle's disease). Subsequent authors have frequently confused the two. A more recent review of this subject is by Gorlin, Spranger and Koszalka (1969).

Inheritance. Most cases appear to be of autosomal dominant inheritance (Rimoin, Woodruff and Holman, 1969), though there is likely also to be an autosomal recessive form of this disease which is clinically indistinguishable (Lehmann, 1957).

Frequency. The disorder is extremely rare. It is not apparent at birth, the first changes in the skull and facial bones perhaps occurring in later infancy or childhood.

Clinical and radiographic features. Although there is generalised hyperostosis of the skull, the frontonasal and occipital parts are mainly affected. There is thickening of the frontal region, a wide ridge of bone over the bridge of the nose, and hypertelorism develops. The air cells and sinuses are small or obliterated, and gradual bony encroachment of the nasal passages leads to their blockage. Obliteration of foramina in the base of the skull causes optic atrophy, facial palsy and deafness. The mandible is often involved in the sclerotic process.

In the infant the long bones show diaphyseal sclerosis with subperiosteal new bone and, at this stage, normal metaphyses. However as the child grows, and in the adult, the metaphyses become club-shaped, rather similar to those seen in osteopetrosis. These changes are more apparent in the lower than in the upper limbs.

Differential diagnosis. This is from familial metaphyseal dysplasia (Pyle's disease), in which the long bones are similarly affected but the skull is much less involved, and the disorder is of autosomal recessive inheritance. Craniodiaphyseal dysplasia has an even more severely affected skull and reveals less and later metaphyseal widening. Progressive diaphyseal dysplasia (Engelmann's disease) may present a similar picture of the long bones during infancy, but these children have marked muscle weakness, the bone dysplasia is always in the diaphyseal region, and the skull is not severely affected.

Progress and complications. Life expectancy in craniometaphyseal dysplasia is usually normal but there are many complications arising from the cranial hyperostosis. Sinus obstruction and cranial nerve palsies occur. Millard *et al* (1967) noted thickened bone encroaching on the medulla with loss of volume in the posterior cranial fossa, and there may be recurrent attacks of unconsciousness due to the raised intracranial pressure.

Treatment. Millard and colleagues (1967) suggest the possibility of surgical enlargement of the foramen magnum if intracranial pressure is rising.

REFERENCES

Gorlin, R. J., Spranger, J. & Koszalka, M. F. (1969). Genetic craniotubular bone dysplasias and hyperostoses. A critical analysis. *Birth Defects Original Article Series 5*, Part 4, 79.

Jackson, W. P. U., Albright, F., Drewry, G., Hanelin, J. & Rubin, M. I. (1954). Metaphyseal dysplasia, epiphyseal dysplasia, diaphyseal dysplasia and related conditions. *Archives of Internal Medicine*, **94**, 871.

Lehmann, E. C. H. (1957). Familial osteodystrophy of the skull and face. *Journal of Bone & Joint Surgery*, **39B**, 313.

Millard, D. R., Maisels, D. O., Batstone, J. H. F. & Yates, B. W. (1967). Craniofacial surgery in craniometaphyseal dysplasia. *American Journal of Surgery*, **113**, 615.

Rimoin, D. L., Woodruff, S. L. & Holman, B. L. (1969). Craniometaphyseal dysplasia (Pyle's disease): Autosomal dominant inheritance in a large kindred. *Birth Defects Original Article Series 5*, Part 4, 96.

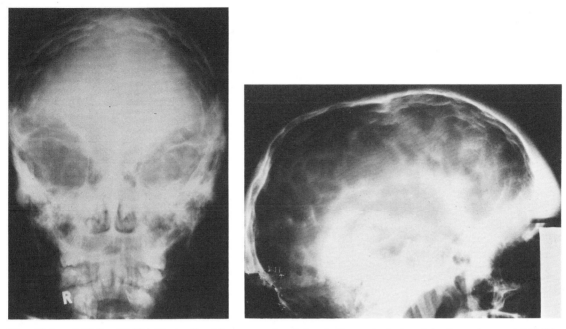

Figs 28.1 and 28.2   (G.W.) Generalised hyperostosis of the skull, particularly of the frontal area. (G.O.S.)

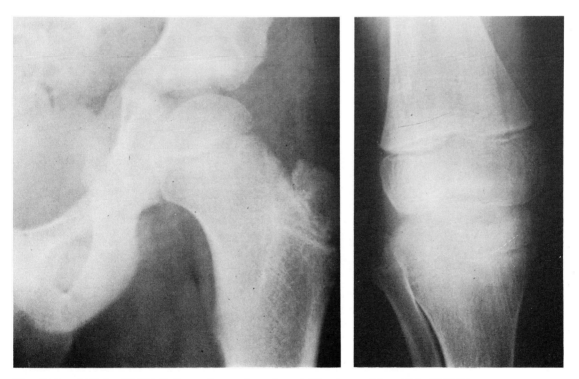

Figs 28.3 and 28.4   (G.W.) Failure of metaphyseal modelling in an older child. (G.O.S.)

29 Familial Metaphyseal Dysplasia
Pyle's Disease

In spite of the name, this is also a craniometaphyseal dysplasia but the skull is only minimally involved. It was first named by Pyle (1931) though he made no mention of a cranial abnormality. The radiographs were later studied by Gorlin, Koszalka and Spranger (1970) who found some thickening of the calvaria and slight frontal bulging.

Inheritance. It is of autosomal recessive inheritance.

Frequency. The population incidence is not known but it is a rare disorder. It is not apparent at birth and indeed the age of onset may not be known. Frew (1961) described three patients each discovered only incidentally.

Clinical and radiographic features. The symptoms are surprisingly few, the main defect being severe genu valgum. Patients are not short in stature and the lower limbs may be disproportionately long. There is sometimes an increased tendency to fracture.

Radiological signs in the skull are only of some supraorbital bulging and mild prognathism. Frew (1961) noticed a diminished facial angle. The ribs and clavicles are thicker than normal, as are the ischium and pubis. The long bone modelling defect is distinctive, in that the widened, splayed metaphyseal area extends far into the diaphysis. It has been called an 'Erlenmeyer flask' or 'paddle-shaped' deformity. The defect is particularly obvious in the upper two-thirds of the humerus, distal half of the radius and ulna, distal half of the femur and both ends of the tibia and fibula (Bakwin and Krida, 1937). The tibiae show a characteristic gentle S-curve, the expanded lower third lying parallel but slightly lateral and posterior to the upper third.

Differential diagnosis. This is from other disorders with some increased bone density and with skull and metaphyseal defects. In both craniometaphyseal and frontometaphyseal dysplasia the skull is more severely involved and cranial nerve palsies develop. In osteopetrosis tarda and pycnodysostosis the bone density is greater and there may be evidence of remissions and exacerbations of the sclerotic process.

Progress and complications. This disorder is not of great severity; life expectancy and height are normal.

REFERENCES

Bakwin, H. & Krida, A. (1937). Familial metaphyseal dysplasia. *American Journal of Diseases in Childhood*, **53**, 1521.

Frew, J. F. M. (1961). Familial metaphyseal dysplasia. *Journal of Bone & Joint Surgery*, **43B**, 188.

Gorlin, R. J., Koszalka, M. F. & Spranger, J. (1970). Pyle's disease (familial metaphyseal dysplasia). *Journal of Bone & Joint Surgery*, **52A**, 347.

Pyle, E. (1931). A case of unusual bone development. *Journal of Bone & Joint Surgery*, **13**, 874.

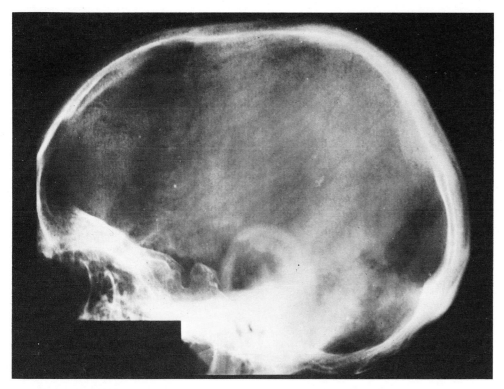

Fig. 29.1 (G.) Minimal signs in the skull with some supraorbital bulging. (H.A.T.F.)

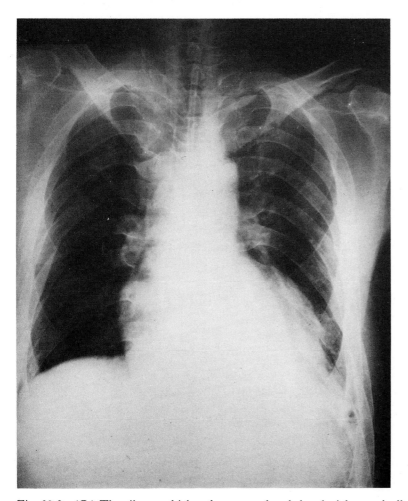

Fig. 29.2 (G.) The ribs are thicker than normal and the clavicles markedly so. (H.A.T.F.)

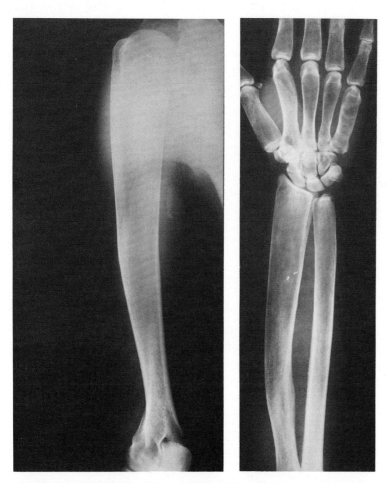

Figs 29.3 and 29.4 (G.) The modelling defect is characteristic in that the widened metaphyseal area extends far down into the diaphysis. (H.A.T.F.)

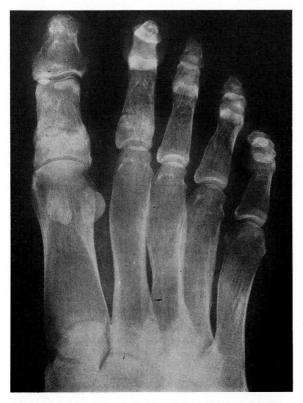

Fig. 29.5 (G.) The modelling defect principally affects the metatarsals. (H.A.T.F.)

30 Craniodiaphyseal Dysplasia
Leontiasis Ossea

This infrequently seen condition is characterised by bizarre and severe cranio-facial hyperostosis and diaphyseal dysplasia with 'straight' long bones. It was differentiated from other 'craniotubular' bone dysplasias by Gorlin, Spranger and Koszalka (1969). Cases previously described in the literature as leontiasis ossea are likely to be examples of this disorder, though it is not certain that only a single entity is involved (Macpherson, 1974).

Inheritance. Certainly one type is likely to be of autosomal recessive inheritance as consanguinous parents have been reported (Halliday, 1949).

Frequency. The disorder is extremely rare. It becomes apparent during infancy.

Clinical and radiographic features. The disorder mainly involves the facial bones and mandible. There is hypertelorism but no frontal bulging. Patients are likely to be short in stature and mentally retarded. Complications arise from blockage of the nasal passages and sinuses, and from involvement of the foramina in the base of the skull, leading to cranial nerve palsies.

On radiography there is very severe sclerosis and overgrowth of the facial bones. The cervical vertebrae may be involved and the ribs and clavicles are thick and dense. Long bones are characteristically straight, with no metaphyseal flare.

The differential diagnosis is from craniometaphyseal dysplasia, but here the skull changes are not so severe and the long bone contour is different, with expanded metaphyses.

The prognosis is poor, with death occurring during the first two decades.

REFERENCES

Gorlin, R. J., Spranger, J. & Koszalka, M. F. (1969). Genetic craniotubular bone dysplasias and hyperostoses. A critical analysis. *Birth Defects Original Article Series 5,* Part 4, 79.

Halliday, J. (1949). A rare case of bone dystrophy. *British Journal of Surgery,* **37,** 52.

Macpherson, R. I. (1974). Craniodiaphyseal dysplasia, a disease or group of diseases? *Journal de L'Association Canadienne des Radiologistes,* **25,** 22.

31 Progressive Diaphyseal Dysplasia
Camurati–Engelmann Disease

In this condition there is limb pain, hypotonia and muscle weakness associated with progressive thickening of the diaphyseal part of the long bones, and sometimes with sclerosis of the skull.

Probably the first patient to be reported was by Cockayne (1920) who presented a case for diagnosis at the Royal Society of Medicine. The disorder was named by Neuhauser et al (1948) and by 1956 Griffiths was able to find 21 cases in the literature.

Inheritance. The condition is often of autosomal dominant inheritance but there is considerable variation in expression and many cases are apparently sporadic: however, without a radiographic survey of relatives it is difficult to know the true picture. Sparkes and Graham (1972) studied 8 individuals in three generations of one family, and Hundley and Wilson (1973) reported 7 cases in three generations, confirming the theory of autosomal dominance.

Frequency. The population incidence is not known but this is one of the rarer of the skeletal dysplasias. Symptoms of muscle weakness develop during childhood, probably after the second year of life. Bony changes have been found at ages varying from a few months old to late adult life.

Clinical and radiographic features. Griffiths (1956) noted the childhood symptoms of failure to thrive, weakness, late age of walking and easy fatigue. The gait is always awkward and there is a reduction of muscle mass. Hundley and Wilson (1973) noted muscle atrophy in about half their patients, and pain and muscle weakness in one-third. In severe cases the pain, particularly in the lower limbs, is progressive.

Radiographic features are of a thickened, sclerotic base and vault of the skull, and perhaps also of the upper cervical vertebrae. Sclerosis of the mandible has been reported, and occasionally the ribs are involved. The chief radiographic sign is in the long bones, where the middle two-quarters are abnormal but neither the metaphysis nor epiphysis is affected.

There is a symmetrical, fusiform enlargement of the shaft of the bone and the thickened cortex is usually of increased density. The surface of the bone is smooth, and on occasion there may be more than one fusiform swelling. In order of frequency, Hundley and Wilson (1973) noted the tibia, femur, fibula, humerus, ulna and radius, with no case of unilateral involvement. The short bones of the hands and feet are not affected, and in most patients the vertebrae and pectoral and pelvic girdles escape involvement.

Pathology. There are diffuse non-specific bony changes with an increase in the fibrous component of the periosteum and marked osteoblastic and osteoclastic activity. Sometimes there is vascular thickening and Sparks and Graham (1972) suggest the non-osseus symptoms of the disease could be related to this feature.

Differential diagnosis. The sclerotic lesions of the metaphyseal and craniometaphyseal disorders are excluded by reason of their primarily metaphyseal involvement, and by the fact that the short bones of the hands and feet are affected. Infantile cortical hyperostosis occurs at a younger age (usually during the first few months of life) and the signs regress. Hyperphosphatasia, chronic osteomyelitis and congenital syphilis are excluded by laboratory tests. Paget's disease is usually asymmetrical.

Progress and complications. The course of the disease is variable, and in some cases there seems to be spontaneous improvement during adolescence. Some cases are so mild as to be discovered only incidentally during adult life. Life expectancy, height and bone healing all appear to be normal.

Treatment. In recent years there have been attempts to treat progressive diaphyseal dysplasia with corticosteroids (Royer et al, 1967; Allen et al, 1970). This results in stimulation of osteoclasis, decreased lamellar bone deposition and a more normal histological picture. Bone pain was relieved almost immediately.

REFERENCES

Allen, D. T., Saunders, A. M., Northway, W. H., Williams, G. F. & Schafer, I. A. (1970). Corticosteroids in the treatment of Engelmann's disease: progressive diaphyseal dysplasia. *Pediatrics*, **46**, 523.

Camurati, M. (1922). Di un raro caso de osteite simmetrica ereditaria degli arti inferiori. *Chirurgia degli Organi di Movimento (Bologna)*, **6**, 662.

Cockayne, E. A. (1920). Case for diagnosis. *Proceedings of the Royal Society of Medicine*, **13**, 132.

Engelmann, G. (1929). Ein Fall von Osteopathia hyperostotica (sclerotisans) multiplex infantilis. *Fortschritte auf dem Gebiete der Roentgenstrahlen und der Nuklearmedezin*, **39**, 1101.

Griffiths, D. L. (1956). Engelmann's Disease. *Journal of Bone & Joint Surgery*, **38B**, 312.

Hundley, J. D. & Wilson, F. C. (1973). Progressive diaphyseal dysplasia. Review of the literature and report of 7 cases in one family. *Journal of Bone & Joint Surgery*, **55A**, 461.

Neuhauser, E. B. D., Schwachman, H., Wittenborg, M. & Cohen, J. (1948). Progressive diaphyseal dysplasia. *Radiology*, **51**, 11.

Royer, P., Vermeil, G., Apostolides, P. & Engelmann, F. (1967). Maladie d'Engelmann, résultat du traitment par le prednisone. *Archives françaises de Pédiatrie*, **24**, 693.

Sparkes, R. & Graham, C. B. (1972). Camurati–Engelmann disease. Genetics and clinical manifestations with a review of the literature. *Journal of Medical Genetics*, **9**, 73.

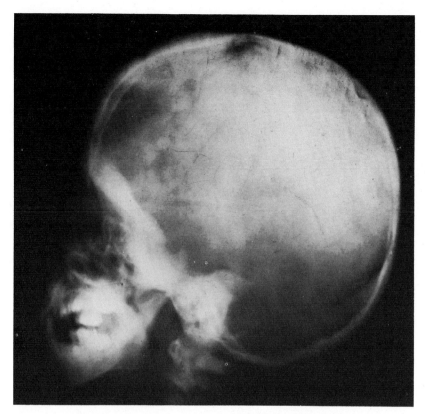

Fig. 31.1 Both the base and vault of the skull are thickened and sclerotic. (H.A.T.F.)

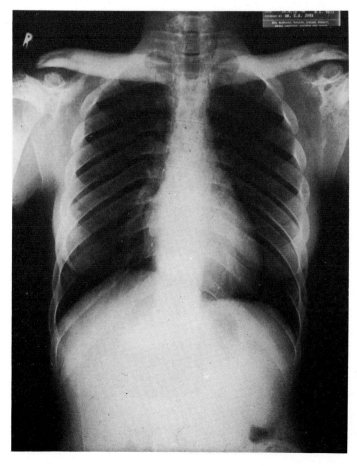

Fig. 31.2 Considerable thickening of the ribs and the modelling defect is even more noticable in the clavicles. (Courtesy of Mr A. G. Apley, Pyrford.)

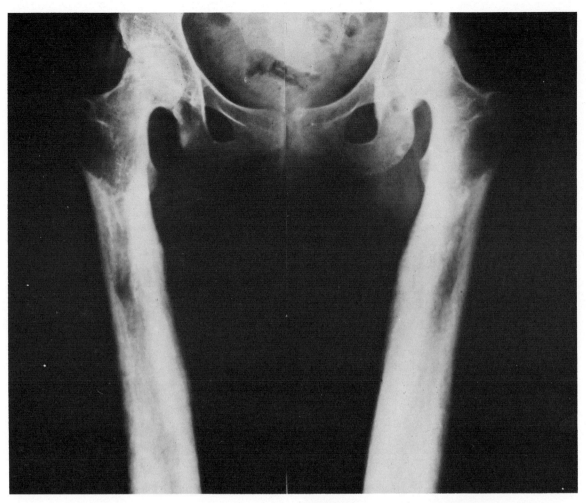

Fig. 31.3 Thickening defect of the shaft of the femora, with normal epiphyseal and metaphyseal areas. (H.A.T.F.)

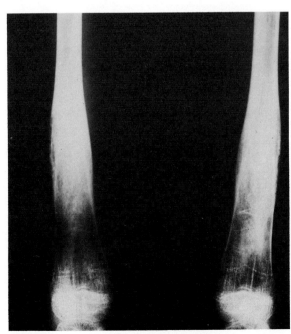

Fig. 31.4 The lower part of the femora confirm the diaphyseal thickening with normal metaphysis and epiphysis. (H.A.T.F.)

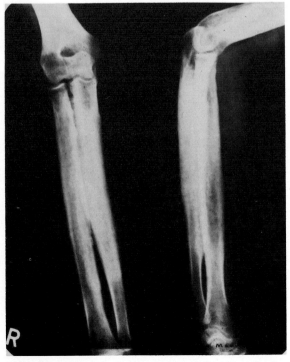

Fig. 31.5 The forearm bones are similarly involved. (H.A.T.F.)

32 Osteodysplasty
Melnick–Needles Syndrome

This rare disorder is characterised by anomalies of the face and skull and some bowing and failure of modelling of the long bones.

It was described first by Melnick and Needles (1966) and subsequently by Maroteaux, Chouraki and Coste (1968).

Inheritance. The original study by Melnick and Needles was of two families, one of four and the other of three generations affected and thus it would seem to be of autosomal dominant inheritance. Kozlowski, Mayne and Danks (1973) have reported affected sibs with normal parents and suggest there is an autosomal recessive form of the disease which is more severe—three babies all failed to thrive and died of respiratory infection.

Frequency. The disorder is extremely rare. The dominant cases reported became apparent during childhood, and those described by Kozlowski and colleagues were diagnosed in infancy.

Clinical and radiographic features. The head and face are characteristic with a high, narrow forehead, exophthalmos, micrognathia and malalignment of the teeth. Scoliosis has developed in several patients and there is cubitus valgus, genu valgum and some bowing of the limbs.

On radiography the skull is abnormal in that the anterior fontanelle is large and closes late. The base of the skull and the frontal region are sclerotic. There is failure of modelling of the ribs and clavicles and the vertebral bodies are characterised by a concave anterior border.

The long bones have metaphyseal flaring, irregularity in density and thickness of the cortex. There is bowing, particularly of the humerus, femur and tibia, and multiple constrictions are present. The iliac bones are also somewhat constricted in the region above the acetabulum.

Differential diagnosis. This is from other disorders with increased bone density which affect the skull, but no other condition is characterised by the irregular bony contours and constrictions which are present in osteodysplasty.

Progress and complications. There seems to be little functional disability and the disorder may only be discovered incidentally. The height is normal.

REFERENCES

Kozlowski, K., Mayne, V. & Danks, D. M. (1973). Precocious type of osteodysplasia. A new autosomal recessive form. *Acta Radiologica*, **14**, 171.

Maroteaux, P., Chouraki, L. & Coste, F. (1968). L'osteodysplastie (syndrome de Melnick et de Needles). *La Presse Médicale*, **76**, 715.

Melnick, J. C. & Needles, C. F. (1966). An undiagnosed bone dysplasia. A 2 family study of 4 generations and 3 generations. *American Journal of Roentgenology*, **97**, 39.

33   The Hyperphosphatasias

HYPERPHOSPHATASIA CONGENITA
(Juvenile Paget's Disease)

This severe form of hyperphosphatasia, with onset in infancy, is characterised by fever, pain and fragility of bone together with dwarfing and thickening of the limb bones.

It was first clearly defined by Bakwin and Eiger (1956) who described the condition in a 7 year old child, although multiple fractures had occurred during the first year of life. The condition described by Choremis et al (1958) of Paget's disease in an 11 year old boy is likely to be the same condition and since then there have been several reports in the literature.

Inheritance. It is of autosomal recessive inheritance, several cases of affected sibs with normal parents having been reported, and also there was parental consanguinity in Bakwin and Eiger's original case.

Frequency. The population incidence is not known but the disorder is extremely rare. This early onset type of hyperphosphatasia, although called 'congenita', becomes apparent during infancy, and is not usually recognisable at birth.

Clinical and radiographic features. Fever, bone pain and fractures are likely to be the first signs of this disease, together with premature shedding of the teeth. The children are dwarfed with large heads and blue sclerae similar to some cases of osteogenesis imperfecta. The limbs are tender, thickened and bowed. The muscle mass is reduced and contractures may develop.

The radiographic signs are characteristic and rather similar to those of Paget's disease in the adult. There is irregular massive thickening of the skull and patchy areas of increased and decreased density. In early infancy the vertebrae are normal, subsequently they become flat and then develop the biconcave appearance of osteoporosis. Scoliosis may be a feature.

The limb bones have a very thin cortex but the overall thickness is much increased and there is bowing and osteoporosis with coarse trabeculation. There may be some thickening of the cortex on the concave side of the bow. The short bones are widened, and the pelvis is characterised by protrusio acetabuli and a 'caving in' of the whole lower pelvis. Coxa vara is severe and the diaphysis of the femur is of greater diameter than the neck and epiphyseal region.

Pathology and clinical chemistry. There appears to be a rapid turnover of lamellar bone with failure to lay down compact cortical bone. Bakwin, Golden and Fox (1964) noted that the marrow spaces were filled with vascular fibrous tissue, quite unlike Paget's disease, and there were numerous thin trabeculae showing both active bone resorption and new bone formation. The serum levels of both alkaline and acid phosphatase are high though they may be normal in early life. There is a massive urinary excretion of hydroxyproline and proline containing peptides (Eyring and Eisenberg, 1968; Thompson et al, 1969).

Differential diagnosis. This includes polyostotic fibrous dysplasia, but here the lesions are usually asymmetrical. Hyperphosphatasia tarda (Van Buchem disease) begins in the second decade of life; the density of bone is increased and bowing and fractures are not features. Osteogenesis imperfecta, progressive diaphyseal dysplasia (Engelmann's disease) and infantile cortical hyperostosis are not characterised by high levels of alkaline phosphatase, or by the symmetrical patchy areas of osteoporosis and sclerosis.

Progress and complications. The severity of the disease is variable. Some children never learn to walk, others may do so and then regress. At its worst these children are severely deformed and incapacitated. Complications may arise from obliteration of the cranial nerve foramina with secondary cranial nerve involvement. The overgrowth of bone may also obliterate the nasal air passages (Marshall, 1962).

Treatment. Woodhouse et al (1972) reported treatment of a 5 year old child with human calcitonin and found that the bone turnover was reduced, as evidenced by a sustained fall in urine hydroxyproline excretion while the calcium and phosphate balance became more positive.

HYPERPHOSPHATASIA TARDA
(Van Buchem's disease)

This disease is similar to hyperphosphatasia congenita but the onset is not until a later age. It was first described by Van Buchem, Hadders and Ubbens (1955), with a subsequent report of 7 cases by Van Buchem et al (1962).

Inheritance. Like the congenital form, it appears also to be of autosomal recessive inheritance. However, there maybe a dominant form of the disease as reported by Maroteaux et al (1971).

Frequency. The population incidence is not known. The age of onset is usually during adolescence.

Clinical and radiographic features. The main clinical signs are of gradual involvement of cranial nerves due to obliteration of foramina in the base of the skull.

On radiography, the calvarium is thick, the base of the skull dense and the body of the mandible is also enlarged and sclerotic. Other areas of bone thickening are the spinous processes of the vertebrae, the ribs and clavicles. Bone strength, however, is normal and fractures are not a feature.

The long bones show symmetrical thickening and sclerosis of the diaphysis, without involvement of the epiphyseal region.

Pathology. The only available reports indicate that although there is an increase in the size of bones, the mineralisation seems comparable with normal.

Differential diagnosis. This is from osteopetrosis tarda, but here there is more generalised bone density including the pelvis and vertebrae, and there is an accompanying metaphyseal modelling defect.

Progress and complications. The main complication in hyperphosphatasia tarda is the gradual involvement of cranial nerves, the 7th being commonest, but the optic and auditory nerves are later involved. There may be some encroachment on the marrow cavities and developing anaemia.

Laboratory investigations. The serum alkaline phosphatase may be raised but, in spite of the name of the disease, this is not a consistent sign.

REFERENCES

Bakwin, H. & Eiger, M. S. (1956). Fragile bones and macrocranium. *Journal of Pediatrics*, **49**, 558.

Bakwin, H., Golden, A. & Fox, S. (1964). Familial osteoectasia with macrocranium. *American Journal of Roentgenology*, **91**, 609.

Buchem, F. S. P., Van., Hadders, H. N. & Ubbens, R. (1955). An uncommon familial systemic disease of the skeleton: hyperostosis corticalis generalisata familiaris. *Acta Radiologica*, **44**, 109.

Buchem, F. S. P., Van., Hadders, H. N., Hansen, J. F. & Woldring, M. G. (1962). Hyperostosis corticalis generalisata. Report of seven cases. *American Journal of Medicine*, **33**, 387.

Choremis, C., Yannakos, D., Papadatos, C. & Baroustou, E. (1958). Osteitis deformans (Paget's disease) in an 11 year old boy. *Helvetica Paediatrica Acta*, **13**, 185.

Eyring, E. J. & Eisenberg, E. (1968). Congenital hyperphosphatasia. *Journal of Bone & Joint Surgery*, **50A**, 1099.

Maroteaux, P., Fontaine, G., Scharfman, W. & Farriaux, J. P. (1971). L'hyperostose corticale généralisée à transmission dominante. *Archives Françaises de Pédiatrie*, **28**, 685.

Marshall, W. C. (1962). A chronic progressive osteopathy with hyperphosphatasia. *Proceedings of the Royal Society of Medicine*, **55**, 238.

Thompson, R. C., Gaull, G. E., Horwitz, S. J. & Schenk, R. K. (1969). Hereditary hyperphosphatasia. Studies of three siblings. *American Journal of Medicine*, **47**, 209.

Woodhouse, N. J. Y., Fisher, M. T., Sigurdsson, G., Joplin, G. F. & MacIntyre, I. (1972). Paget's disease in a 5 year old: acute response to human calcitonin. *British Medical Journal*, **4**, 267.

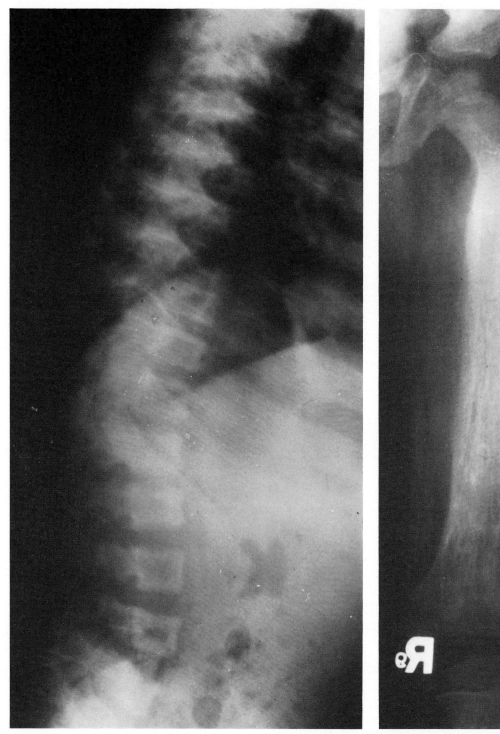

Fig. 33.1 (M.S.) The spine and ribs show irregular thickening with patchy areas of increased and decreased density. Some of the vertebrae are flattened. (G.O.S.)

Fig. 33.2 (M.S.) The shaft of the femur is much thickened with a thin cortex and there is osteoporosis with coarse trabeculation. (G.O.S.)

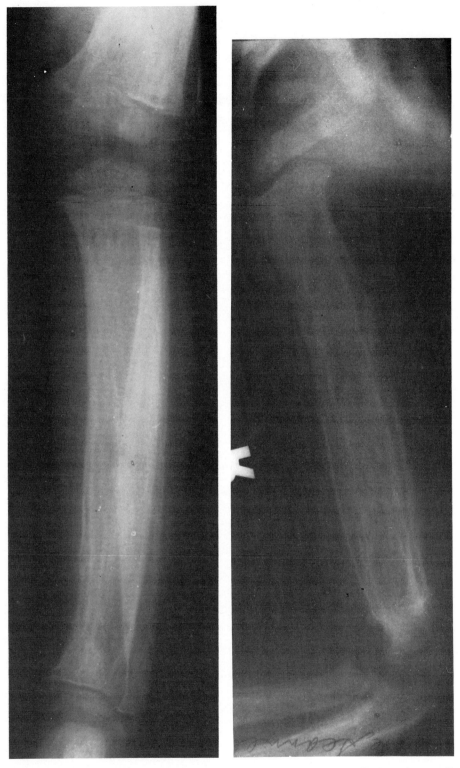

Figs 33.3 and 33.4   (M.S.) Similar changes are shown in the tibia, fibula and upper limb bones. (G.O.S.)

34 Pachydermoperiostitis
Idiopathic Hypertrophic Osteoarthropathy

This familial disease is characterised by soft tissue thickening, clubbing of the fingers and periosteal new bone formation. In the past it has been confused with secondary ('pulmonary') hypertrophic osteoarthropathy (Chapter 65) but this is often associated with intrathoracic disease, and is not familial.

There have been occasional reports in the literature over the past 100 years, but pachydermoperiostitis was most clearly defined by Touraine, Solenti and Gole (1935). More recent reports are by Rimoin (1965) and Harbison and Nice (1971).

Inheritance. Both autosomal dominant and recessive forms of the disorder appear to exist, the former being rather more common. Males are affected more frequently and more severely than females. The disorder becomes apparent during adolescence.

Clinical and radiographic features. Seborrhoeic hyperplasia of the skin with deep furrowing and oiliness of the face and forehead is probably noticed first. The facial features become coarse and thick and there is hyperhidrosis of the hands and feet. There is clubbing of the fingers and toes, caused by soft tissue hyperplasia, and the extremities may be disproportionately long, although the overall height is within normal limits. Rimoin (1965) suggested that hereditary finger clubbing may be an incompletely expressed form of the dominant disease. The distal parts of particularly the forearm and leg may be diffusely thickened and have a raised skin temperature associated with the underlying periostitis. These areas are not tender, but sometimes there is local joint pain and easy fatigue.

On radiography, there is thickening of both the calvarium and base of the skull with enlarged frontal and paranasal sinuses. The osteosclerosis may result in deafness and other cranial nerve lesions. The vertebral bodies show a mixture of rarefaction and sclerosis, some of the trabeculae becoming markedly sclerotic in the lines of tension and pressure, giving an appearance not unlike angioma. Narrowing of the vertebral foramina may produce neurological symptoms.

The generalised periostitis of the long bones usually affects the distal ends of radius, ulna, tibia and fibula, and the degree of periosteal reaction is matched by the overlying skin thickening. The new bone laid down is thick and rough, and the radiographic outline is very irregular and spiculated. In the long term there is no differentiation between the cortex and overlying periosteal new bone.

Differential diagnosis. This is chiefly from secondary (pulmonary) hypertrophic osteoarthropathy, the distinguishing features being the association of the latter with intrathoracic disease, together with the absence of a family history.

Harbison and Nice (1971) pointed out that the facial changes of pachydermoperiostitis may be confused with acromegaly but this disease is not associated with clubbing and periosteal new bone formation.

Hyperphosphatasia of late onset has some similar features but here the mandible is much enlarged, there is *cortical* thickening of the long bones, and no clubbing of the fingers or skin changes.

Progress and complications. The disorder is very slowly progressive and tends to become stationary about ten years after the onset. Complications reported are thickened eyelids obstructing vision, occasional cranial nerve palsies due to obstruction of foramina in the base of the skull and neurological signs related to narrowing of intervertebral foramina. Life expectancy and height are normal.

REFERENCES

Harbison, J. B. & Nice, C. M. (1971). Familial pachydermoperiostosis presenting as an acromegaly-like syndrome. *American Journal of Roentgenology*, **112**, 532.
Rimoin, D. (1965). Pachydermoperiostosis (idiopathic clubbing and periositis). *New England Journal of Medicine*, **272**, 923.
Touraine, A., Solente, G. & Golé, L. (1935). Un syndrome ostéodermatopathique. La pachydermie plicaturée avec pachypériostose des extrémités. *La Presse Médicale*, **43**, 1820.

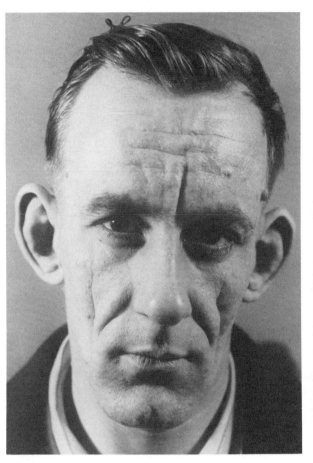

Fig. 34.1 (E.B. aged 31 years.) Facial features are thickened and there is deep furrowing of the forehead and cheeks. (H.A.T.F.)

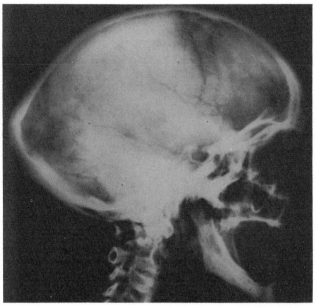

Fig. 34.2 (D.S. aged 57 years.) There is some thickening both of the calvarium and base of the skull. (H.A.T.F.)

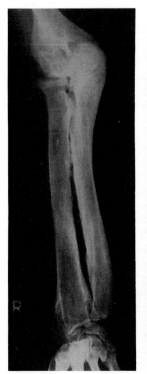 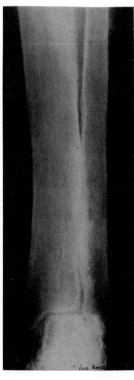

Fig. 34.3 (*Left*) (F.H. aged 47 years.) There is generalised periosteal reaction of most of the radius and ulna, matched by overlying skin thickening. The outline of the new bone is irregular and spiculated. (H.A.T.F.)

Fig. 34.4 (*Right*) (F.H.) The tibia and fibula show osteosclerosis and some irregular periosteal reaction. The distinction between cortex and medulla is lost. (H.A.T.F.)

35 Paget's Disease
Osteitis Deformans

This well known, fairly common disease of the middle aged and elderly is characterised by much thickening and enlargement of bone together with softening and bending at first. In the later stages there is a much increased density of bone with a liability to pathological fractures. It may affect only one or several bones, and is usually asymmetrical.

The description of the severe form of the disease by Sir James Paget in 1877 was not the first account but it remains a classical and accurate description. There have been recent reviews by Barry (1969) and Woodhouse (1972).

Aetiology and inheritance. The aetiology of this disease is still completely unknown. There are occasional reports of more than one case in a family, indicating possible autosomal (not X-linked) dominant inheritance (Jones and Reed, 1967; Evens and Bartter, 1968; and McKusick, 1972). However, since mild cases of the disease will pass unnoticed and family surveys to be of value would require radiography of all relatives, there are currently no reliable figures relating to genetic factors in Paget's disease.

Frequency. The disease is very rare before the age of 40 years and thus incidence figures have been based on various populations over this age. Schmorl (1932) found Paget's disease in 3 per cent of 4,614 autopsies in Germany. In a radiological study, Pygott (1957) found a similar proportion in the spine or pelvis of patients aged 45 or over, the proportion rising from less than 0·5 per cent (at ages 45 to 54 years), to approximately 5 per cent over the age of 75 years. The condition is somewhat commoner in males than females in a ratio of about 4:3.

There are racial and geographical differences in incidence, the disease being relatively common in Europe, North America and Australia but not in Africa or China. However, Lawrence (1970) found the disease was almost as common amongst negroes in Jamaica as amongst the Europeans there.

Clinical and radiographic features. The disease may exist for some years before symptoms present, if indeed they ever do. Any bone in the body may be affected, but the commonest areas are the lumbo-sacral vertebrae, skull, pelvis, femur and tibia. The upper limb bones are less commonly involved and the hand and foot even more rarely. The disease may remain monostotic for many years, and is virtually always asymmetrical. Although the vault and base of the skull are frequently involved, the facial bones usually escape. The mandible may be affected and also the teeth.

The presenting symptom of Paget's disease may be pain in the region of an affected bone, including headache, when the skull is affected, deformity from a bone that bends, enlargement of a bone may be noticed by the patient, or, frequently, a pathological fracture is the first indication of the disease. The cause of the pain in Paget's disease is unknown but it is clearly not related to the severity of the radiological changes and may spontaneously remit even though the disease apparently remains unchanged. When the disease is extensive, the skin over the affected bone may be warm and sometimes a bruit can be heard. The classical deformities that may occur are enlargement of the skull, anterior and lateral bowing of the femur and anterior bowing of the tibia. Thickening of bone with blunting of edges may easily be felt. In the later stages of severe Paget's disease many bones are affected and there is considerable reduction in stature from deformities and curvature of bone. However, individual bones affected by the disease may be increased in length as well as much thickened.

The radiographic appearances vary with the stage of the disease. In the early stages bone density is decreased and sometimes the osteolytic activity is seen as a 'V' shaped advancing lesion in or adjacent to the cortex of a long bone. In the later stages of the disease, sclerosis with increased bone density predominates. The trabeculae are coarse and disorganised, the cortex is thickened and may show micro-fractures along the convex side of a bent bone. The medullary cavity is usually enlarged, or more rarely, reduced in size.

In between these two main stages of osteolysis and sclerosis, there is a combined phase in which both these aspects are apparent at the same time, in the same or different bones. Cystic areas are sometimes seen; the sclerotic lesions may have a striated appearance or the denseness may be more evenly distributed. In the skull there is thickening of the outer table and irregular increased density with coarse mottling.

Pathology. In the first phase of abnormal destruction of bone, the 'vascular' stage, there appears to be an excessive number of osteoclasts, seen best in the skull and in the region of the 'V' shaped advancing edge of disease in a long bone. The spaces left fill with vascular fibrous tissue and there is a very vascular fibrous marrow. In the sclerotic phase there are irregular trabeculae, unorientated and separated by irregular cement lines and at this stage the marrow becomes less vascular. The 'lytic' and 'sclerotic' phases are noted separately, but in fact they co-exist.

Differential diagnosis. This is not usually in doubt, the thickened, bent and often painful bone in a middle-aged individual being quite characteristic. Polyostotic fibrous dysplasia occasionally has a similar appearance but does not usually have the thickened cortex of Paget's disease and also occurs in younger individuals. Metastatic neoplasm, particularly in the pelvis, may be similar to some stages of Paget's disease and a biopsy may be needed to distinguish the two.

Progress and complications. Most patients with Paget's disease have no symptoms, and between 10 and 40 per cent (in various series) have only mono-stotic lesions (Suchett-Kaye, 1970). Even when the disease is widespread it is never symmetrical, nor does it involve the whole skeleton.

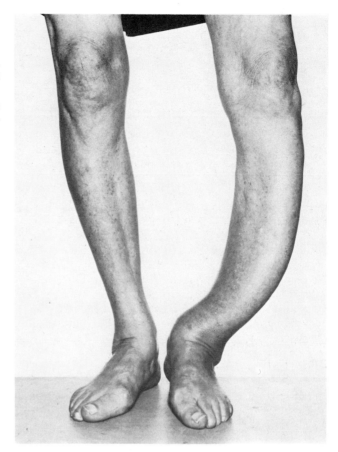

Fig. 35.2 (E.L.) Deformity of left tibia with lengthening and bowing. (Courtesy of Mr A. G. Apley, Pyrford.)

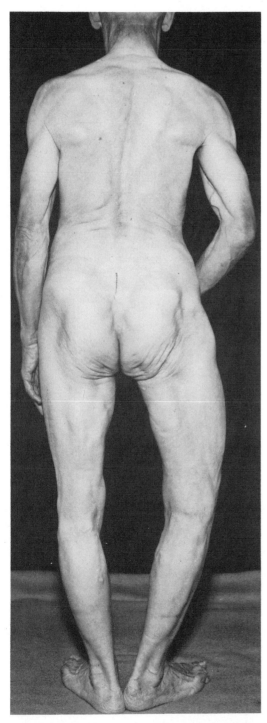

Fig. 35.1 (H.R.) Disease principally affecting the right femur, with lengthening and bowing. (Courtesy of Mr A. G. Apley, Pyrford.)

Pathological fracture is a common complication, sometimes in the early osteolytic stage, but more commonly in the later sclerotic phase when the bone becomes brittle—however, it is of frequent occurrence at any phase of the disease. The usual sites affected are the vertebrae, femur, tibia and pelvis. The fractures form callus and usually heal well, but management of them may be difficult because of the bending of bone. In the later sclerotic stage union may be long delayed.

Secondary osteoarthritis, due to the deformed bone and altered joint mechanics, is a likely complication particularly in the hip and knee joints.

Neoplastic change occurs in Paget's disease, though it is difficult to know the true proportion since many individuals with the disease pass unnoticed. Various surveys have reported up to 11 per cent of cases with malignant change. The tumour is usually a sarcoma but giant cell tumours also occur. Malignant change should be suspected with the onset of pain and swelling in a patient with pre-existing Paget's disease. Metastatic deposits may be found in affected bone at a distance from the primary growth, as well as in normal bone and in the lungs or elsewhere.

Neurological complications in Paget's disease arise from pressure on cranial nerves or spinal nerve roots. The thickened, abnormal bone encroaches on the foramina in the base of the skull, not infrequently causing optic atrophy or deafness (Henkin, Lifschitz and Larson, 1972). Root symptoms, particularly in the lower limbs, arise from the disease process affecting the vertebrae. Deafness may be due not only to 8th nerve paralysis but also to sclerosis of the stapes, and may be improved by stapedectomy. In spite of the frequent involvement of the skull in Paget's disease, platybasia is uncommon but long tract signs and hydrocephalus have been reported.

Cardiovascular complications in Paget's disease occur only occasionally, but are of a serious nature. The enormous increase in the bone capillaries with increased blood flow can lead to high output cardiac failure.

In spite of all these possible complications, provided the bone lesions do not turn malignant, most patients are surprisingly fit and have a normal expectation of life.

Laboratory investigations. A greatly increased bone turnover in Paget's disease is reflected in the very high serum alkaline phosphatase and urinary hydroxyproline. The serum calcium and phosphorus levels are generally normal though hypercalcaemia occurs if the patient is immobilised during treatment of a fracture or for any other reason.

Treatment. Until recent years there was no effective specific treatment for Paget's disease but there are now various agents which undoubtedly have an effect in reducing bone turnover. Treatment is only indicated when the disease is causing symptoms of bone pain or compression of cranial, spinal or other nerves.

Calcitonin (porcine, salmon and human). All reduce the high levels of serum alkaline phosphatase and urinary hydroxyproline. However, some patients respond only initially or with a limited response due to the development of antibodies (Bijvoet, Sluys Veer and Jansen, 1968; Goldfield et al, 1972; and Singer et al, 1974). The relief of bone pain is usually dramatic, though not that due to nerve compression.

Diphosphonates have the advantage of being administered by mouth. They are thought to act by blocking the growth and dissolution of apatite crystals. The serum alkaline phosphatase and urinary hydroxyproline levels are reduced and there is some success in the relief of bone pain (Smith et al, 1973; Russell et al, 1974). The bone however does not become normal, there being often an excessive quantity of osteoid.

Symptomatic treatment in Paget's disease is related to the care of fractures and secondary osteoarthritis. Fractures occurring in the elderly with sclerotic bone lesions are likely to heal slowly and internal fixation is usually employed, although likely to be technically difficult. Osteotomies may be required to straighten the bone in relation to weight-bearing joints, and sometimes advantage can be taken of pathological fractures to achieve this.

REFERENCES

Barry, H. C. (1969). *Paget's disease of bone*. Edinburgh, Livingstone.
Bijvoet, O. L. M., Sluys Veer, J. van der & Jansen, A. P. (1968). Effects of calcitonin on patients with Paget's disease, thyrotoxicosis or hypercalcaemia. *Lancet*, **1**, 876.
Evens, R. G. & Bartter, F. C. (1968). The hereditary aspects of Paget's disease (osteitis deformans). *Journal of American Medical Association*, **205**, 900.
Goldfield, E. B., Braiker, B. M., Prendergast, J. J. & Kolb, F. O. (1972). Synthetic salmon calcitonin. Treatment of Paget's disease and osteogenesis imperfecta. *Journal of American Medical Association*, **221**, 1127.
Henkin, R. I., Lifschitz, M. D. & Larson, A. L. (1972). Hearing loss in patients with osteoporosis and Paget's disease of bone. *American Journal of Medical Sciences*, **263**, 383.
Jones, J. V. & Reed, M. F. (1967). Paget's disease: a family with six cases. *British Medical Journal*, **4**, 90.
Lawrence, J. S. (1970). Paget's disease in population samples. *Annals of the Rheumatic Diseases*, **29**, 562.
McKusick, V. A. (1972). *Heritable Disorders of Connective Tissue*. 4th edition, Mosby, St. Louis.
Paget, J. (1877). *Medico-chirurgical transactions*, London, **60**, 37.
Pygott, F. (1957). Paget's disease of bone: the radiological incidence. *Lancet*, **1**, 1170.
Russell, R. G. G., Smith, R., Preston, C., Walton, R. J. & Woods, C. G. (1974). Diphosphonates in Paget's disease. *Lancet*, **1**, 894.
Schmorl, G. (1932). Uber osteitis deformans Paget. *Virchows Archiv für Pathologische Anatomie*, **283**, 694.
Singer, F. R., Neer, R. M., Golzman, D., Krane, S. M. & Potts, J. T. (1974). Treatment of Paget's disease of bone with salmon calcitonin. In *Endocrinology*, 1973, ed. Taylor, S. London: Heinemann.
Smith, R., Russell, R. G. G., Bishop, M. C., Woods, C. G. & Bishop, M. (1973). Paget's disease of bone. Experience with a diphosphonate (disodium etidronate) in treatment. *Quarterly Journal of Medicine*, **42**, 235.
Suchett-Kaye, A. I. (1970). Paget's disease of bone. *Gerontologia Clinica*, **12**, 241.
Woodhouse, N. Y. J. (1972). Paget's disease of bone. *Clinics in Endocrinology and Metabolism*, **1**, 125.

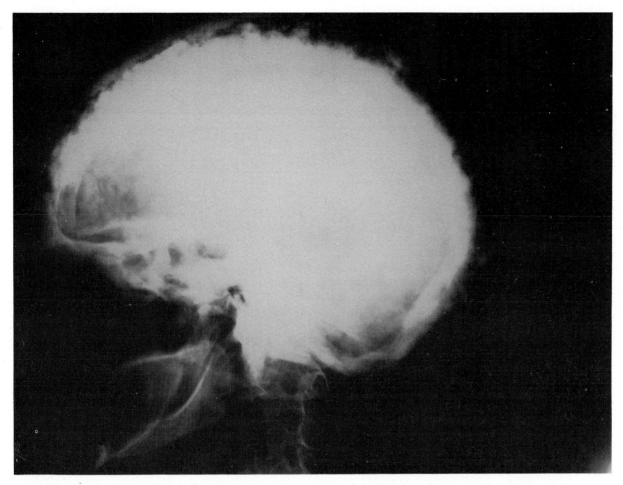

Fig. 35.3 (A.) Severe involvement of the whole vault and base of skull with patchy areas of sclerosis and much thickening. (A.H.)

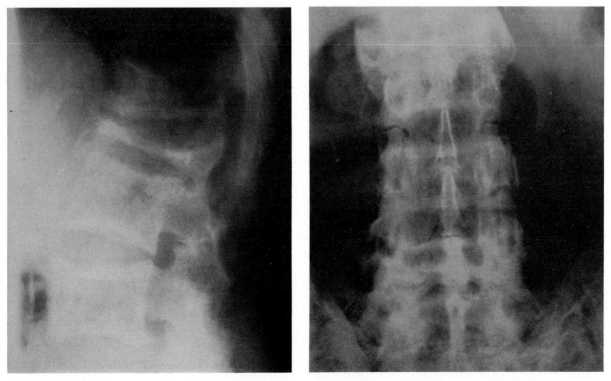

Figs 35.4 and 35.5 (W.J.) Involvement of lumbar vertebrae with collapse of L2. (Courtesy of Dr D. J. Tudor, Cambridge.)

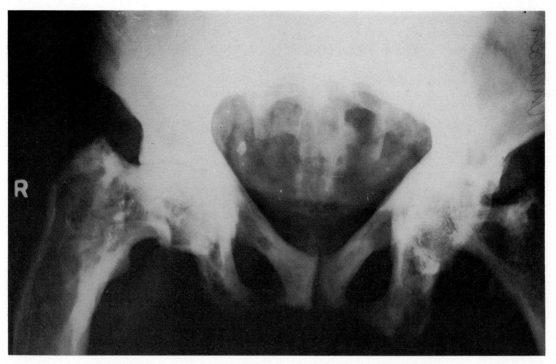

Fig. 35.6   (A.) Irregular increased bone density with mottling, much thickened cortex and bending of the right femur. (A.H.)

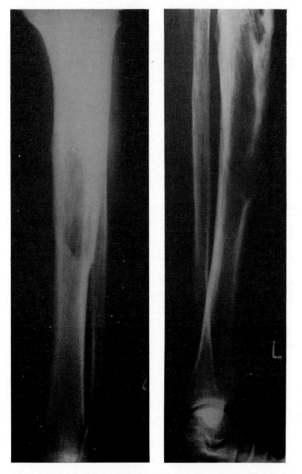

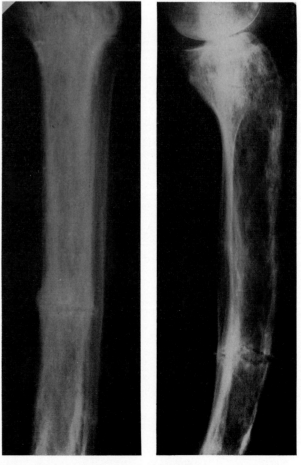

Figs 35.7 and 35.8   (W.J.) The early stage of Paget's disease with principally an osteolytic lesion and 'V' shaped advancing lesion. (Courtesy of Dr D. J. Tudor, Cambridge.)

Figs 35.9 and 35.10   (C.J.) The late stage of Paget's disease with sclerosis predominating, a thickened cortex and transverse pathological fracture. (A.H.)

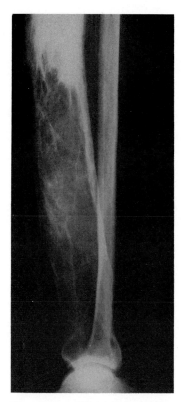

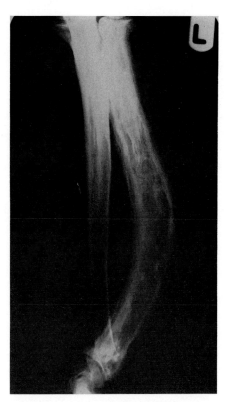

Fig. 35.11 (W.A.) Principally osteolytic lesion involving the tibia only. (A.H.)

Fig. 35.12 (E.C.) Severe involvement of the radius with patchy sclerosis and thickened lesions, lengthening and bending of the bone. (A.H.)

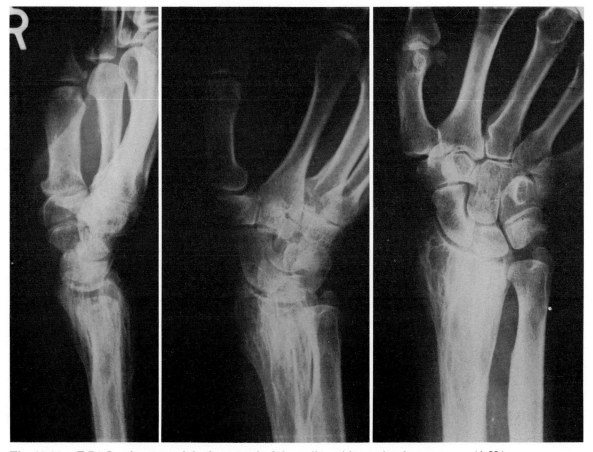

Fig. 35.13 (E.P.) Involvement of the lower end of the radius with a striated appearance. (A.H.)

36 Diaphyseal Aclasis
Multiple Hereditary Exostoses

In this condition there are multiple exostoses which are limited to bone developed in cartilage. They arise, not, as the name suggests, in the diaphysis but in the junctional area between the epiphysis and metaphysis, most commonly at the ends of the long bones. There were numerous references to the disorder in the last century, but the term 'diaphyseal aclasis' was introduced by Keith (1919).

Inheritance. The condition is of autosomal dominant inheritance and there have been several family studies illustrating this (Stocks and Barrington, 1925; Krooth, Macklin and Hilbish, 1961; and Solomon 1964).

Frequency. The population incidence is not known but this is one of the commoner of the skeletal dysplasias. The sex ratio is probably nearly equal, earlier statements that the condition was commoner in males having been made without carrying out radiography of females in the families. However, the condition does appear to be rather less severe in women and thus presents less frequently in clinical practice. The age of onset, or of diagnosis, is variable. Usually the first exostosis presents around the age of 5 years but has clearly been there before this age.

Clinical and radiographic features. The degree of severity of this disorder and the number of exostoses is very variable. Many patients are below average in height but shortness of stature is never marked. The exostoses tend to be bilateral and are often symmetrical, a typical site being around the knee where they may be clinically visible and palpable. The forearm may be obviously deformed on clinical examination, with a severely affected shortened ulna and bowed radius, with ulnar deviation of the wrist.

On radiography the skull is hardly ever affected and the vertebrae are not usually so, though lesions can develop here and cause problems from spinal cord compression. The ribs, scapula and clavicle may all develop exostoses but the commonest and most characteristic sites are the ends of the long bones, where cartilage-capped exostoses arise in the juxta-epiphyseal region and grow pointing away from the epiphysis. The outgrowths may be sessile or pedunculated and may lead to asymmetrical growth of the bone. The carpal and tarsal bones are not usually affected, nor is the patella, but the metacarpals and phalanges may be involved with small projections from the surface of the cortex.

Pathology. It is thought that the lesions arise from a displaced portion of the growth plate which then continues to grow separately from the main shaft. The marrow invades the new bone and the primary and secondary spongiosa are continuous with the main shaft.

Differential diagnosis. The fully developed condition is quite characteristic and unlikely to be mistaken for any other. In Ollier's dyschondroplasia there is often a similar deformity of the forearm but the disease tends to be asymmetrical and has no associated family history. A recently described disorder, the tricho-rhino-phalangeal syndrome (Chapter 47) may be associated with multiple exostoses, but other features differentiate it (microcephaly, mental retardation, a characteristic face and generalised joint laxity).

Progress and complications. Some three-quarters of patients are below average height, depending upon the severity of the lesions. The exostoses continue growing with the rest of the skeleton and stop at skeletal maturity. Occasionally, particularly in the hands, they may regress completely. Complications arising from the exostoses are surprisingly few. The deformed forearm has been referred to. Radiohumeral dislocation can occur (Solomon, 1961), synostosis of the tibia and fibula may be a feature and this rarely occurs between the radius and ulna. There may be a valgus deformity at the ankle and knee due to obliquity of the tibial articular surfaces.

Other complications relate to compression of nerves by the exostoses, particularly of the lateral popliteal nerve, and there have been reports of spinal cord compression from vertebral exostoses (Vinstein and Franken, 1971; Crowell and Wepsic, 1972; Madigan, Worrall and McClain, 1974). An associated aneurysm of the popliteal artery has been reported (Clark and Keokarn, 1965, and Hershey and Lamsden, 1972).

The most serious complication of diaphyseal aclasis is the development of a chondrosarcoma, usually estimated to occur in between 5 and 10 per cent of patients—though this figure is probably too high since many patients with simple diaphyseal aclasis will never attend hospital for treatment (Barnes and Catto, 1966). Malignant change tends to occur in an exostosis of a proximal 'flat' bone such as the scapula or pelvis but may occur in any lesion. It should be suspected if there is pain or discomfort and an unexpected increase in the size of a previously symptomless exostosis, particularly in an adult.

Treatment. Removal of a benign exostosis is usually only indicated for cosmetic reasons or if there are complications due to pressure on surrounding structures. Because of the relatively high risk of malignant change in proximal lesions, however, it is probably as well to remove these, if possible, at the end of skeletal growth.

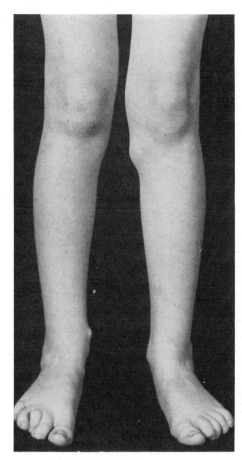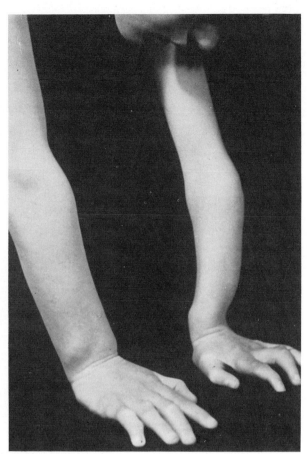

Figs 36.1 and 36.2   (R.C. & E.C.) Clinical appearance of exostoses of the tibia and forearm bones, with some bowing of the latter. (Courtesy of Mr A. G. Apley, Pyrford.)

REFERENCES

Barnes, R. & Catto, M. (1966). Chondrosarcoma of bone. *Journal of Bone & Joint Surgery*, **48B,** 729.

Clark, P. M. & Keokarn, T. (1965). Popliteal aneurysm complicating benign osteocartilaginous exostosis. *Journal of Bone & Joint Surgery*, **47A,** 1386.

Crowell, R. M. & Wepsic, J. G. (1972). Thoracic cord compression due to chondrosarcoma in two cousins with hereditary multiple exostoses. *Journal of Neurosurgery*, **36,** 86.

Hershey, S. L. & Lansden, F. (1972). Osteochondroma as a cause of false popliteal aneurysm. *Journal of Bone & Joint Surgery*, **54A,** 1765.

Keith, A. (1919). Studies on the anatomical changes which accompany certain growth disorders of the human body. *Journal of Anatomy (London)*, **54,** 101.

Krooth, R. S., Macklin, M. T. & Hilbish, T. F. (1961). Diaphyseal aclasis (multiple exostoses) on Guam. *American Journal of Human Genetics*, **13,** 340.

Madigan, R., Worrall, T. & McClain, E. J. (1974). Cervical cord compression in hereditary multiple exostosis. *Journal of Bone & Joint Surgery*, **56A,** 401.

Solomon, L. (1961). Bone growth in diaphyseal aclasis. *Journal of Bone & Joint Surgery*, **43B,** 700.

Solomon, L. (1964). Hereditary multiple exostosis. *American Journal of Human Genetics*, **16,** 351.

Stocks, P. & Barrington, A. (1925). Hereditary disorders of bone development. Part I. *Treasury of Human Genetics*, Vol. 3, Cambridge.

Vinstein, A. L. & Franken, E. A. Jun. (1971). Hereditary multiple exostoses. Report of a case with spinal cord compression. *American Journal of Roentgenology*, **112,** 405.

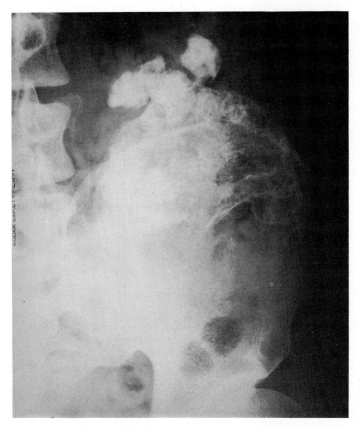

Fig. 36.3   (J.C.) Large exostosis of the ilium; removal is indicated because of the risk of malignant change. (A.H.)

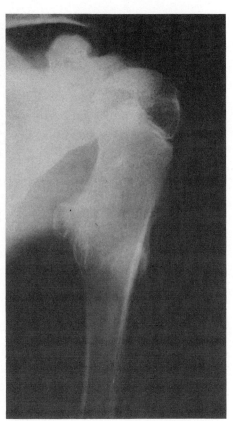

Fig. 36.4   (L.D.) Exostosis at the upper end of the humerus, apparently moving down the shaft with growth. (H.A.T.F.)

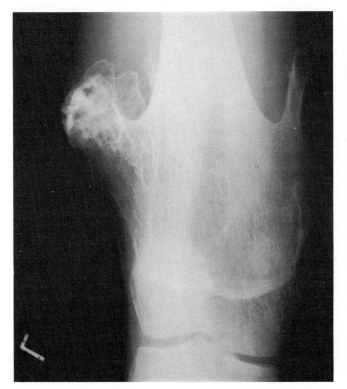

Fig. 36.5   (M.R.) Typical upward growing exostoses at the lower end of the femur. (A.H.)

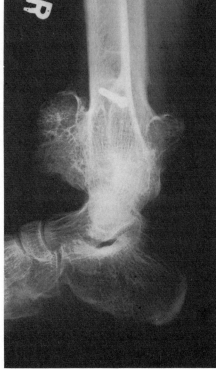

Fig. 36.6   (M.R.) Large exostosis involving the lower end of the fibula. (A.H.)

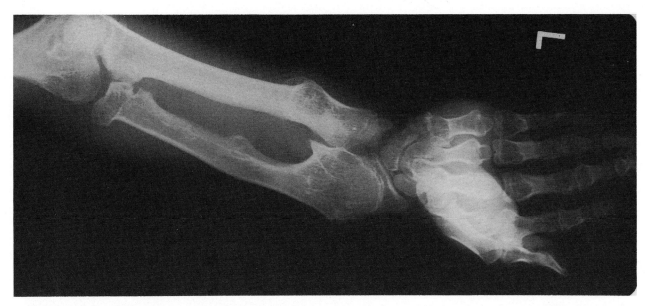

Fig. 36.7 (M.R.) Involvement of forearm bones and hand, with shortening of both radius and ulna. (A.H.)

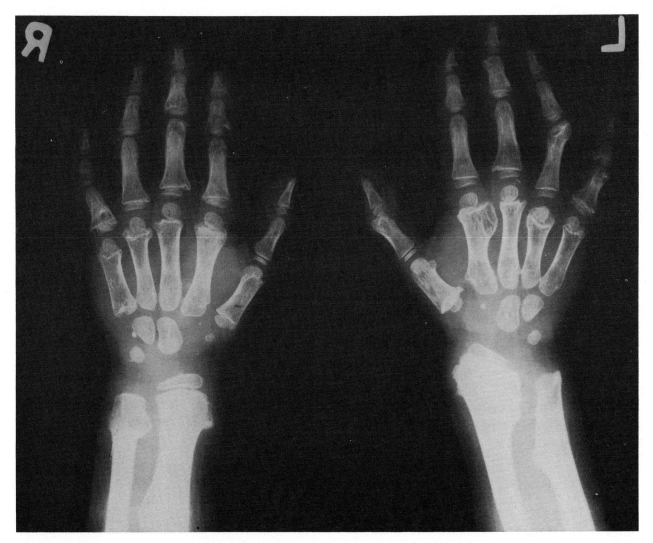

Fig. 36.8 (M.R.) Appearance of lesion at an earlier age, with involvement of many of the short bones of the hand as well as the lower radius and ulna. (A.H.)

OLLIER'S DISEASE

In Ollier's disease the characteristic feature is unossified areas of cartilage remaining in the metaphysis and diaphysis, sometimes expanding to form huge tumour masses. The term 'Ollier's disease' originally referred only to the unilateral or monosseous condition, but the enchondromatosis is frequently bilateral, though usually asymmetrical.

The first description was by Ollier (1900) and there have been many reports since then.

Aetiology. There is no evidence for any genetic factor in this disease; all reported cases have been sporadic.

Frequency. The population incidence is not known but it is a very rare disorder. The sexes are equally affected and the age of onset is during childhood.

Clinical and radiographic features. The presenting sign is swelling of bone in the metaphyseal region, often of one bone only, or unilaterally. Those chiefly involved are the long bones formed in cartilage, and particularly common sites are around the knee joint and at the lower end of the radius and ulna. However, any of the long bones may be affected, the pelvis is often involved and lesions in the hands, particularly of the phalanges, are common. Fractures may occur through the abnormal bone, and the lesions increase in size as the child grows, sometimes to such an extent that amputation is required for functional and cosmetic reasons. The affected limb fails to grow in length and there may be a considerable discrepancy between it and its fellow. Involvement principally of one side of a metaphysis gives rise to deformities such as genu valgum as well as the shortening. There is often a forearm deformity which is similar to that seen in diaphyseal aclasis, with a markedly shortened ulna, a curved radius and dislocation of the radial head.

On radiography the irregular translucent areas and streaks of cartilage seen in the metaphyseal region are quite distinctive and the density of bone between the streaks is often increased. The shafts of the major long bones are not usually extensively involved but lesions in the metacarpals and phalanges tend to expand over the whole length of the bone. As the child grows, the metaphyseal lesions spread to the diaphysis and may expand to form huge cartilaginous masses.

In childhood the epiphyses are usually normal but later, areas of irregular density and mottling occur. If the pelvis is affected, translucent columns are seen radiating in a fan-like manner towards the iliac crest.

Pathology. In Ollier's disease the defect is of the cartilage cells of the growth plate which fail to mature and are left behind in the metaphysis; apparently they fail to develop an extracellular matrix which can mineralise. The periosteal sleeve fails to remodel and longitudinal bone growth is slowed.

Differential diagnosis. The diagnosis of Ollier's disease is not usually in doubt, but a recently described condition, metachondromatosis (Maroteaux, 1971) also exhibits multiple enchondromatous lesions, particularly in the short bones of the hands and feet. It differs from Ollier's disease in that it is of dominant inheritance, and also the bony lesions may regress.

Progress and complications. The lesions of Ollier's disease continue to appear during growth, but new ones do not usually develop after puberty. Asymmetrical limb shortening is common and fractures through affected areas may occur. The chief disability is from the massive swellings. Malignant degeneration is not usually a feature though chondrosarcoma has been reported on rare occasions.

Treatment. This is directed to the fractures, deformities, limb length discrepancies and to the removal of unsightly lesions.

MAFFUCCI'S DISEASE
(Enchondromatosis with haemangiomata)

This disorder is an enchondromatosis associated with multiple haemangiomata of the soft tissues. It was described by Maffucci (1881) and many cases have been reported since then. There have been reviews by Carleton et al (1942) and Lewis and Ketcham (1973).

Aetiology. As in Ollier's disease, there is no evidence for any genetic factor and the aetiology is obscure.

Frequency. The population incidence is not known but the condition is extremely rare, more so than Ollier's disease. The sexes are equally affected. The disorder becomes apparent during infancy, childhood or adolescence, the average age being 5 years (Lewis and Ketcham, 1973).

Clinical and radiographic features. The presenting features may be either skeletal or vascular, and about one-quarter of cases present at birth or during the first year of life. 88 per cent of patients have bony lesions in the hand and 61 per cent in the feet, but almost any bone may be affected.

Radiographic features are similar to Ollier's disease with the addition of phleboliths associated with the vascular lesions. These and the bony lesions do not necessarily affect the same areas of the body.

Pathology. There may be cavernous or capillary haemangiomata, or, rarely lymphangiomata (Strang and Rannie, 1950; Lewis and Ketcham, 1973) and all these types of lesions may occur in the same patient.

Progress and complications. In the Maffucci syn-

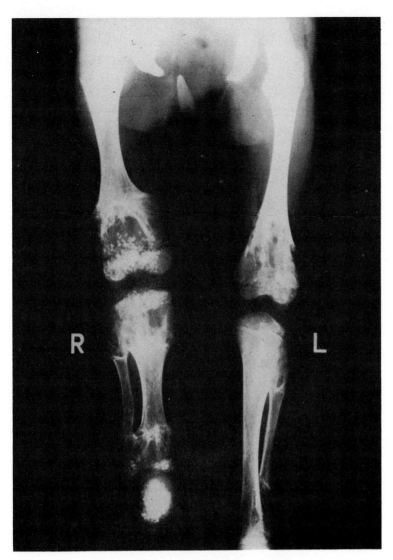

Fig. 37.1 A severely affected child with asymmetrical areas of mottling and streaking of bone in the metaphyseal regions. The epiphyses also contain irregular areas of increased density and there is considerable limb shortening on the right side. (H.A.T.F.)

drome there may be some progression of lesions after skeletal growth has ceased. The main complication of this disorder is malignant change, in either the bony or the vascular lesions. This was reported as 18·6 per cent of cases by Elmore and Cantrill (1966) and 15·2 per cent by Lewis and Ketcham (1973). Multiple primary growths may occur and malignancy may appear in other regions, for example in the brain, ovary or pancreas.

Treatment. This is related to the fractures, the deformities and to the malignant change, should it occur.

REFERENCES

Carleton, A., Elkington, J. St.C., Greenfield, J. G. & Robb-Smith, A. H. T. (1942). Maffucci's syndrome (dyschondroplasia with haemangiomata). *Quarterly Journal of Medicine*, **11**, 203.

Elmore, S. M. & Cantrill, W. C. (1966). Maffucci's syndrome. Case report with a normal karyotype. *Journal of Bone & Joint Surgery*, **48A**, 1607.

Lewis, R. J. & Ketcham, A. S. (1973). Maffucci's syndrome: functional and neoplastic significance. Case report and a review of the literature. *Journal of Bone & Joint Surgery*, **55A**, 1465.

Maffucci, A. (1881). Di un caso di enchondroma ed angioma multiplo. *Morgagni*, **3,** 399.

Maroteaux, P. (1971). Metachondromatosis. *Zeitschrift für Kinderheilkunde*, **109,** 246.

Ollier, L. X. E. L. (1900). *Lyons Médical*, **93,** 23.

Strang, C. & Rannie, I. (1950). Dyschondroplasia with haemangiomata. *Journal of Bone & Joint Surgery*, **32B,** 376.

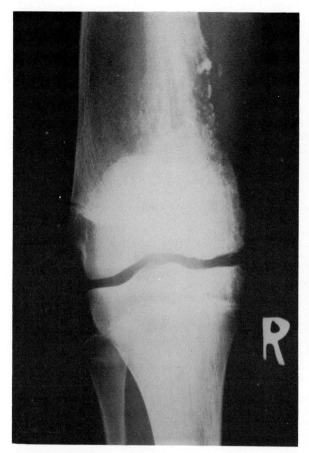

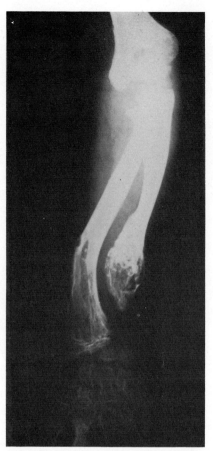

Fig. 37.2 (J.S.) A less severe lesion in an older child, involving the cortex of the bone. (A.H.)

Fig. 37.3 The forearm deformity is characteristic with shortening of the ulna and the radius curving round it. (H.A.T.F.)

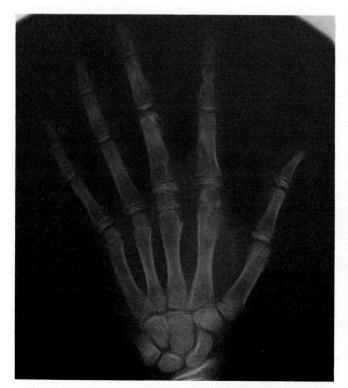

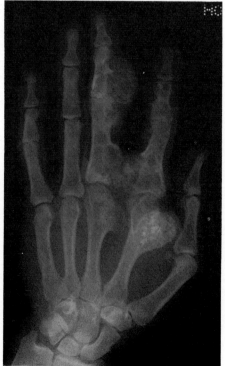

Figs 37.4 and 37.5 (J.S.) The second and third rays are both involved, with the exception of the terminal phalanges; 12 years had elapsed between the two radiographs. (A.H.)

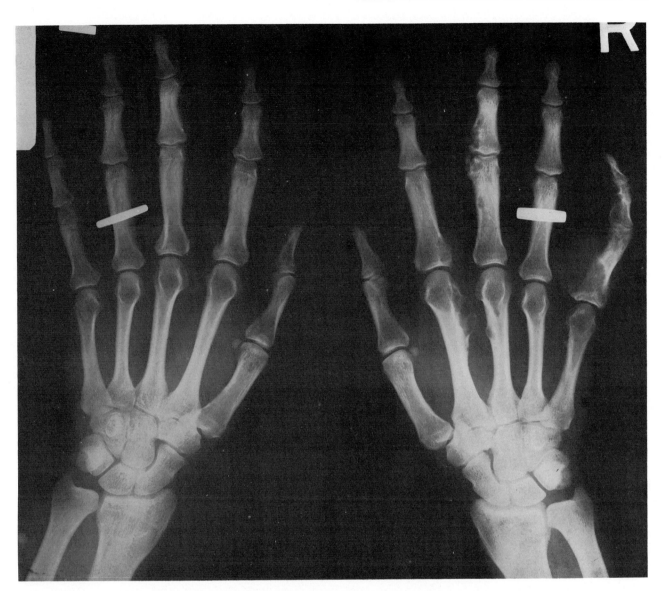

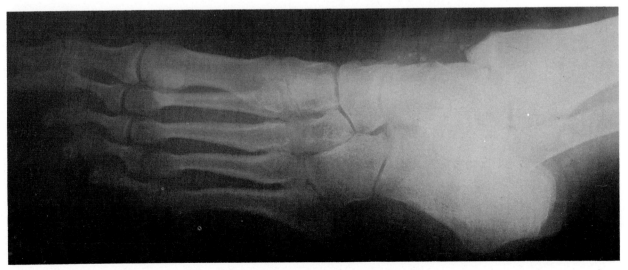

Figs 37.6 and 37.7 (F.G.) An example of the Maffucci syndrome, where the bony lesions in the hand are identical with Ollier's disease; in addition there are areas of soft tissue swelling, particularly at the left wrist and right ankle, where there were vascular lesions; phleboliths can be seen. (Courtesy of Mr A. G. Apley, Pyrford.)

38 Melorheostosis

Melorheostosis is characterised by usually asymmetrical linear streaks of hyperostosis developing along the major axes of long bones, together with soft tissue contractures, fibrosis and abnormalities of the skin. It was first clearly described by Léri and Lièvre (1928) since when many cases have been reported. By 1968, Campbell, Papademitriou and Bonfiglio were able to review 151 cases of their own and from the literature.

Aetiology. The cause of the condition is quite unknown; it does not appear to be genetically determined as all reported cases have been sporadic.

Frequency. The population incidence is not known but the disorder is an extremely rare one. The usual age of onset is during childhood, when either the soft tissue contractures or pain and swelling associated with hyperostosis around the joints is noticed, but it may be discovered only incidentally in adult life. The sexes are equally affected.

Clinical and radiographic features. This is one of the few generalised affections of the skeleton in which pain is a presenting and continuing feature. The skin is often involved and may be tense, shiny, erythematous and indurated. Soft tissue thickening and contractures of several joints may occur, including contractures of the palmar and plantar fascia. Other presenting signs of the disease may be limb stiffness or palpable bone enlargement. Muscles gradually become atrophic and weak, and the affected limbs wasted.

On radiography, the bony lesions are most frequently seen in the long bones, the skull, vertebrae and ribs being least often affected. The sclerotic linear streaks are usually likened to wax flowing down the side of a candle. The disease process frequently involves only one bone or one limb, though this is not invariably so, and often only one side of a long bone is affected, the other half being apparently normal. The main characteristic is the longitudinal arrangement of the sclerotic areas involving both inner and outer aspects of the cortex. The scapula or other 'flat' bones are affected by dense patches and spots rather than by linear areas of sclerosis.

Streaks and spots can affect the epiphyses, though bone in the region of a joint tends to remain uninvolved. Deposits of bone in the soft tissues around joints add to the stiffness and limitation of movement.

Pathology. Bone formation exceeds destruction and sclerotic, thick, irregular laminae almost obliterate the Haversian systems. Hoshino and Murakami (1971) investigated the mineral content of bone per unit volume and found it was not higher than that of normal bone. Morris, Samilson and Corley (1963) suggested a progression from vasculitis to vascular obliteration, associated with muscular degeneration and atrophy. They also noted metaplastic cartilage formation and cartilage degeneration with calcification and later ossification. The skin lesions showed a nonspecific fibrosis.

Differential diagnosis. When melorheostosis is fully developed there is no mistaking the diagnosis, but the first signs in infancy may be the soft tissue lesions and joint contractures, which have been confused with arthrogryposis multiplex congenita. However, this condition is immediately apparent at birth, is not painful and the limbs characteristically lack the usual contours. In osteopetrosis and similar dysplasias with increased bone density the disease is generalised and symmetrical, unlike melorheostosis.

Progress and complications. The lesions of melorheostosis progress during childhood and more slowly in adult life. In nearly every patient there is pain, limitation of joint movement and increasing contracture of joints. It is a serious disorder in the amount of deformity and disability that is produced, but malignant change has not been reported. An association with arteriovenous aneurysm has been described (Murray, 1951; Patrick, 1969).

Treatment. This is related to the relief of pain and attempts to control soft tissue contractures.

REFERENCES

Campbell, C. J., Papademitriou, T. & Bonfiglio, M. (1968). Melorheostosis. A report of the clinical, roentgenographic and pathological findings in fourteen cases. *Journal of Bone & Joint Surgery*, **50A**, 1281.
Hoshino, T. & Murakami, Y. (1971). Melorheostosis. *Acta Orthopaedica Scandinavica*, **42**, 28.
Léri, A. & Lièvre, J. A. (1928). La melorhéostose. *La Presse Médicale*, **36**, 801.
Morris, J. M., Samilson, R. L. & Corley, C. L. (1963). Melorheostosis. *Journal of Bone & Joint Surgery*, **45A**, 1191.
Murray, R. O. (1951). Melorheostosis associated with congenital arteriovenous aneurysms. *Proceedings of the Royal Society of Medicine*, **44**, 473.
Patrick, J. H. (1969). Melorheostosis associated with arteriovenous aneurysm of the left arm and trunk. *Journal of Bone & Joint Surgery*, **51B**, 126.

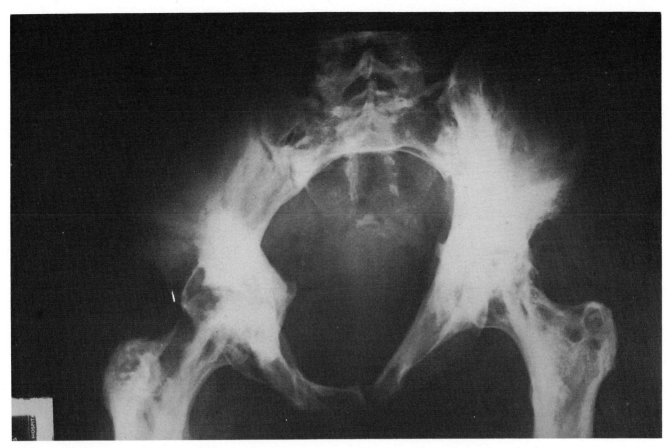

Fig. 38.1 (I.S.) There is blotchy sclerosis of most of the pelvis. The linear streaking is best seen in the necks of the femora. (A.H.)

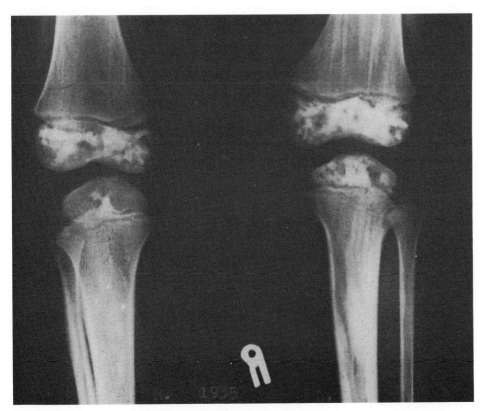

Fig. 38.2 Linear streaks in the lower femora and upper tibae, but the striking feature is the patchy sclerotic areas confined to the epiphyses. (H.A.T.F.)

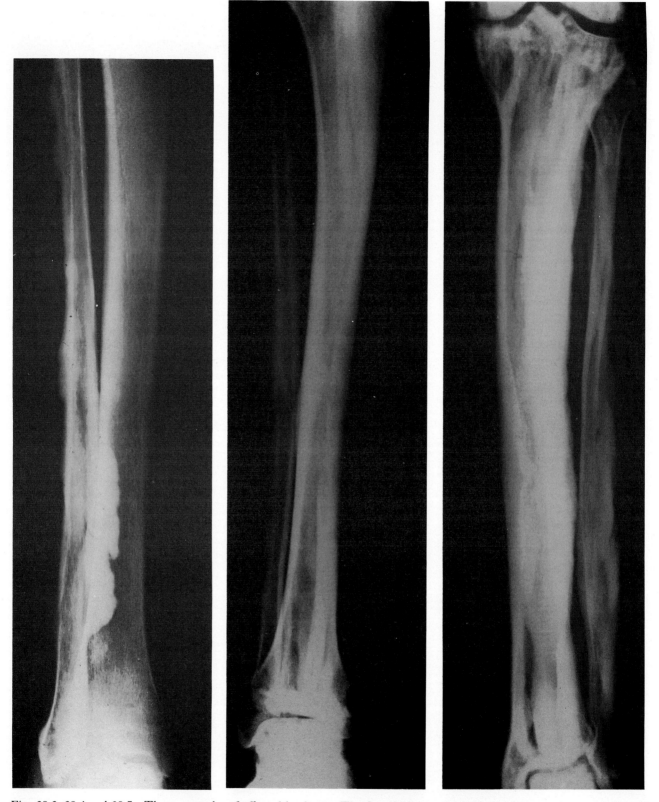

Figs 38.3, 38.4 and 38.5   Three examples of affected leg bones. The first illustrates the sclerotic streaks likened to wax flowing down the side of a candle whereas the others show different degrees of sclerosis, thickening and linear streaking. (H.A.T.F. and A.H.)

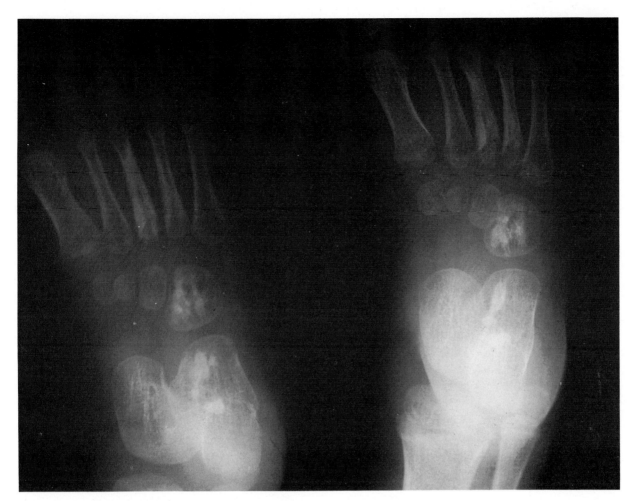

Fig. 38.6 (K.D.) A child with early signs of the disease in the tarsus and metatarsals. (A.H.)

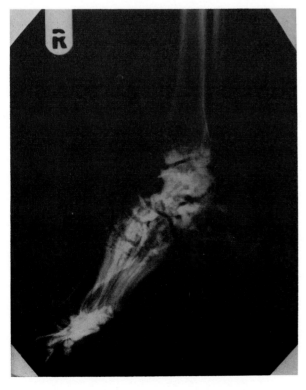

Fig. 38.7 A more advanced lesion involving most of the foot and distal end of the tibia. (H.A.T.F.)

39 Polyostotic Fibrous Dysplasia
McCune–Albright

The main features of this condition were described in 1937 both by McCune and Bruch, and by Albright *et al*. It is characterised by fibrous tissue spreading within the bony medullary space, eroding and replacing bone. It is a disease which progresses throughout childhood and is frequently associated with skin pigmentation and sometimes (particularly in girls) with endocrine problems such as precocious sexual development and occasional hyperthyroidism.

By 1962 Harris, Dudley and Barrie were able to report on 37 patients and more were reported in a general review of fibrous dysplasia of bone by Stewart, Gilmer and Edmonson (1962).

Aetiology. There appears to be no genetic basis for this curious disorder, all cases reported being sporadic. The aetiology is obscure, though it is clearly developmental in origin (Lichtenstein, 1970).

Frequency. Polyostotic fibrous dysplasia is extremely rare, unlike the monostotic form (not discussed here). The full syndrome described by Albright and colleagues in which the fibrous dysplasia of bone was accompanied by skin pigmentation and sexual precocity, is present usually only in girls and only in 2 to 3 per cent of all cases. The age of onset of symptoms is variable but Harris, Dudley and Barrie (1962) noted that two-thirds of patients were under the age of 10 years.

Clinical and radiographic features. The presenting signs of the disorder are usually those of pain and deformity from a pathological fracture, although the skin pigmentation may have been present from birth. In girls the first symptom may be vaginal bleeding. Other presenting features include, asymmetrical bone enlargement or pain and stiffness of a limb, but pain is not usually a prominent feature of this disorder. The pigmented areas of skin are smooth, common on the trunk and thighs, and may be very extensive. Pigmentation of mucous membranes in the mouth, for example, may be a feature.

The radiographic appearance of the bone in polyostotic fibrous dysplasia is usually quite characteristic, with patches of rarefaction and sclerosis. The bone is sometimes described as having a 'ground glass' appearance of uniform density, but unaffected bones, or parts of them, are quite normal in appearance. The condition is essentially one of multiple localised lesions, not a generalised bone disease such as hyperparathyroidism. The size of the individual lesion is very variable, some being only small and cyst-like, and at the other extreme the whole shaft of a major limb bone may be involved with patchy rarefaction and sclerosis. The epiphyses are rarely involved.

The skull and mandible are frequently affected unilaterally, giving rise sometimes to marked facial asymmetry and obliteration of the air sinuses. Involvement of ribs with fractures is common, but the most serious deformities are in the long bones. Radiographs of the pelvis and femur often show coxa vara and lateral curving of the femur, and, since the disorder is frequently asymmetrical, there may be leg length discrepancies—the limb with fibrous dysplasia being sometimes the longer of the two.

Pathology. The picture is of a fibrous replacement of bone, beginning as a proliferation of connective tissue in the medullary spaces and gradually encroaching upon and destroying the cancellous trabeculae. Multiple bone cysts occur and the areas of skin pigmentation have some connection with these.

Differential diagnosis. The fully developed picture of polyostotic fibrous dysplasia is unlikely to be mistaken for any other disease, the most similar to it being severe primary hyperparathyroidism. However, this is uncommon in childhood, is not typically asymmetrical, is not accompanied by skin pigmentation and has an associated hypercalcaemia. Melorheostosis is differentiated by the skin changes, contractures and typically sclerotic bone lesions. In histiocytosis X the bone lesions appear sharply outlined and punched out, unlike the diffuse rarefaction of polyostotic fibrous dysplasia.

Progress and complications. The lesions progress in size until the epiphyses close, and these may fuse early leading to some degree of short stature. The appearance of new lesions or the enlargement of old ones after puberty is not common, but the fibrous tissue remains together with the deformities and the continuing risk of fracture. Very occasionally bone lesions may resolve. The skull lesions may progress to obliterate cranial nerve foramina and paralysis particularly of the 2nd, 7th and 8th nerves may occur.

In addition to the early onset of menstruation in girls, polyostotic fibrous dysplasia has also been reported in association with gigantism, diabetes mellitus, and hyperthyroidism. There has also been one report of fibrous dysplasia associated with hyperparathyroidism (Ehrig and Wilson, 1972).

Laboratory investigations. There are no consistent changes in blood chemistry but the alkaline phosphatase is raised in about one-third of cases.

Treatment. This is related to the control of fractures and prevention and correction of deformity so far as possible. The obliteration of these extensive lesions by bone grafting may be difficult to accomplish and recurrent fractures and bowing tend to occur. The effect of calcitonin in treatment is being evaluated (Bell, Avery and Johnston, 1970; and Morii *et al*, 1971).

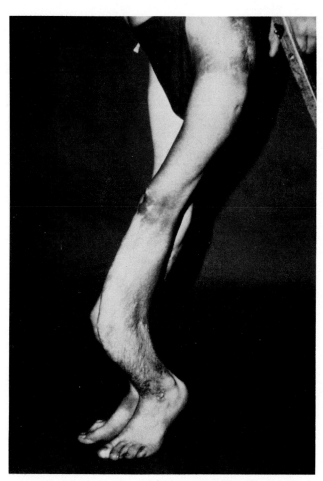

Fig. 39.1 (K.B.) Gross deformity associated with this disease, together with skin pigmentation. (Courtesy of Professor J. I. P. James, Edinburgh.)

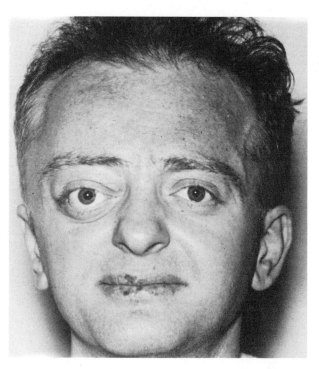

Fig. 39.2 (L.M.) This man has gross involvement of the skull (radiograph Figure 39.4) with asymmetrical involvement and proptosis on the right side. Note also pigmentation of the lips.

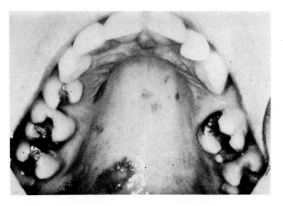

Fig. 39.3 (A.H.) Spots of pigmentation seen on the membrous membrane of the mouth. (Courtesy of Mr A. G. Apley, Pyrford.)

REFERENCES

Albright, F., Butter, A. M., Hampton, A. O. & Smith, P. (1937). Syndrome characterised by osteitis fibrosa disseminata, areas of pigmentation and endocrine dysfunction, with precocious puberty in females. *The New England Journal of Medicine*, **216**, 727.

Bell, N. H., Avery, S. & Johnston, C. C. (1970). Effects of calcitonin in Paget's disease and polyostotic fibrous dysplasia. *Journal of Clinical Endocrinology and Metabolism*, **31**, 283.

Ehrig, U. & Wilson, D. R. (1972). Fibrous dysplasia of bone and primary hyperparathyroidism. *Annals of Internal Medicine*, **77**, 234.

Harris, W. H., Dudley, R. & Barry, R. J. (1962). The natural history of fibrous dysplasia. *Journal of Bone & Joint Surgery*, **44A**, 207.

Lichtenstein, L. (1970). *Disease of Bones and Joints*. St Louis: C. V. Mosby.

Morii, H., Tanae, A., Ibayashi, H. & Nakao, K. (1971). Effects of calcitonin in metastatic bone carcinoma, osteoporosis, polyostotic fibrous dysplasia and hypercalcaemia. *Endocrinologia Japonica*, **18**, 81.

McCune, D. J. & Bruch, H. (1937). Osteodystrophia fibrosa. Report of a case in which the condition was combined with precocious puberty, pathologic pigmentation of the skin and hyperthyroidism, with a review of the literature. *American Journal of Diseases of Children*, **54**, 806.

Stewart, M. J., Scott Gilmer, W. & Edmonson, A. S. (1962). Fibrous dysplasia of bone. *Journal of Bone & Joint Surgery*, **44B**, 302.

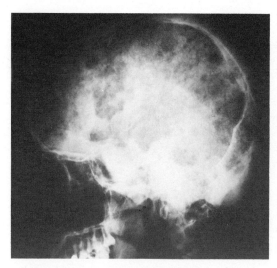

Fig. 39.4 (L.M.) Typical involvement of the vault of the skull, patchy areas of sclerosis and rarefaction.

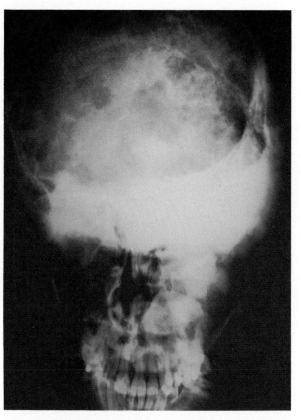

Fig. 39.5 (B.) Areas of patchy sclerosis and rarefaction are seen, irregular in size and asymmetrical. (H.A.T.F.)

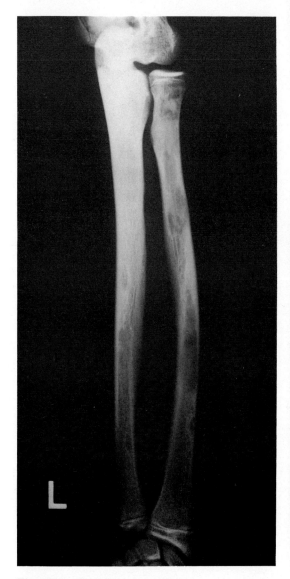

Fig. 39.6 (B.) Multiple localised lesions are seen in the radius and ulna. (H.A.T.F.)

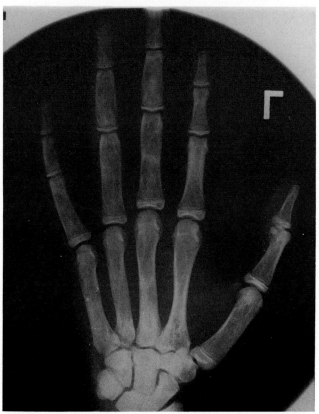

Fig. 39.7 (B.) There are lesions in most of the phalanges with loss of definition and modelling. (H.A.T.F.)

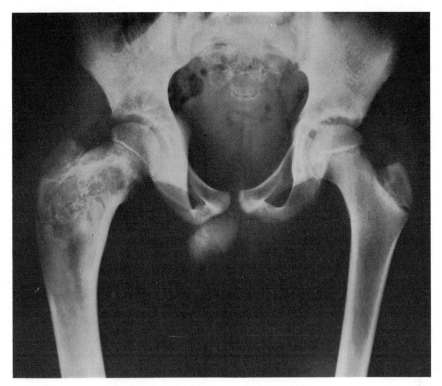

Fig. 39.8 (T.M.) Asymmetrical involvement of the upper femur with lateral curvature. (H.A.T.F.)

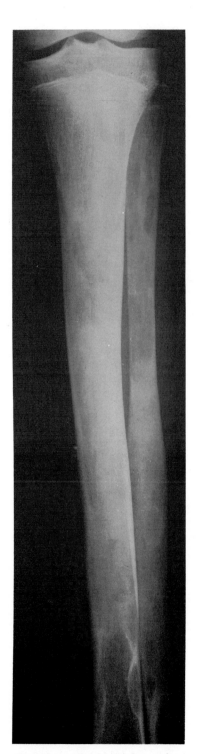

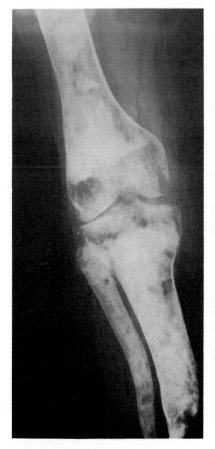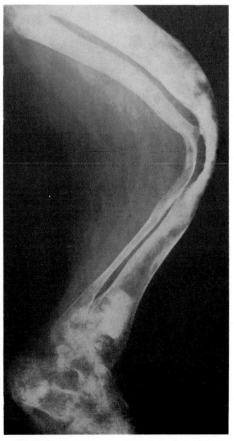

Fig. 39.9 (B.) Multiple patchy early lesions of decreased bone density throughout the length of the tibia and fibula. (H.A.T.F.)

Figs 39.10 and 39.11 (J.P.) The gross deformity caused by long standing bone lesions, with marked areas of sclerosis. (H.A.T.F.)

40 Osteopoikilosis

In this condition there are circumscribed sclerotic areas near the ends of the long bones and small sclerotic, but not calcified, nodules of connective tissue in the skin.

It was first described by Stieder (1905) and since then there have been many reports (Albers-Schönberg, 1915; Ledoux-Lebard, Chabanix and Dessane, 1916). By 1971 Szabo was able to find 300 cases in the literature.

Inheritance. It is of autosomal dominant inheritance, many affected families having been described (Melnick, 1959; Raque and Wood, 1970).

Frequency. The population incidence is not known since the condition is of little clinical importance, and may only be an incidental finding on radiography. The sexes are equally affected, and the age of onset is variable—though it is rarely noticed in infancy.

Clinical and radiographic features. There are no clinical findings in the majority of cases. In 10 to 15 per cent of patients there is a skin lesion (dermato-fibrosis lenticularis disseminata), in which small, slightly elevated, whitish-yellow fibrous cutaneous and subcutaneous nodules develop (Green, Ellswood and Collins, 1962).

The radiographic findings are usually found incidentally. The sclerotic areas of bone are 3 to 5 mm in diameter, mostly symmetrical and affecting the epiphyses, although the adjacent metaphyses can also be involved. The diaphysis is unaffected and it is unusual for the skull, face, ribs, sternum or vertebrae to be involved (Green, Ellswood and Collins, 1962).

Pathology. The bony lesion is a focal condensation of cancellous tissue subject to the same metabolic changes as the surrounding bone.

Differential diagnosis. There is no other condition quite similar to this. The sclerotic bone of melorheostosis involves the shaft of the long bones rather than the ends.

Progress and complications. The condition is of no great importance and the bony condensations have been variably reported as disappearing or becoming denser with growth.

REFERENCES

Albers-Schönberg, H. E. (1915). Einer seltene, bisher nicht bekannte Strukturanomalie de Skelettes. *Fortschritte auf dem Gebiete der Roentgenstrahlen und der Nuklearmedezin*, **23**, 174.

Green, A. E., Ellswood, W. H. & Collins, J. R. (1962). Melorheostosis and osteopoikilosis. *American Journal of Roentgenology*, **87**, 1096.

Ledoux-Lebard, R. Chabanix & Dessane (1916). L'osteopoecilie, form nouvelle d'osteite condensante generalisée. *Journal de Radiologie et d'Electrologie*, **2**, 133.

Melnick, J. C. (1959). Osteopathia condensans disseminata (osteopoikilosis). Study of a family of 4 generations. *American Journal of Roentgenology*, **82**, 229.

Raque, C. J. & Wood, M. G. (1970). Connective tissue naevus. Dermatofibrosis lenticularis disseminata with osteopoikilosis. *Archives of Dermatology*, **102**, 390.

Stieda, A. (1905). Uber umschriebene Knochenvernichtungen in Bereich der Substantia spongiosa im Roentgenbilde. *Beitrage zur Klinischen Chirurgie*, **45**, 700.

Szabo, A. D. (1971). Osteopoikilosis in a twin. *Clinical Orthopaedics and Related Research*, **79**, 156.

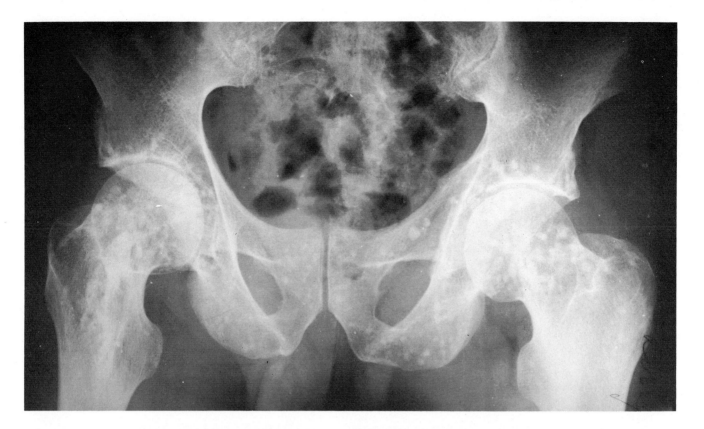

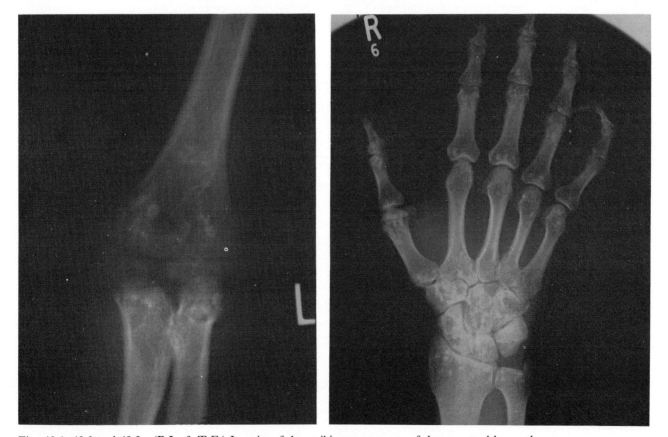

Figs 40.1, 40.2 and 40.3   (B.L. & T.F.) In spite of the striking appearance of these spotted bones they are of no clinical importance. (Courtesy of Mr A. G. Apley, Pyrford.)

41 Osteopathia Striata

In this condition linear bands of dense vertical striations are found in variable portions of the long bones and pelvis.

It was first described by Voorhoeve (1924) who noted the condition in a father and his two children. The case described by Fairbank (1925) was similar and the condition was named osteopathia striata by him in 1935. Since these original patients (in whom there were no symptoms) were described, other writers have noted an associated osteosclerosis of the skull, face and pelvis (Bloor 1954, Rucker and Alfid 1964).

Inheritance. This is not fully established, but certainly some cases appear to be of autosomal dominant inheritance.

Frequency. The population incidence is not known, neither is the age of onset, since the findings are usually incidental.

Clinical and radiographic features. There are no symptoms or physical signs related to the condition.

On radiography the striation of the skeleton affects particularly the metaphyses of the long bones, the dense lines running parallel to the long axis, and sometimes extending into the epiphyses. In the ilia they are distributed in a fan-like manner. Sometimes the epiphyses are mottled with dense and clear spots. In Bloor's patient (a girl of 3 years) the skull was large with a dense base and frontal region, and the antra and ethmoids were obscured.

Differential diagnosis. The diagnosis is not usually in doubt but osteopathia striata can be found in combination with other forms of bony condensation such as osteopoikiloisis or melorheostosis (Spranger, Langer and Wiedemann 1974).

Progress and complications. There are no complications, and the bone striations do not change appreciably with age.

REFERENCES

Bloor, D. U. (1954). A case of osteopathia striata. *Journal of Bone & Joint Surgery*, **36B,** 261.
Fairbank, H. A. T. (1925). A case of unilateral affection of the skeleton of unknown origin. *British Journal of Surgery*, **12,** 594.
Fairbank, H. A. T. (1935). Generalised disorders of the skeleton. *Proceedings of the Royal Society of Medicine (Clinical Section)*, **28,** 1611.
Rucker, T. N. & Alfidi, R. J. (1964). A rare familial systematic affection of the skeleton: Fairbank's disease. *Radiology*, **82,** 63.
Spranger, J. W., Langer, L. O. & Wiedemann, H. R. (1974). *Bone Dysplasias. An Atlas of Constitutional Disorders of Skeletal Development.* W. B. Saunders Company, Philadelphia: Toronto.
Voorhoeve, N. (1924). L'image radiologique non encore décrite d'une anomalie du squelette. *Acta Radiologica*, **3,** 407.

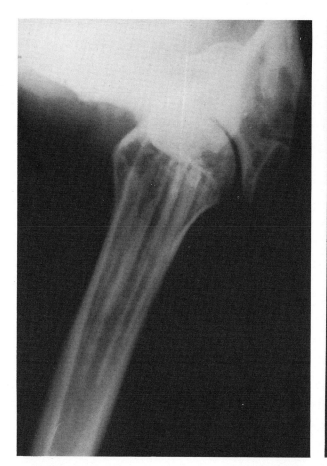
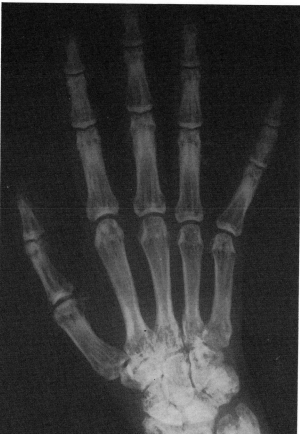
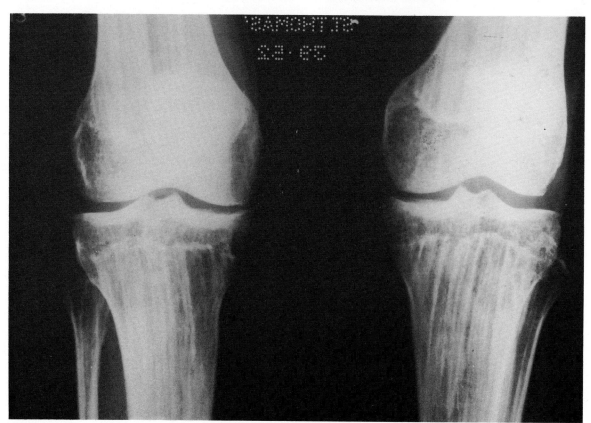

Figs 41.1, 41.2 and 41.3   The linear striations run parallel to the long axis of the bones, principally affecting the metaphyseal areas but also extending into the epiphyses. Occurring as an isolated feature they are of no clinical significance. (Courtesy of Mr A. G. Apley, Pyrford.)

SECTION II

MISCELLANEOUS DYSPLASIAS AND MALFORMATION SYNDROMES WITH MAJOR BONY INVOLVEMENT

42 Neurofibromatosis

This disease is often called Von Recklinghausen's disease since he first clearly defined it in 1882, although there are probably earlier reports than this. It is a bizarre syndrome characterised by protean manifestations of which the major ones are café au lait skin patches, nerve tumours and (not invariably) skeletal abnormalities.

There have been major reviews of the subject by Crowe, Schull and Neel (1956), Fienman and Yakovac (1970) and Brasfield and Das Gupta (1972).

Inheritance. The condition is of autosomal dominant inheritance with very variable clinical manifestations. Various surveys have shown between 20 and 50 per cent of first degree relatives with the disease, sometimes with four or five generations involved. However, the true proportion of affected relatives is difficult to arrive at since minor degrees of the disease may pass unnoticed. The most frequent manifestations are the café au lait skin patches, and an arbitrary decision has to be made as to how many and how large they must be before they provide evidence that any one individual has neurofibromatosis. Crowe and colleagues considered that the presence of six or more, each greater than 1·5 cm in diameter was evidence of the disease. More recently, Whitehouse (1966) examined 365 normal children under the age of 5 years and found that whereas 19 per cent of them showed one patch, less than one per cent had two (though the figure for negroes was higher than this). Of the three children with four or more spots, two had other manifestations of neurofibromatosis.

Frequency. The same problem relating to diagnosis arises when attempting to estimate the frequency of neurofibromatosis. Crowe and colleagues estimated one in 2 to 3,000 live births in the State of Michigan. However, the number of individuals with serious manifestations and skeletal involvement must be very much less than this figure.

The sexes are equally affected. The age when the disease is first diagnosed is very variable, ranging from birth to late adult life. Café au lait patches are unusual at birth, but develop during the first decade. Nerve tumours are also uncommon at birth and develop in later childhood or adolescence.

Clinical and radiographic features. The café au lait patches are usually the first sign of the disease and in mild cases may be the only manifestation. Crowe (1964) has referred to axillary freckling as a diagnostic aid in neurofibromatosis. Fibromatous skin tumours and multiple tumours of nerve trunks are typical features, varying in size from a few millimetres to several centimetres, together with hypertrophy of one limb, or part of it, or of other areas, such as the skull. This local gigantism may affect the underlying bone as well as the soft tissues. A single or perhaps two or three digits only may be hypertrophied. Plexiform neurofibromata are another feature; tumours may arise in other soft tissue structures, and haemangiomata and lymphangiomata have also been described. These plexiform neuromata may reach an enormous size, especially in the scalp and buttocks.

In a few cases neurofibromatosis presents at birth with pseudarthrosis of the tibia, or occasionally with fibrous replacement of other bones such as the ulna (Wellwood, Bulmer and Graff, 1971; Sprague and Brown, 1974).

There are not invariably any radiographic signs to be found in neurofibromatosis but the following skeletal anomalies may occur: the plexiform tumours or other soft tissue lesions may be associated with overgrowth of limb or other bones, including the skull; the texture of bone is sometimes abnormal, with a streaky medullary pattern; pseudarthrosis of the tibia (or more rarely of other bones) is usually associated with dense sclerotic bone and a narrowed or absent medullary cavity at this site; pressure from neurofibromata (whether of cranial, spinal or peripheral nerves) may cause erosion of adjacent bone. A rare manifestation is the development of subperiosteal or cortical bone cysts, associated with intramedullary neurofibromata, or one arising from a periosteal nerve (Hensley, 1953; Sane, Yunis and Greer, 1970). The radiographic features of neurofibromatosis have been reviewed by Holt and Wright (1948) and by Hunt and Pugh (1961).

Pathology. The tumours arise from the nerve sheath and may be encapsulated or diffuse (Heard, 1963).

Differential diagnosis. There is no condition similar to the fully developed syndrome.

Progress and complications. Scoliosis is one of the main complications of this disease. The curvature usually starts in early childhood and characteristically is short, involving only a few vertebrae, and severe. The reason for its development is obscure since there are not usually any congenital vertebral anomalies, nor any demonstrable neurological defect. Most surveys report that scoliosis occurs in about 25 per cent of all cases.

When pseudarthrosis of the tibia is present there are invariably problems of treatment, particularly when the defect is associated with dense sclerotic bone. Repeated bone grafts may fail and some patients come to amputation.

One of the main dangers of neurofibromatosis is the development of nerve tumours in an enclosed space, for example in the auditory canals causing deafness, or in the spinal canal where pressure effects may be serious. Curtis *et al* (1969) were able to find 40 cases of paraplegia associated with neurofibromatosis in the literature, and noted that this complication is liable to occur at any time during the patient's life. Other areas where the pressure of a nerve tumour in a confined space causes problems are the wrist and hand, and both median and ulnar nerve palsies occur.

Malignant change in the nerve tumours has been variously reported as occurring in between 5 and 20 per cent of all cases (Hunt and Pugh, 1961), though the true proportion is difficult to assess since mild cases of the syndrome do not attend for treatment.

An occasional feature of neurofibromatosis is an associated osteomalacia which develops in middle age, presumably from a renal tubular defect (Hernberg and Edgren, 1949; Dent, 1952; Swann, 1954; Saville *et al*, 1955).

Treatment. This can only be directed to the various features and complications of the syndrome: that is to the congenital pseudarthrosis, scoliosis, limb inequality, nerve tumours where pressure symptoms arise and to malignant tumours should they develop.

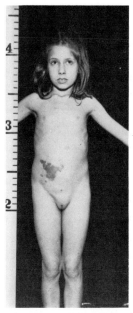

Fig. 42.1 (S.P.) Skin pigmentation of the trunk. (Courtesy of Mr A. G. Apley, Pyrford.)

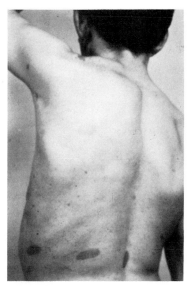

Fig. 42.2 (M.W.) Café au lait patches on the trunk. (Courtesy of Professor J. I. P. James, Edinburgh.)

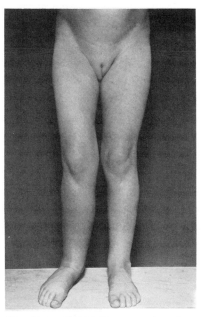

Fig. 42.3 (D.H.) Hypertrophy of the whole right lower limb. Skin pigmentation can also be seen on the left aspect of the trunk. (A.H.)

REFERENCES

Brasfield, R. D. & Das Gupta, T. K. (1972). Von Recklinghausen's Disease: A clinicopathological study. *Annals of Surgery*, **175**, 86.

Crowe, F. W., Schull, W. J. & Neel, J. V. (1956). *A Clinical, Pathological and Genetic Study of Multiple Neurofibromatosis*. C. Thomas, Springfield, Illinois.

Crowe, F. W. (1964). Axillary freckling as a diagnostic aid in neurofibromatosis. *Annals of Internal Medicine*, **61**, 1142.

Curtis, B. H., Fisher, R. L., Butterfield, W. L. & Saunders, F. P. (1969). Neurofibromatosis with paraplegia. Report of 8 cases. *Journal of Bone & Joint Surgery*, **51A**, 843.

Dent, C. E. (1952). Rickets and osteomalacia from renal tubular defects. *Journal of Bone & Joint Surgery*, **34B**, 266.

Fienman, N. L. & Yakovac, W. C. (1970). Neurofibromatosis in childhood. *Journal of Pediatrics*, **76**, 339.

Heard, G. (1963). Nerve sheath tumours and Von Recklinghausen's disease of the nervous system. *Annals of the Royal College of Surgeons*, **31**, 229.

Hensley, C. D. (1953). The rapid development of a 'subperiosteal bone cyst' in multiple neurofibromatosis. *Journal of Bone & Joint Surgery*, **35A**, 197.

Hernberg, C. A. & Edgren, W. (1949). Looser Milkman's syndrome with neurofibromatosis Recklinghausen and general decalcification of the skeleton. *Acta Medica Scandinavica*, **136**, 26.

Holt, J. F. & Wright, E. M. (1948). The radiologic features of neurofibromatosis. *Radiology*, **51**, 647.

Hunt, J. C. & Pugh, D. G. (1961). Skeletal lesions in neurofibromatosis. *Radiology*, **76**, 1.

Recklinghausen, F. von (1882). *Uber die multiplen Fibrome der Haut und ihre Beziehung zu den multiplen Neuromen*, Hirschwald, Berlin.

Sane, S., Yunis, E. & Greer, R. (1971). Subperiosteal or cortical cyst and intramedullary neurofibromatosis—uncommon manifestations of neurofibromatosis. *Journal of Bone & Joint Surgery*, **53A**, 1194.

Saville, P. D., Nassim, J. R., Stevenson, F. H., Mulligan, L. & Carey, M. (1955). Osteomalacia in von Recklinghausen's neurofibromatosis. Metabolic study of a case. *British Medical Journal*, **1**, 1311.

Sprague, B. L. & Brown, G. A. (1974). Congenital pseudarthrosis of the radius. *Journal of Bone & Joint Surgery*, **56A**, 191.

Swann, G. F. (1954). Pathogenesis of bone lesions in neurofibromatosis. *British Journal of Radiology*, **27**, 623.

Wellwood, J. M., Bulmer, J. H. & Graff, D. J. C. (1971). Congenital defects of the tibia in siblings with neurofibromatosis. *Journal of Bone & Joint Surgery*, **53B**, 314.

Whitehouse, D. (1966). Diagnostic value of the café au lait spot in children. *Archives of Diseases in Childhood*, **41**, 316.

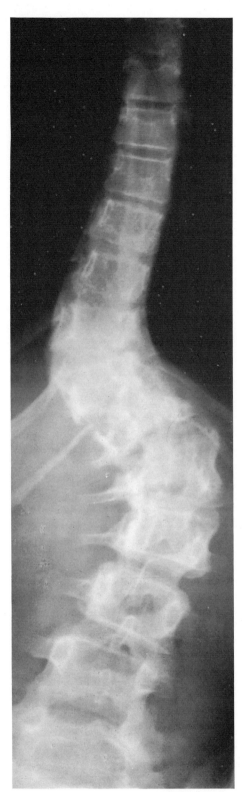

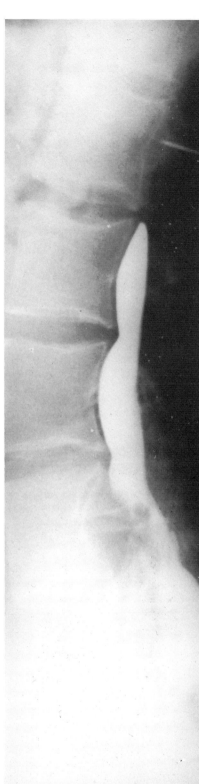

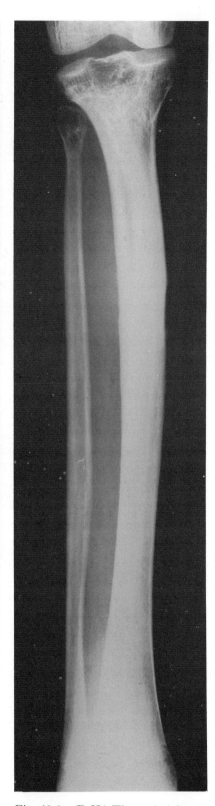

Fig. 42.4 (S.P.) Thoraco-lumbar scoliosis, characteristically a short sharp curve. (Courtesy of Mr A. G. Apley, Pyrford.)

Fig. 42.5 (D.M.) Scalloping of the posterior borders of the lower lumbar vertebrae, with a filling defect indicating a neurofibroma. (A.H.)

Fig. 42.6 (D.H.) The underlying bone changes in the tibia and fibula of the patient shown in Figure 42.3. Changes are not marked but there is some thickening of the tibial cortex and deformity of the bone. (A.H.)

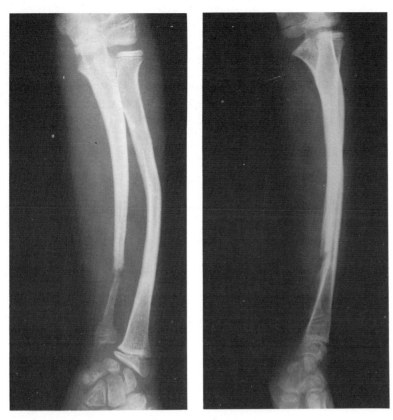

Figs 42.7 and 42.8 (S.P.) A congenital bony defect at the lower end of the ulna. (Courtesy of Mr A. G. Apley, Pyrford.)

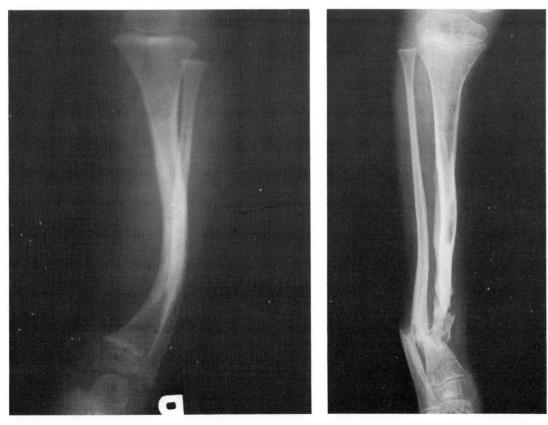

Figs 42.9 and 42.10 (S.J.) Congenital bowing of the tibia with dense sclerotic bone in the region of the deformity; 6 months later fracture and pseudarthrosis developed, with the inevitable problems of treatment. (A.H.)

43 The Marfan Syndrome

The Marfan syndrome is characterised by increased length of the limbs particularly in the distal part, dislocated lens, generalised joint laxity with muscle hypotonia and frequently, as growth develops, scoliosis, herniae, and aortic dilatation and aneurysm.

It was first described by Marfan (1896), and a recent very full review of the subject has been given by McKusick (1972).

Inheritance. The disorder is of autosomal dominant inheritance, though like so many other dominant syndromes it has a very wide range of expression and mild cases may go unrecognised. Murdoch, Walker and McKusick (1972) have shown that there is a paternal age effect, the fathers being significantly older than average in sporadic cases, the presumption being that a new mutation has occurred in the sperm.

Frequency. A population incidence of 1·46 per million has been estimated, and the sexes are equally affected. The disorder is not apparent at birth but becomes so usually during the first few years of life. However there are likely to be many mild cases in which diagnosis of the disease is uncertain even in adult life.

Clinical and radiographic features. The most striking feature of the Marfan syndrome is the excessive height of patients, though unequal body proportions are of greater significance in the diagnosis. The lower segment measurement (pubis to heel) is greater than the upper (head to pubis) whereas in normal individuals the two are nearly equal. The upper limbs are also abnormally long in the Marfan syndrome and the arm span (that is, the measurement between left and right finger tips with the arms horizontal) is markedly greater than the height, whereas in the normal individual, arm span and height measurements are approximately equal (Sinclair, Kitchin and Turner, 1960).

Apart from the body proportions, the most characteristic feature of the Marfan syndrome is ectopia lentis, and there are frequently other eye signs such as myopia, detached retina, cataract, and strabismus. A high arched palate is common. The chest is frequently deformed (pectus carinatum or excavatum) and the shoulder girdle narrow. Generalised joint laxity is often a feature and associated with this connective tissue defect are a number of other anomalies, for example: herniae, (inguinal, femoral, umbilical or diaphragmatic) recurrent dislocation of the patella, and congenital or later dislocation of the hips, clavicle, head of radius or other joints. Genu recurvatum or severe genu valgum are common, as are flat feet, or sometimes talipes equinovarus. Severe

scoliosis develops in perhaps half these patients and is likely also to be associated with the generalised joint laxity (Robbins, Winter and Moe, 1974).

Patients with the Marfan syndrome have poor musculature and a reduced amount of subcutaneous tissue. Some joints, particularly those not affected by the generalised joint laxity, may show contractures, and this is particularly a feature in the hands.

The most serious non-skeletal defects are of the cardiovascular system, a characteristic feature being aortic dilatation and aneurysm. However, pulmonary dilatation may occur and cardiac arrhythmias are common (auricular fibrillation or paroxysmal tachycardia).

On radiography the signs are not striking although there is clearly overgrowth of the long bones, particularly in the distal segments (hands and feet), together with some general lack of modelling. Scoliosis may be present, but there is no apparent bony cause for the curvature. On lateral radiography of the spine sometimes abnormally tall vertebrae are seen. In some instances the pelvis has a characteristic shape with a wide cavity and vertical ilia. Coxa valga is also a frequent feature.

Differential diagnosis. The only two disorders with similar body proportions which are likely to be confused with the Marfan syndrome are homocystinuria and congenital contractural arachnodactyly. Homocystinuria (Chapter 51) is of autosomal recessive inheritance, mental retardation is common and homocystine can be found in the urine. A comparison of the two diseases was given by Brenton et al (1972). Congenital contractural arachnodactyly is, like the Marfan syndrome, of autosomal dominant inheritance but it is characterised by congenital symmetrical contractures of many joints and is without generalised joint laxity, dislocation of the lens or heart disease (Beals and Hecht, 1971).

Progress and complications. Many individuals with the Marfan syndrome are not severely affected and in them life expectancy is normal. The most serious complications of the syndrome relate to the cardiovascular defects, the development of aortic aneurysm in early middle age being of frequent occurrence. If scoliosis is present, it may be very severe and, untreated, will lead to a reduction in the vital capacity and cardiorespiratory problems. Some individuals with the Marfan syndrome suffer from herniae, perhaps at several sites, and their treatment may cause problems in that repair is difficult and recurrence common. Treatment of the disorder can only be that of its various manifestations.

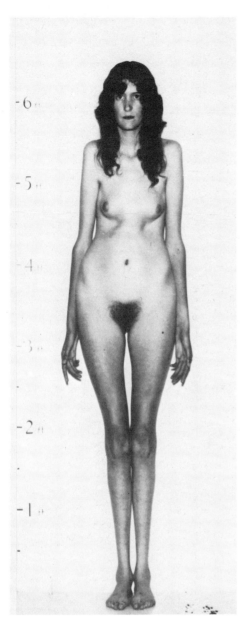

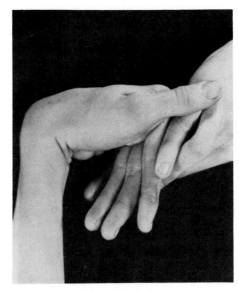

Fig. 43.2 (R.L.) Marked joint laxity in an adult patient. (Courtesy of Professor J. I. P. James, Edinburgh.)

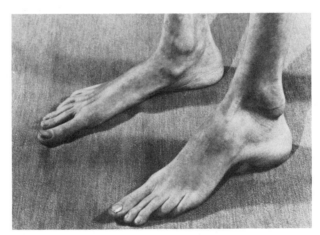

Fig. 43.1 (A.G.) The patient is over 6' in height, with the typical long thin build, an arm span exceeding her height and body disproportion (the head to pubis measurement being less than pubis to heel). (A.H.)

Fig. 43.3 The typical long thin feet of the Marfan syndrome. (H.A.T.F.)

REFERENCES

Beals, R. K. & Hecht, F. (1971). Congenital contractural arachnodactyly. A heritable disorder of connective tissue. *Journal of Bone & Joint Surgery,* **53A,** 987.

Brenton, D. P., Dow, C. J., James, J. I. P., Hay, R. L. & Wynne-Davies, R. (1972). Homocystinuria and Marfan's syndrome. A comparison. *Journal of Bone & Joint Surgery,* **54B,** 277.

Marfan, M. A. B. (1896). Un cas de déformation congénitale des quatres membres, plus prononcée aux extremités, caractérisée par l'allongement des os avec un certain degré d'amincissement. *Bulletin de la Société médicale des Hôpitaux de Paris.*

Murdoch, J. L., Walker, B. A. & McKusick, V. A. (1972). Parental age effects on the occurrence of new mutations for the Marfan syndrome. *Annals of Human Genetics,* **35,** 331.

McKusick, V. A. (1972). *Heritable Disorders of Connective Tissue.* 4th Edition, Mosby, St Louis.

Robins, P. R., Winter, R. B. & Moe, J. H. (1974). Scoliosis in patients with Marfan's syndrome. *Journal of Bone & Joint Surgery,* **56A,** 1540.

Sinclair, R. J. G., Kitchin, A. H. & Turner, R. W. D. (1960). The Marfan syndrome. *Quarterly Journal of Medicine,* **53,** 19.

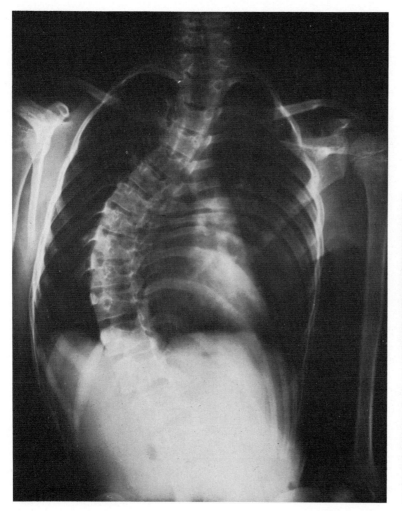

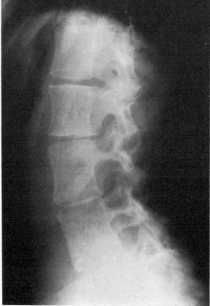

Fig. 43.4   (A.W.) Scoliosis is a frequent complication of
the Marfan syndrome. (Courtesy of Professor J. I. P.
James, Edinburgh.)

Fig. 43.5   (J.H.) Unusual height of
the vertebral bodies is sometimes a
feature. (Courtesy of Professor
J. I. P. James, Edinburgh.)

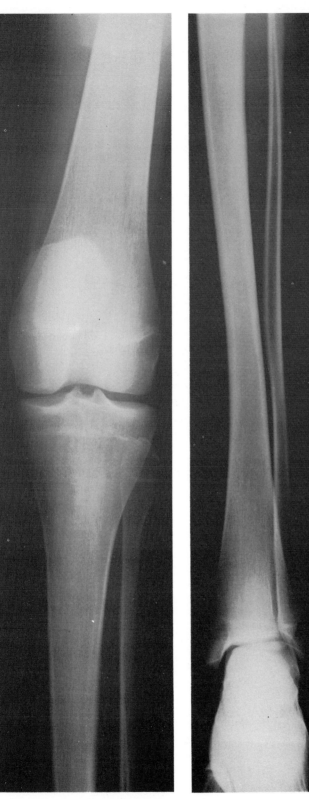

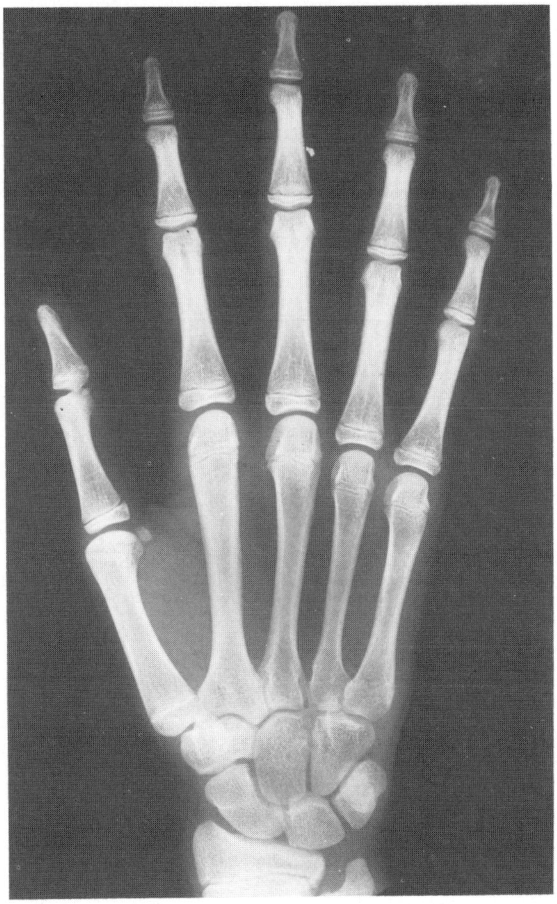

Fig. 43.8 The long thin metacarpals and phalanges are usually a feature of the Marfan syndrome. (A.H.)

Figs 43.6 and 43.7 (A.G.) Radiographs of patient shown in Figure 43.1. Apart from the increased length of bones and some lack of metaphyseal modelling there is no abnormality. (A.H.)

44 Cleido-Cranio-Dysplasia
Cranio-Cleido-Dysostosis

This disorder is a generalised bone dysplasia affecting principally the skull and clavicles, but the scapulae, pelvis, vertebrae, phalanges and teeth are also usually involved.

The disorder has been known for over 200 years as a hereditary condition and there have been recent reviews by Forland (1962), and Fauré and Maroteaux (1973).

Inheritance. The disorder is of autosomal dominant inheritance, about 20 per cent of cases being new mutations (Lasker, 1946).

Frequency. The population incidence is not known, but this is an uncommon disorder. The sexes are equally affected. It usually becomes apparent during infancy, though the dysplastic lesions are present at birth. However, patients with the condition may escape notice until adult life.

Clinical and radiographic features. There may be some shortness of stature but this is not very marked. Patients are usually of slender build with a characteristic head, being large with prominent frontal and parietal regions and delayed fusion of cranial sutures. Intelligence is normal. There is disordered eruption of teeth and the deciduous teeth are long persisting. The most characteristic clinical sign of the disorder is the absence or reduced size of the clavicles which allow the shoulder joints to be approximated anteriorly. Other features are a funnel chest, drooping shoulders with small scapulae, a waddling gait due to the coxa vara and malformed pelvis, and short terminal phalanges with hypoplastic nails. In infancy there is hypotonia with increased joint mobility.

On radiography, signs in the skull are characteristic, with imperfect ossification, delayed fusion and Wormian bones in the suture lines. There may be absence of the mastoid or other air cells. An enlarged or deformed foramen magnum has been reported due to a median cleft of the occipital bone, and there may be failure of fusion at the mandibular symphysis. Ossification of vertebrae is retarded and they remain biconvex for longer than usual, also spina bifida occulta may be found at a number of levels.

The clavicles are absent either completely or in the lateral part, though sometimes two separate fragments are present with the ends overlapping. The scapulae tend to be small and deformed.

Radiographs of the pelvis are characteristic, particularly in childhood. The pubic bones ossify late and

the symphysis pubis, sacro-iliac joint and Y-shaped cartilage are all wide. Ossification does occur eventually, but is markedly delayed. Coxa vara is likely to be a feature.

Both the carpus and tarsus show retarded ossification and short terminal phalanges are nearly always present, sometimes accompanied by dysplasia of the

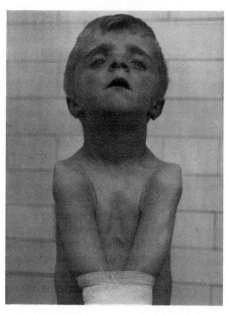

Fig. 44.1 (B.B. aged 7 years.) The frontal and parietal regions of the head are prominent and absent clavicles allow the shoulders to come unusually far forward. (H.A.T.F.)

middle phalanges also. Epiphyses at both ends of the metacarpals and metatarsals have been described.

Differential diagnosis. Cleido-cranio-dysplasia must be differentiated from pycnodysostosis which also has Wormian bones and dysplastic terminal phalanges, but here the bones are abnormally dense, the pelvis is normal and the condition is of autosomal recessive inheritance. Another condition in which Wormian bones are present is osteogenesis imperfecta, but the fragile bones and normal clavicles and pelvis should distinguish the condition.

Progress and complications. The expectation of life is normal and there are no major complications. Those that do arise are likely to be associated with the generalised joint laxity, and scoliosis has also been reported.

REFERENCES

Forland, M. (1962). Cleidocranial dysostosis. A review of the syndrome. *American Journal of Medicine*, **33**, 792.
Fauré, C. & Maroteaux, P. (1973). Cleidocranial dysplasia. *Progress in Paediatric Radiology*, 4. Intrinsic Diseases of Bones, Krager, Basel, 211.
Lasker, G. W. (1946). The inheritance of cleidocranial dysostosis. *Human Biology*, **18**, 103.

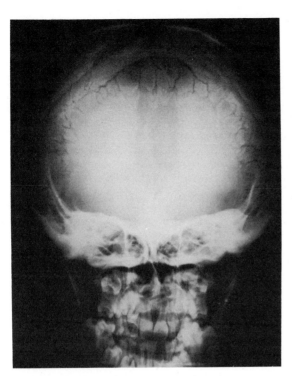

Fig. 44.2 (K.N.) Wormian bones in the suture lines. (A.H.)

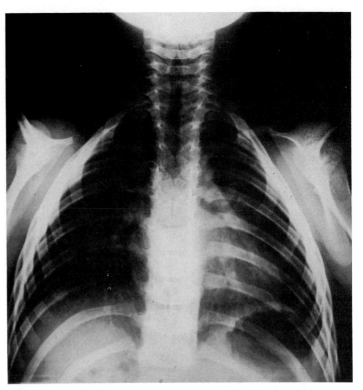

Fig. 44.3 (K.N.) Spina bifida is seen at several levels in the upper thoracic region; the vertebral bodies are biconvex; the clavicles are completely absent in the lateral part and there is only attenuated bone medially; the scapulae are rather small and stubby. (A.H.)

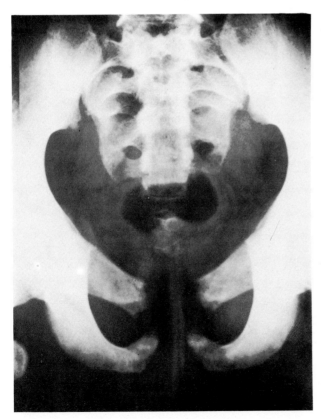

Fig. 44.4 (R.T.) Ossification of the anterior part of the pelvis is retarded and the sacro-iliac joints wide (A.H.)

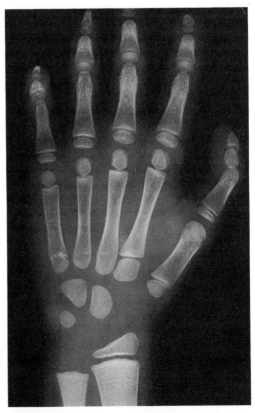

Fig. 44.5 (B.B. aged 7 years.) Ossification of the carpus is retarded and the terminal phalanges short; there is also dysplasia of some of the middle phalanges. (H.A.T.F.)

45 Nail-Patella Syndrome
Hereditary Osteo-Onycho Dysplasia

This rare, but clear-cut and well recognised syndrome is characterised by hypoplastic or absent patellae and small, split or dysplastic nails. There may be other structural defects of the skeleton, for example iliac horns and subluxation of the radial heads but these signs are not invariably present.

Little (1897) first noted a family with hereditary absent patellae and thumb nails; Turner (1933) also described the condition and since then there have been many reports, the most recent by Beals and Eckhardt (1969), Aggarwal and Mittal (1970) and Valdueza (1973).

Inheritance. The nail-patella syndrome is of autosomal dominant inheritance and like most dominant disorders, shows considerable clinical variation. There are many families reported with affected members of both sexes, in several generations. The mutant gene is linked to the locus determining the ABO blood groups (Renwick and Lawler, 1955; Renwick and Schulze, 1965), thus a particular blood group is inherited with the syndrome.

Frequency. Renwick and Izaat (1965) noted a birth frequency of 1 in 50,000. The sexes are equally affected. Diagnosis is not usually made until the 2nd or 3rd decade.

Clinical and radiographic features. The signs most consistently present are the hypoplastic, split or absent nails on several or all digits, and small or absent patellae. The presenting feature of the syndrome may be recurrent dislocation of the patella. Iliac horns, when present, may be palpable in infancy.

The chief radiographic findings are around the knee, where the abnormal (or absent) patellae are accompanied by hypoplasia of the lateral femoral condyle and head of the fibula. The iliac horns, if present, are diagnostic of this condition. Other features sometimes present are hypoplasia of the capitellum with dislocation or subluxation of the

radial head; and a small scapula with convexity and thickening of the lateral border.

Differential diagnosis. The fully developed syndrome is unlikely to be confused with any other disorder.

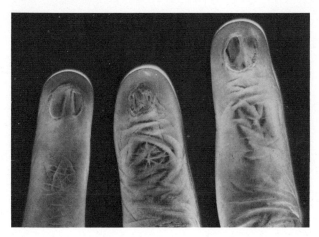

Fig. 45.1 (P.C. aged 19 years.) The fingernails are absent or dysplastic. (A.H.)

Progress and complications. Apart from the possibility of dislocating patellae, most of these patients have little disability and the expectation of life is normal. However, in about one-third or more of cases the syndrome is associated with renal dysfunction, proteinuria and subsequent renal failure. This is rare before middle age (Hawkins and Smith, 1950), though Eisenberg, Potter and Bovill (1972) reported nephropathy and renal osteodystrophy in a boy of 11 years old. Histological findings in the kidney show diffuse hyaline thickening of the glomerular basement membrane.

Treatment. This is directed to the dislocating patellae, if present, and to the renal disorder.

REFERENCES

Aggarwal, N. D. & Mittal, R. L. (1970). Nail patella syndrome. *Journal of Bone & Joint Surgery*, **52B**, 29.

Beals, R. K. & Eckhardt, A. L. (1969). Hereditary onycho-osteodysplasia (nail-patella syndrome). *Journal of Bone & Joint Surgery*, **51A**, 505.

Eisenberg, K. S., Potter, D. E. & Bovill, E. G. (1972). Osteo-onychodystrophy with nephropathy and renal osteodystrophy. A case report. *Journal of Bone & Joint Surgery*, **54A**, 1301.

Hawkins, C. F. & Smith, O. E. (1950). Renal dysplasia in a family with multiple hereditary abnormalities including iliac horns. *Lancet*, **1**, 803.

Little, E. M. (1897). Congenital absence or delayed development of the patella. *Lancet*, **ii**, 781.

Renwick, J. H. & Lawler, S. D. (1955). Genetical linkage between the ABO and nail-patella loci. *Annals of Human Genetics*, **19**, 312.

Renwick, J. H. & Izatt, M. M. (1965). Some genetical parameters of the nail-patella locus. *Annals of Human Genetics*, **28**, 369.

Renwick, J. H. & Schulze, J. (1965). Male and female recombination fractions for the nail-patella ABO linkage in man. *Annals of Human Genetics*, **28**, 379.

Turner, J. W. (1933). A hereditary arthrodysplasia associated with hereditary dystrophy of thumb nails. *Journal of the American Medical Association*, **100**, 882.

Valdueza, A. F. (1973). The nail-patella syndrome. A report of 3 families. *Journal of Bone & Joint Surgery*, **55B**, 145.

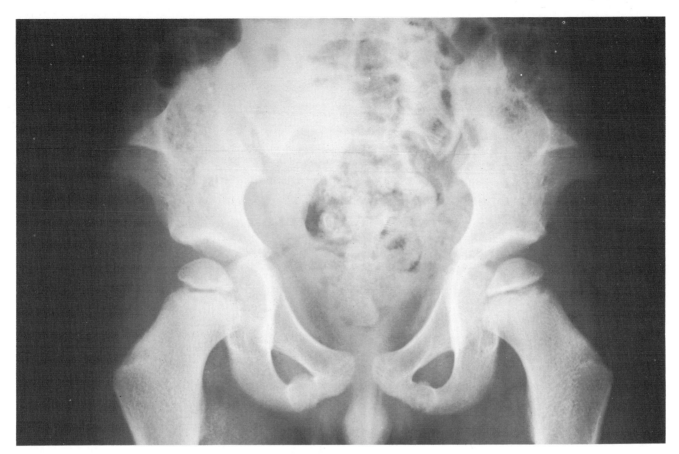

Fig. 45.2 (M.C.) The iliac horns are well formed—in early infancy they may even have been palpable. (A.H.)

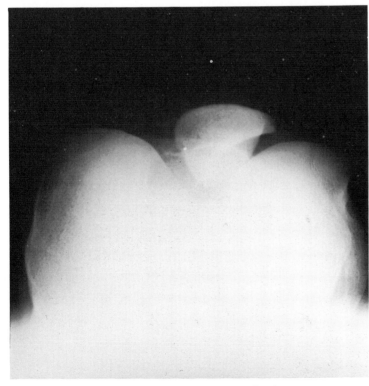

Fig. 45.3 (A.C.) This skyline view of the patella shows a small dysplastic bone and hypoplasia of the lateral femoral condyle. Recurrent dislocation is a feature, or the patellae may be absent. (A.H.)

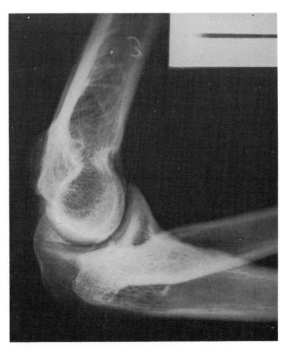

Fig. 45.4 (A.C.) The head of the radius is dysplastic and dislocated. (A.H.)

46 Fibrodysplasia Ossificans Progressiva
Myositis Ossificans Progressiva

In this rare developmental disorder there is progressive calcification followed by ossification of fasciae, aponeuroses and tendons, accompanied by a short hallux and (less often) a short thumb.

The condition has been known for a very long time; a review of 23 patients was reported by Tünte, Becker and Knorr (1967).

Inheritance. Most cases described are sporadic but since the disorder is likely to be lethal before the affected individual has children, the genetics are uncertain. It is probably of autosomal dominant inheritance since more than one affected generation has been reported. Tünte and colleagues noted an increased paternal age in their sporadic cases, which may indicate that a new (dominant) mutation had occurred in the sperm. The condition has also been reported in both of identical twins (Vastine, Vastine and Oriel, 1948; and Eaton, Conkling and Daeschner, 1957).

Frequency. The population incidence is not known but this is an extremely rare disorder. The usual age of onset is in late childhood but in some instances it has been reported at birth, or it may be delayed until adult life.

Clinical and radiographic features. The short hallux (and sometimes thumb) is present at birth and its presence should alert the examiner to the possibility of this rare disease. On radiography of the hands and feet hypoplasia of the terminal phalanx is seen and there may be synostosis of the phalanges of the first digit. Less commonly the first metatarsal and metacarpal are also short. Other abnormalities of the digits can occur, for example hypoplasia of the middle phalanx of the little finger.

The initial sign of the ectopic calcification is swelling of aponeuroses, fascia and intermuscular septa usually in the region around the shoulder girdle and thorax. These swellings are usually painless and without tenderness. Initially they are small, and may at first subside, only to be replaced by others. On palpation they may be hard from the outset, or cyst-like, and on occasion may break down and discharge.

The symptoms are at first only of some discomfort with limitation of movement, though occasionally there is slight pyrexia. The neck tissues are frequently affected and so torticollis may be the presenting sign. The masseter muscle may be involved early and this interferes with mandibular movements and feeding.

As the disease progresses, irregular masses of bone develop, usually along the course of a muscle, and ossification of a tendon near its attachment gives rise to an appearance not unlike an exostosis. Thick bars of bone may develop between bony masses—for example between the trunk and humerus—further immobilising the patient.

The areas involved invariably include the trunk, particularly the dorsal muscles, and often the neck, scalp muscles and proximal part of the limbs, upper more often than lower. Tissues below the elbow and knee are rarely affected. Certain muscles seem to be exempt, namely those of the larynx and eye; the tongue and facial muscles other than the masseter; also the diaphragm, levator ani, sphincters and heart muscle.

There is progressive replacement of the fascia and intermuscular septa by calcification and later ossification. The changes may be rapid and within a few months of the first signs of the disease plates of bone have developed in many areas. The lesions progress to secondary involvement of the muscles themselves (hence the original name of myositis ossificans progressiva) and degeneration of muscle fibre occurs.

The later stages of the disease are extremely serious: the chest becomes rigid, major joints ankylose, and ultimately the individual becomes completely immobile and dies of respiratory failure. Where the onset of this disease is early, patients usually die in their teens, though milder cases may continue with exacerbations and remissions over many years.

Surgical excision of the bars or masses of bone is unsatisfactory, since they quickly reform. There is not as yet any certain form of drug therapy (Smith, Russell and Woods, 1976).

REFERENCES

Eaton, W. L., Conkling, W. S. & Daeschner, C. W. (1957). Early myositis ossificans progressiva occurring in homozygotic twins; a clinical and pathologic study. *Journal of Pediatrics*, **50,** 591.

Smith, R., Russell, R. G. G. & Woods, C. G. (1976). Myositis ossificans progressiva. *Journal of Bone & Joint Surgery,* **58B,** 48.

Tünte, W., Becker, P. E. & Knorr, G. V. (1967). Zur Genetik der myositis ossificans progressiva. *Human Genetics,* **4,** 320.

Vastine, J. H., Vastine, M. F. & Oriel, A. (1948). Myositis ossificans progressiva in homozygotic twins. *American Journal of Roentgenology,* **59,** 204.

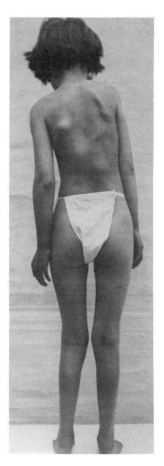

Fig. 46.1 (R.G.) Plaques of bone on the posterior aspect of the trunk. (H.A.T.F.)

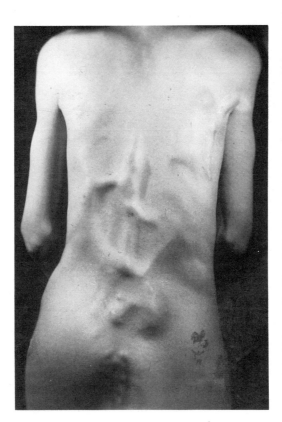

Fig. 46.2 (H.G.) Irregular masses of bone underlying the skin of the trunk. (H.A.T.F.)

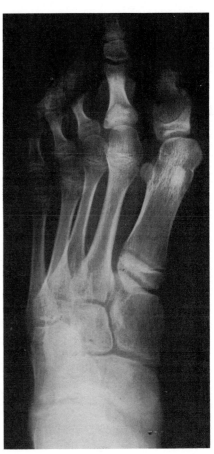

Fig. 46.3 (S.) The first metatarsal is nearly normal but there is only one short phalanx. (H.A.T.F.)

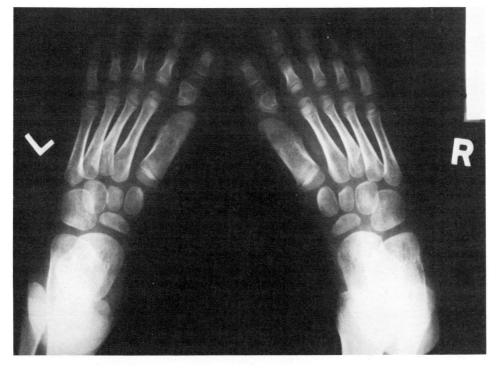

Fig. 46.4 (M.M. aged 4 years.) Both metatarsals are thickened and distorted at their distal end. The two terminal phalanges are dysplastic and shortened. (H.A.T.F.)

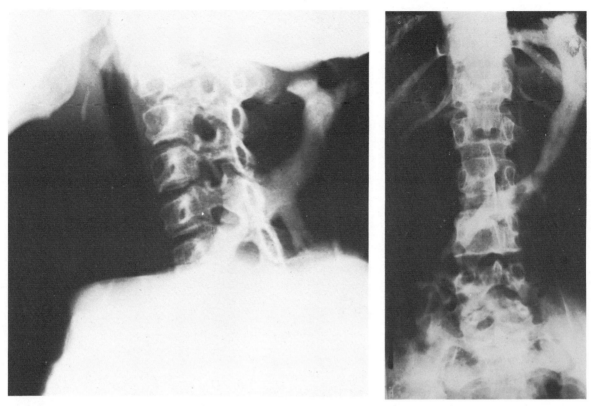

Figs 46.5 and 46.6   Irregular bars of bone showing in the posterior part of the neck and adjacent to the vertebral column. (H.A.T.F.)

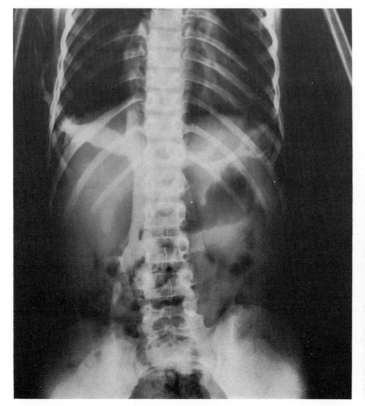

Fig. 46.7   (M.B.) Extensive ossification adjacent to the erector spinae, spreading laterally. (H.A.T.F.)

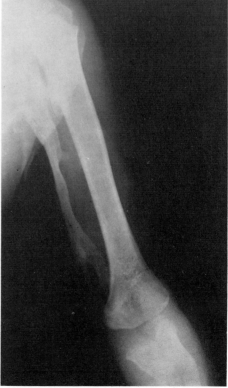

Fig. 46.8   (M.M.) An irregular bar of bone extending from the thorax down the medial aspect of the humeral shaft. (H.A.T.F.)

47 Tricho-Rhino-Phalangeal Syndrome

Langer, Spranger and Wiedemann (1974) describe tricho-rhino-phalangeal dysplasia Types I and II. Both have fine sparse hair and a characteristic face with a prominent nose and long philtrum.

Type I was first described by Giedeon (1966). The patients have brachydactyly (which may include both phalanges and metacarpals) and there are epiphyseal deformities in many regions, particularly the capital femoral epiphyses which have been likened to the deformities produced by Perthes' disease. Cone-shaped epiphyses in the hands are a characteristic finding. There have been recent reports by Beals (1973) and Weaver, Cohen and Smith (1974). The disorder is probably of autosomal dominant inheritance (McKusick, 1972).

Type II patients are of short stature and have microcephaly and mental retardation in addition to the other defects. Generalised joint laxity has been noted and also multiple exostoses, similar to those seen in diaphyseal aclasis (Gorlin, Cohen and Wolfson, 1969).

The genetics are unknown. Radiographic diagnosis can only be made after the cone-shaped epiphyses and exostoses have appeared—during the third year of life or later.

REFERENCES

Beals, R. K. (1973). Tricho-rhino-phalangeal dysplasia: Report of a kindred. *Journal of Bone & Joint Surgery*, **55A,** 821.

Giedion, A. (1966). Das tricho-rhino-phalangeal syndrom. *Helvetica Paediatrica Acta*, **21,** 475.

Gorlin, R. J., Cohen, M. & Wolfson, J. (1969). Tricho-rhino-phalangeal syndrome. *American Journal of Diseases in Children*, **118,** 595.

McKusick, V. A. (1972). *Heritable Disorders of Connective Tissue*. 4th Edition, Mosby, St Louis.

Spranger, J. W., Langer, L. O. & Wiedemann, H. R. (1974). *Bone Dysplasias: An Atlas of Constitutional Disorders of Skeletal Development*. W. B. Saunders Company: Philadelphia, Toronto.

Weaver, D. D., Cohen, M. M. & Smith, D. W. (1974). The tricho-rhino-phalangeal syndrome. *Journal of Medical Genetics*, **11,** 312.

SECTION III

INBORN ERRORS OF METABOLISM

48 The Mucopolysaccharidoses

The mucopolysaccharidoses and the mucolipidoses (Chapter 49) are a group of storage diseases, most of which have a marked effect on skeletal growth and development. Many of them have distinctive clinical and biochemical features but the radiological signs, sometimes collectively called 'dysostosis multiplex', are similar throughout the group, differing mainly in the degree of severity and in the age of onset. Thus, in most instances radiographic examination will indicate whether a patient has one of the mucopolysaccharidoses or mucolipidoses, but differentiation between types is not always possible on radiographic signs alone. The individual diseases are listed, with their inheritance, in Table I p. 172, and the most significant features of 'dysostosis multiplex' are illustrated in Figures 48.5–48.12.

A more precise diagnosis of the mucopolysaccharidoses and mucolipidoses is made on a combination of clinical, genetic, radiological and laboratory findings, related to the excretion of mucopolysaccharides in the urine. In a few cases the precise enzyme deficiency has been identified and it is likely in the future that further subdivisions of the group will be made. However, the similarity of skeletal findings in all the mucopolysaccharidoses and mucolipidoses remains, and our purpose has been to illustrate the main radiographic features rather than describe possibly insignificant findings in individual patients. The whole subject has been recently reviewed by McKusick (1972) and Grossman and Dorst (1973).

HURLER SYNDROME
(Mucopolysaccharidosis I H)

This disease was first described by Hurler (1919). The main features are a coarse facies, shortness of stature, mental retardation, enlarged liver and spleen and stiffness of joints.

In 1952 Brante classified it as a mucopolysaccharide disorder, and in 1957 Dorfmann and Lorincz, and Meyer, Hoffman and Linker reported the urinary excretion of dermatan sulphate and heparan sulphate. Numerous necropsy reports have shown an accumulation of these same mucopolysaccharides in many tissues, particularly the liver, spleen, nervous system, and in cartilage and bone marrow. Finally, Bach and colleagues (1972) showed that the basic enzyme deficiency was of α-L-iduronidase.

Inheritance. The Hurler syndrome is of autosomal recessive inheritance. There are many reports of affected sibs with normal parents, and also a higher than expected proportion of consanguinity of parents.

On fibroblast culture metachromatic granules are found on staining cells with toluidine blue (Danes and Bearn, 1967), both in (homozygous) patients and (heterozygous) parents.

Frequency. This is the commonest of the mucopolysaccharide disorders but is still a rare disease. It is not a congenital disorder, infants appearing normal at birth. Coarsening of the face and hepato-splenomegaly begin to develop around 3 to 6 months of age, mental retardation becomes apparent soon after and the fully developed syndrome is usually present by the age of 18 months.

Clinical and radiographic features. The first sign of this syndrome is a distinctive facial appearance (the former name of the disease was 'gargoylism'), the features are coarse and the tongue protruding. The head is large with frontal bossing, protruding eyes and thickened soft tissues. Due to maldevelopment of the skull the nasal passages are narrowed and this, together with the thickening of soft tissues and large tongue and adenoids causes stertorous breathing and chronic upper respiratory infection. These infants are not small at birth, indeed being described as rather large babies for the first few months of life. However, growth slows and after infancy they are of markedly short stature.

The joints become increasingly stiff; mental retardation is usually severe and appears to be progressive. Other clinical features are hepatosplenomegaly, umbilical and other herniae, corneal opacities and cardiovascular anomalies due to thickening of mitral and aortic valves and also of the coronary vessel walls.

Radiographic changes are marked and illustrate well the type of skeletal abnormalities found throughout this group of diseases. The skull is normal at 6 months of age, but by 2 years the deformities are striking. The sagittal suture closes first, giving the head its scaphocephalic shape, and it is unusually large with thickening of the diploë, the base and the orbital roofs. The sella turcica is usually enlarged, sometimes being 'J-shaped'. Hydrocephalus may be present due to obstruction of the subarachnoid space by thickened meninges. Neuhauser et al (1968) have suggested that arachnoid cysts are a frequent cause of this obstruction.

In comparison with the enlarged skull the facial bones appear small, with a short wide mandible and deformed or missing condyles. The coronoid process is large. The molar teeth are abnormally sited sometimes even within the mandibular ramus.

Within the first few months of life there are radiological signs in the vertebral column. On lateral view, the infantile biconvex shape may persist for longer than usual and the last thoracic and first lumbar vertebrae may be unduly small causing a mild kyphosis in this region. By 1 to 2 years of age the characteristic picture of a marked thoracolumbar kyphus with one or more hypoplastic vertebrae at the apex is present. The anterosuperior portion of the vertebral bodies is under-developed, the inferior part projecting forwards giving the appearance of a broad hook. The anterior and posterior surfaces of all vertebrae are concave, while the superior and inferior surfaces are slightly convex.

The shape of the pelvis is distinctive, changes being apparent by the age of 6 months and progressing thereafter. The iliac wings are described as 'flared' with an oblique acetabular roof. This, together with the associated coxa valga, accounts for the frequent subluxation or dislocation of the hips in the Hurler syndrome. The ischial and pubic bones are less abnormal, but may be thick and undermodelled. The femoral capital epiphyses are late in appearing.

The most characteristic of all radiological signs in this disease are in the thorax, where the ribs are seen to widen considerably towards their anterior ends, giving a paddle-shaped appearance. The clavicles are short and thick, particularly at the medial ends; the lateral ends may be hypoplastic or even missing. The scapulae are high, short and thick. Since there are often cardiovascular problems the heart shadow may be enlarged. Upper respiratory infections are common and so radiological signs in the thorax often include those of pneumonia and atelectasis.

The long bones are abnormal, particularly in the upper limb, where lack of diaphyseal modelling leads sometimes to the shaft being thicker than the metaphyseal area. A varus deformity of the neck of the humerus and a tilting towards each other of the distal ends of the radius and ulna are characteristic signs. The radiographic appearance of the hands in this, and many of the other mucopolysaccharide disorders, is typical. Signs are present by 6 months of age and, as in the other long bones, the metacarpals and phalanges show lack of diaphyseal modelling and a thick shaft. The 2nd to 4th metacarpals are pointed at their proximal ends. The phalanges are short and stubby, described as 'bullet-shaped'. Ossification centres for the carpal bones are late and when they do appear, are small and irregular.

The long bones of the lower limb and of the feet show similar changes but to a lesser degree.

Differential diagnosis. This is from the other mucopolysaccharidoses and mucolipidoses, and indeed it may not be possible on radiological grounds alone to distinguish them from the Hurler syndrome. The two severe mucolipidoses (mucolipidosis II and gangliosidosis I), unlike the Hurler syndrome, have skeletal signs present at birth. The Maroteaux–Lamy syndrome (mucopolysaccharidosis VI) has very similar skeletal findings, but these individuals are not mentally retarded.

Progress and complications. The Hurler syndrome is a progressive disease, both mental and physical abnormalities increasing with the years and numerous complications occur from deposition of mucopolysaccharides in many different tissues. Thus, there may be a raised intracranial pressure and hydrocephalus associated with meningeal deposits; blockage of the nasal passages and chronic respiratory infection, and cardiovascular disease, including coronary artery and valvular obstruction. Death usually occurs by the age of 10 years from pneumonia or coronary disease.

Laboratory investigations. There is increased urinary excretion of dermatan sulphate and heparan sulphate. The abnormal mucopolysaccharide depositions occur in many cells, including the leucocytes and in the bone marrow. On fibroblast culture metachromasia is shown on staining with toluidine blue. The specific enzyme deficiency of the Hurler syndrome is α-L-iduronidase, and low or absent activity can be identified in various tissues. Mixed fibroblast cultures from patients with the Hurler and Scheie syndromes do not correct each other's metachromasia, whereas this does occur with the other (enzymatically different) mucopolysaccharidoses.

Treatment. This can only be symptomatic and is related to the chronic respiratory infection, herniae and dislocated hips (if present).

SCHEIE SYNDROME (Mucopolysaccharidosis I-S: formerly mucopolysaccharidosis V)

This was first described by Scheie, Hambreck and Barness (1962). It has been shown by Bach et al (1972) that the Scheie syndrome has the same deficient enzyme (α-L-iduronidase) as the Hurler syndrome, but the clinical features of the two diseases are markedly dissimilar. In the Scheie syndrome there may be no radiological signs, the typical features being a coarse face (though not similar to the Hurler syndrome), multiple joint contractures, clouding of the cornea, herniae and sometimes heart disease. These individuals are of normal intelligence and height, and life expectancy is probably normal.

If radiological signs are present, the most likely ones are broadening of the medial end of the clavicles and hypoplasia of the small bones of the hands and feet.

Like the Hurler syndrome it is of autosomal recessive inheritance and there is increased urinary excretion of mucopolysaccharide, mainly of dermatan sulphate.

HUNTER SYNDROME
(Mucopolysaccharidosis II)

This disease was described before the Hurler syndrome, by Hunter in 1917. It is less common and the only one of the mucopolysaccharidoses which is of X-linked recessive inheritance—thus all patients are male (Njå, 1946).

In general the disease is of later onset and is less severe than the Hurler syndrome, but the differences are quantitative not qualitative. The main clinical distinctions are: a lesser degree of mental retardation, no clouding of the cornea, absence of kyphosis, and progressive deafness occurring in about half the patients. The similarities are: the presence of hepatosplenomegaly, herniae, joint stiffness, and sometimes cardiovascular complications. Patients with the Hunter syndrome have a longer life span than those with Hurler's, living perhaps to the second or third decade.

Radiographic findings are similar to the Hurler syndrome but less severe and more slowly progressive. The most obvious findings are in the skull, ribs, scapulae, clavicles, and to a lesser extent in the hand bones. The shape of the pelvis may be indistinguishable from the Hurler syndrome, or it may be almost normal.

Mucopolysaccharides accumulate in a variety of tissues and both dermatan and heparan sulphate are excreted in the urine.

SANFILIPPO SYNDROME
(Mucopolysaccharidosis III)

This was first described by Harris (1961). Two years later Sanfilippo et al (1963) reported two affected sib pairs.
Inheritance. It is of autosomal recessive inheritance, affected sibs with normal parents having been reported several times (Maroteaux and Lamy, 1964 and Wallace et al, 1966). Consanguinous parents have also been noted.
Clinical and radiographic features. These patients are apparently normal for the first few years of life but subsequently mental retardation develops, and is severe. They are not dwarfed, the face is not markedly coarse-featured and there is only minimal clouding of the cornea. As with other forms of mucopolysaccharidosis the joints are stiff and there may be hand contractures.

Radiographic changes are mild, and may even be absent. The most striking feature is the skull, where the posterior part is unusually thick and dense. The vertebral bodies may be slightly biconvex on lateral view, but the typical hook shape is not usually present. A thickening of the medial end of the clavicles and minimal changes in the pelvis, similar but less severe than in the Hurler syndrome, may also be present.
Laboratory investigations. There is increased urinary excretion of heparan sulphate, and this is also present to excess in various tissues. There are two probably clinically indistinguishable types of this disease, one caused by a deficiency of N-heparan-sulfatase and the other by deficiency of α-acetyl-glucosaminidase.
Progress and complications. From appearing to be normal individuals during the first few years of life, the mental retardation in this syndrome eventually becomes very severe. The skeletal involvement, which in any case is minimal, tends to revert to normal during later childhood.

THE MAROTEAUX–LAMY SYNDROME
(Mucopolysaccharidosis VI)

This was first described by Maroteaux et al as 'polydystrophic dwarfism' in 1963. By 1970, Spranger et al were able to review 19 cases. These patients are mentally normal but the skeletal and soft tissue changes may be as severe as those of the Hurler syndrome.

Inheritance. It is of autosomal recessive inheritance, several affected sibs born to unrelated parents having been reported as well as consanguinous parents. It is likely that there is more than one form of the disease, one mild and the other severe. The deficient enzyme is N-Ac-Ga/-4-sulfatase.
Clinical and radiographic features. The syndrome becomes apparent probably during early childhood and at its most severe shows all the features of the Hurler syndrome, apart from mental retardation. The eventual height of these children is only between three and four feet. All patients have poor vision due to corneal opacities and cardiovascular complications are common. Hepatomegaly is more common than splenomegaly, herniae occur and also hydrocephalus in some patients.

The radiographic features vary in severity, but are qualitatively the same as the Hurler syndrome involving the skull, mandible, teeth and vertebral column. The pelvis is usually abnormal with flared iliac wings and a sloping acetabular roof. Disorders of ossification in the femoral capital epiphysis are marked and coxa valga is present. The scapulae, clavicles and ribs show the same deformities as the Hurler syndrome and the long bones have some failure of modelling with thickening of the shaft and a constriction in the metaphyseal region.

THE MORQUIO SYNDROME
(Mucopolysaccharidosis IV)

This mucopolysaccharide disorder is described last since it has a number of features which distinguish it both clinically and radiographically from others in this group of storage diseases. It was described in 1929 both by Brailsford and by Morquio, though it is likely that there were earlier reports than this, labelled 'atypical achondroplasia'. Since 1929 the condition has been considerably over-diagnosed, being confused not only with achondroplasia but with several of the spondylo-epiphyseal dysplasias. Maroteaux, Lamy and Focher (1963) defined the syndrome more clearly, and there is a more recent description by Grossman and Dorst (1973).

The main features are: normal intelligence, marked dwarfing with platyspondyly, pectus carinatum and generalised joint laxity.
Inheritance. It is of autosomal recessive inheritance, the largest survey being reported by Lamy and Maroteaux (1961) who found the expected 1 in 4 ratio of affected sibs.
Clinical and radiographic features. As with the other mucopolysaccharide disorders, these infants are normal at birth, the disease not usually becoming manifest until the first year of life. They are of normal intelligence. There is no coarsening of the face as in the Hurler syndrome, but the maxilla is prominent and the mouth broad. Dwarfing is severe, the height rarely exceeding 122 cm (4 ft). In infancy the trunk is not unduly short; it is only at a later age that platyspondyly develops and the typical Morquio 'short-trunk' type of dwarfism becomes apparent.

Unlike other mucopolysaccharide disorders in which stiff joints and contractures are a feature, in Morquio's disease there is usually generalised joint laxity—which probably accounts for the severe genu valgum, another almost constant clinical feature. The thorax is practically immobile, with marked pectus carinatum. Corneal opacities are only mild and late in developing. Hepatosplenomegaly may or may not be present.

On radiography the skull is normal, apart from some flattening of the mandibular condyles. The teeth have thin enamel and the cusps are small and sharp pointed. During infancy the vertebral bodies are biconvex, sometimes with a small central beak protruding anteriorly, and at this age the thoraco-lumbar region has the same broad-hooked appearance seen in other types of mucopolysaccharide disease. Subsequently, the vertebrae increase little in height and the final picture is of platyspondyly, with a central tongue protruding from the anterior surface. Flattening of the cervical vertebrae becomes apparent early in childhood. One of the characteristic features of this disease is a small or absent odontoid process, which gives rise to instability in this region and spinal cord compression (Blaw and Langer, 1969).

The pelvis shows flaring of the iliac wings, oblique acetabular roofs and coxa valga. Grossman and Dorst (1973) note that the flaring of the iliac wings is unlike the Hurler syndrome by being greatest immediately above the anterior inferior iliac spines. In infancy the capital femoral epiphyses are well formed; subsequently, between the ages of 3 and 6 years, they become irregular and finally, by adolescence or early adult life, they disappear altogether.

One of the most striking features of this disease and one of the first to develop, is the protruding sternum with a manubrio-sternal angle of about 90°. There is premature fusion of the sternal segments and severe limitation of chest movement with a reduced vital capacity.

The hand is early affected in Morquio's disease with small, irregular carpal bones in which ossification is delayed—though up to one year of age they are normal. The bases of the 2nd to 5th metacarpals are pointed and the shafts of both metacarpals and phalanges have a marked central constriction (unlike the Hurler syndrome). The forearm bones are normal in infancy; later, shortening is apparent, particularly of the ulna, and the radius curves round it causing ulnar deviation of the hand and wrist.

The ends of the shafts of the long bones in both upper and lower limbs become bulbous and irregular after infancy. A striking sign in the lower limb is delay in ossification of the lateral side of the upper tibial epiphysis and metaphysis, perhaps connected with the generalised joint laxity and severe genu valgum.

The feet are similar to the hands in showing much irregularity of tarsal ossification and diaphyseal constriction of the metatarsals and phalanges.

Progress and complications. The prognosis of Morquio's disease is variable and some of these individuals live for many years, though others die of respiratory or cardiovascular disease before the age of 20.

The complication of atlanto-axial instability has been referred to, and spinal cord compression at the thoracolumbar junction can also develop. Premature osteoarthritis in affected joints is common. Cardiovascular complications may occur and McKusick (1966) has noted that aortic regurgitation is relatively common. Patients develop deafness during adolescence or later.

Laboratory investigations. All true cases of Morquio's disease excrete excess keratan sulphate, but this tends to decrease with age and by adult life may reach normal levels.

Treatment. This is related to the possible atlanto-axial instability, the severe genu valgum and the premature osteoarthritis.

REFERENCES

Bach, G., Friedmann, R., Weissmann, B., & Neufeld, E. F. (1972). The defect in the Hurler and Scheie syndromes: deficiency of α-L-iduronidase. *Proceedings of the National Academy of Sciences,* **69,** 2048.

Blaw, M. E. & Langer, L. O. (1969). Spinal cord compression in Morquio–Brailford's disease. *Journal of Pediatrics,* **74,** 593.

Brailsford, J. F. (1929). Chondro-osteodystrophy. Roentgenographic and clinical features of a child with dislocation of vertebrae. *American Journal of Surgery,* **7,** 404.

Brante, G., (1952). Gargoylism—a mucopolysaccharidosis. *Scandinavian Journal of Clinical and Laboratory Investigation,* **4,** 43.

Danes, B. S. & Bearn, A. G. (1967). Cellular metachromasia: a genetic marker for studying the mucopolysaccharidoses. *Lancet,* **i,** 241.

Dorfman, A. & Lorincz, A. E. (1957). Occurrence of urinary acid mucopolysaccharides in the Hurler syndrome. *Proceedings of the National Academy of Sciences,* **43,** 443.

Grossman, H. & Dorst, J. (1973). The Mucopolysaccharidoses and Mucolipidoses. In *Progress in Pediatric Radiology,* **4,** Intrinsic Diseases of Bones, 495. Karger, Basel.

Harris, R. C. (1961). Mucopolysaccharide disorder. A possible new genotype of Hurler's syndrome (abstract). *American Journal of Diseases of Children,* **102,** 741.

Hunter, C. (1917). A rare disease in two brothers. *Proceedings of the Royal Society of Medicine,* **10,** 104.

Hurler, G. (1919). Über einen Typ multipler Abartungen, vorwiegend am Skelett-system. *Zeitschrift für Kinderheilkunde,* **24,** 220.

Lamy, M. & Maroteaux, P. (1961). *Les Chondrodystrophies génotypiques.* In L'expansion scientifique française, Paris.

Maroteaux, P., Lamy, M. & Focher, M. (1963). La Maladie de Morquio. Etudes clinique, radiologique et biologique. *Presse Médicale,* **71,** 2091.

Maroteaux, P., Lévêque, B., Marie, J. & Lamy, M. (1963). Une nouvelle dysostose avec élimination urinaire de chondroïtine sulfate B. *La Presse Médicale*, **71,** 1849.

Maroteaux, P. & Lamy, M. (1964). L'oligophrénie polydystrophique (mucopolysaccharidose HS). *La Presse Médicale*, **72,** 2991.

McKusick, V. A. (1972). In *Heritable Disorders of Connective Tissue*, 4th edition. Mosby, St. Louis.

Meyer, K., Hoffman, P. & Linker, A. (1957). Chondroitin sulfate B and heparin sulfate (abstract). *Annals of Rheumatic Diseases*, **16,** 129.

Morquio, L. (1929). Sur une forme de dystrophie osseuse familiale. *Archives de médicine des enfants*, **32,** 129.

Neuhauser, E. B. D., Griscom, N. T., Gilles, F. H. & Crocker, A. C. (1968). Arachnoid cysts in the Hurler–Hunter syndrome. *Annales de Radiologie*, **11,** 453.

Njå, A. (1946). A sex-linked type of gargoylism. *Acta Paediatrica*, **33,** 267.

Sanfilippo, S. J., Podosin, R., Langer, L. & Good, R. A. (1963). Mental retardation associated with acid mucopolysacchariduria (heparin sulphate type). *Journal of Pediatrics*, **63,** 837.

Scheie, H. G., Hambrick, G. W. & Barness, L. A. (1962). A newly recognised forme fruste of Hurler's disease (gargoylism). *American Journal of Ophthalmology*, **53,** 753.

Spranger, J. W., Koch, F., McKusick, V. A., Natzschka, J., Wiedemann, H. R. & Zellweger, H. (1970). Mucopolysaccharidosis VI (Maroteaux–Lamy's disease). *Helvetica Paediatrica Acta*, **25,** 337.

Wallace, B. J., Kaplan, D., Adachi, M., Schneck, L. & Volk, B. W. (1966). Mucopolysaccharidosis Type III. *Archives of Pathology*, **82,** 462.

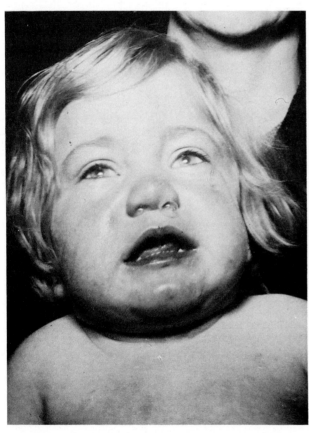

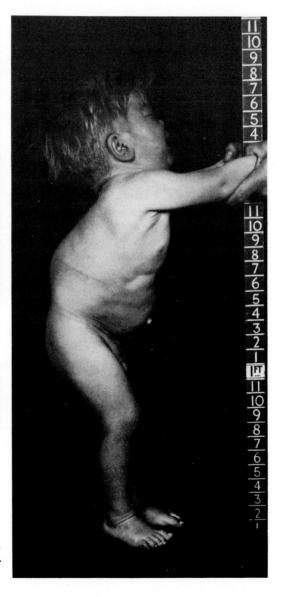

Fig. 48.1   (P.W. aged 2 years.) Female with Hurler syndrome. The face is coarse and the head large. The nasal passages are narrowed and mouth breathing and chronic upper respiratory infection common. (H.A.T.F.)

Fig. 48.2   (D.B.) Male with Hurler syndrome. There is a thoraco-lumbar kyphos, umbilical hernia and enlarged abdomen due to hepato-splenomegaly. (H.A.T.F.)

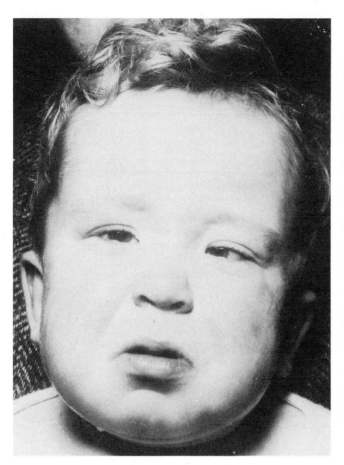

Fig. 48.3 (D.R. aged 2½ years.) Male with Hunter syndrome. The features are somewhat coarse but this is not so marked as in Hurler syndrome. (H.A.T.F.)

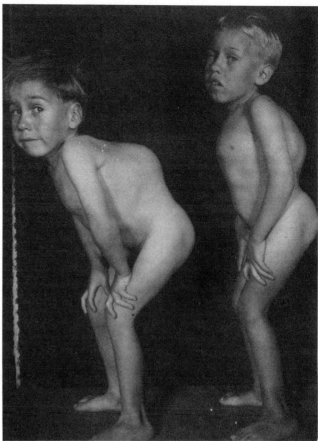

Fig. 48.4 (R. & T.T.) Two brothers with Morquio disease. Although the mouth is somewhat broad the face is otherwise normal, as is intelligence. The trunk is short and the manubrio-sternal angle prominent. (H.A.T.F.)

TABLE I

Storage Diseases with Skeletal Involvement

	Enzyme	Inheritance	Age of onset	Clinical features	Acid mucopolysaccharide in urine
Mucopolysaccharidoses					
Hurler syndrome (MPS I.H.)	Deficient α-L iduronidase	Autosomal recessive	First few months	Severe skeletal changes; dwarfing; mental retardation; death by 10–15 yrs.	Dermatan and heparan sulphate
Scheie syndrome (MPS I.S.)	Deficient α-L iduronidase	Autosomal recessive	Later childhood	Normal intelligence, joint contractures, maybe without radiographic signs; normal life expectancy.	Dermatan and heparan sulphate
Hunter syndrome	Low sulphoiduronate sulphatase	X-linked recessive	6–12 months	As Hurler, but less severe; all patients male.	Dermatan and heparan sulphate
Sanfilippo syndrome	Low N-heparan-sulphatase or α-acetyl-glucosaminidase	Autosomal recessive	Early childhood	Mental retardation; joint contractures; may be without radiographic signs.	Heparan sulphate
Maroteaux–Lamy syndrome	N-Ac-Gal-4-sulfatase	Autosomal recessive	Early–late childhood	Normal intelligence; skeletal changes as severe as Hurler.	Dermatan sulphate (some heparan)
Morquio syndrome	?	Autosomal recessive	2–4 years	Normal intelligence; dwarfing with platyspondyly; joint laxity.	Keratan sulphate
Mucolipidoses					
GM^1 gangliosidosis Type I	Deficient β-galactosidase	Autosomal recessive	Birth–early infancy	Skeletal signs as Hurler but with periosteal cloaking of long bones. Death in infancy.	Nil
Mucolipidosis II (I cell disease)	?	Autosomal recessive	Early infancy	As GM^1 gangliosidosis Type I.	Nil
Others	?	Autosomal recessive	Late infancy–childhood	May be no skeletal findings, only slowly progressive.	Nil
Sphingolipidoses					
Gaucher disease	Reduced glucocerebrosidase	Autosomal recessive	Childhood or adulthood	Osteoporosis, osteolytic areas, bone infarction and necrosis.	Nil

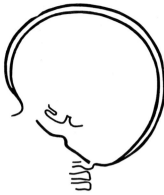

Fig. 48.5   The skull is thick and sella turcica enlarged.

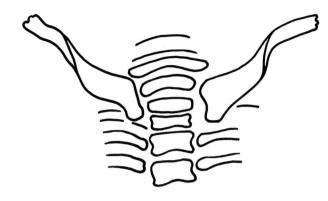

Fig. 48.6   The clavicles are broad, particularly at the medial end.

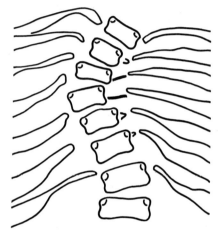

Fig. 48.7   The ribs are narrow and attenuated posteriorly, widening towards their anterior ends. Scoliosis is common.

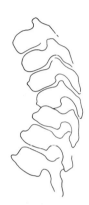

Fig. 48.8   The antero-superior portion of the bodies is under-developed, giving the appearance of a broad hook.

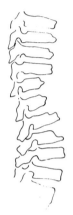

Fig. 48.9   In Morquio's disease, after infancy, the appearance of the vertebrae changes to platyspondyly with a central tongue.

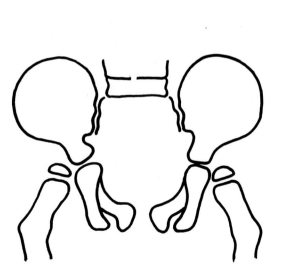

Fig. 48.10   The iliac wings are flared and the acetabular roof oblique. Coxa valga is usual. (In Morquio's disease, after infancy, the capital femoral epiphyses become irregular and finally disappear.)

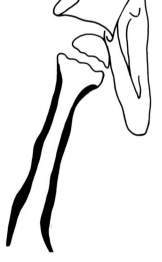

Fig. 48.11   Long bones show lack of diaphyseal modelling, sometimes the shaft being thicker than the metaphysis. Scapula is short and stubby.

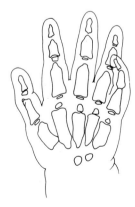

Fig. 48.12   The 2nd to 5th meta-carpals are pointed at their proximal ends, carpal ossification centres are late and the phalanges bullet-shaped, (in Morquio's disease metacarpals and phalanges have a marked central constriction).

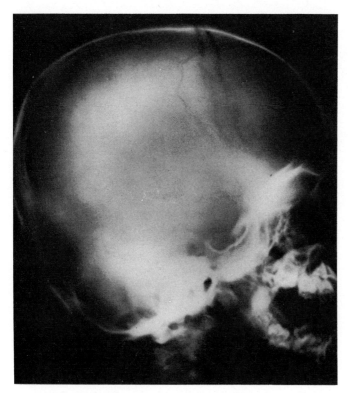

Fig. 48.13 (G.L.) The skull is thickened and sella turcica enlarged. (H.A.T.F.)

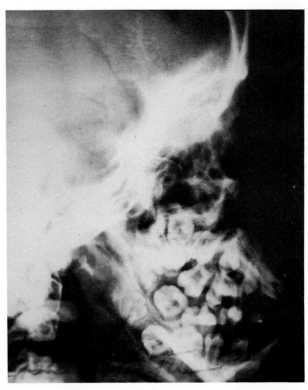

Fig. 48.14 The coronoid process of the mandible is enlarged and the molar teeth sited within the mandibular ramus. (H.A.T.F.)

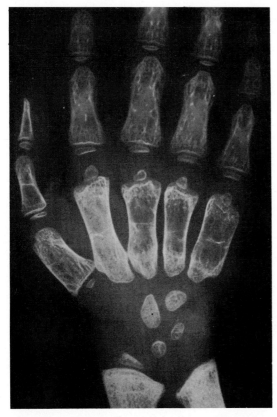

Fig. 48.15 (G.L.) The 2nd to 5th metacarpal bases are pointed: the phalanges short and stubby and there is coarse trabeculation throughout. (H.A.T.F.)

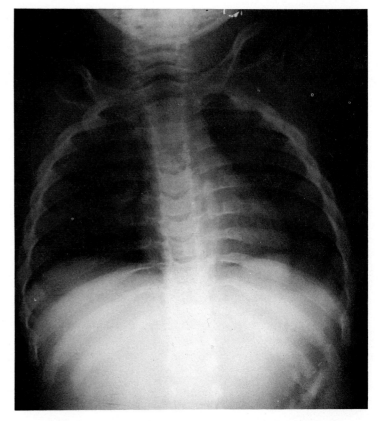

Fig. 48.16 (W.) The medial part of the clavicle is much broadened, the scapulae small and the posterior ends of the ribs very narrow, widening anteriorly. (H.A.T.F.)

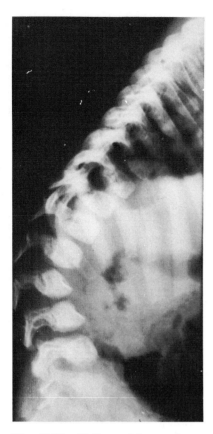

Fig. 48.17 (D.R. aged 3 years.) A thoraco-lumbar kyphos and failure of development of the upper anterior part of the vertebral bodies. (H.A.T.F.)

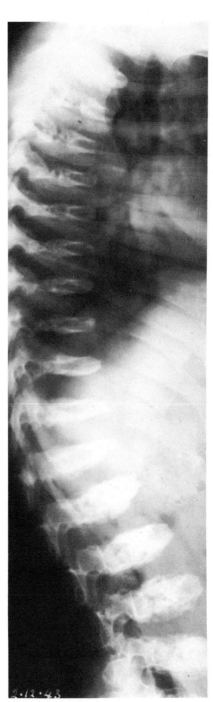

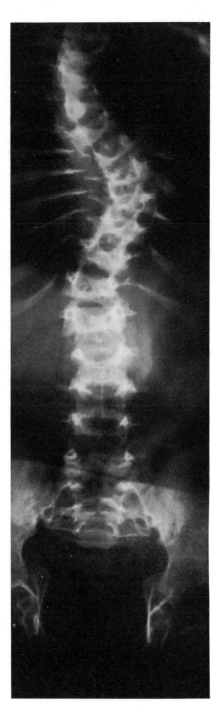

Fig. 48.18 (I.M.) In Morquio's disease after infancy platyspondyly develops. The lower thoracic and upper lumbar vertebrae show an anterior tongue. (H.A.T.F.)

Fig. 48.19 (J.G.) Scoliosis is not uncommon. The dysplastic posterior part of the ribs is well shown here. (H.A.T.F.)

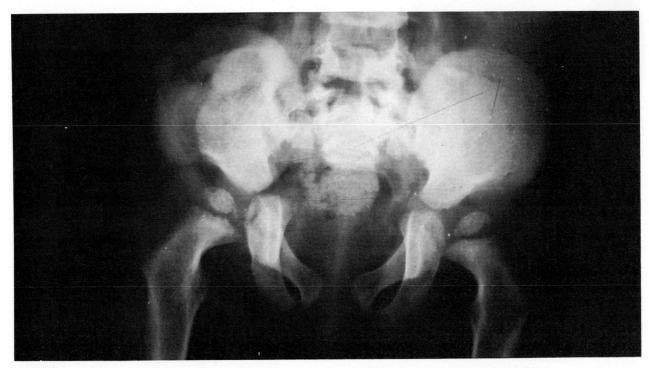

Fig. 48.20 (J.G.) The iliac wings are broad and flared and the acetabular roofs oblique. Coxa valga is present. (H.A.T.F.)

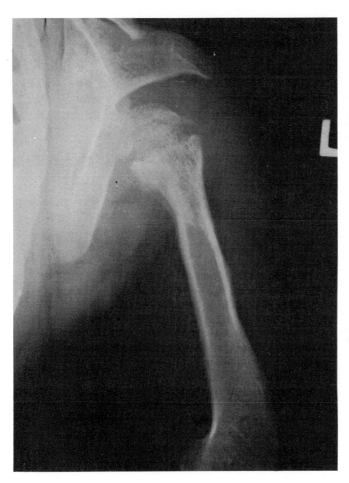

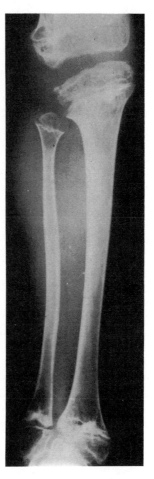

Fig. 48.21   (H.G.) There is lack of diaphyseal modelling and thickening of the shaft. (H.A.T.F.)

Fig. 48.22   (D.B.) Delay in ossification and dysplasia of the lateral side of the upper tibial epiphysis and metaphysis. This occurs in Morquio's disease, perhaps connected with the generalised joint laxity and genu valgum. (H.A.T.F.)

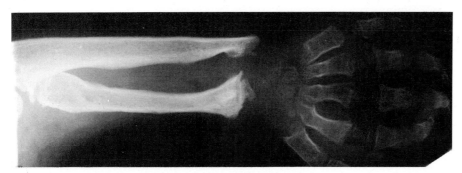

Fig. 48.23   (J.G.) Shortening of the radius and ulna with irregular modelling at the lower end. This, together with the constriction in the shaft of the metacarpals is characteristic of Morquio's disease. (H.A.T.F.)

49 The Mucolipidoses

In this group of storage diseases many of the skeletal and other findings are similar to those of the mucopolysaccharide disorders (Chapter 48), presumably as a result of the deposition of similar compounds in a variety of tissues in both types of disease, but the mucolipidoses do not have any excess MPS in the urine. Spranger and Wiedemann (1970) regard mucolipidosis as a category intermediate between mucopolysaccharidosis and sphingolipidosis (Chapter 50), with their excessive storage of glycolipids and sphingolipids in a number of body tissues. The subject has been reviewed by Spranger (1969) and Grossman and Dorst (1973).

GM₁ GANGLIOSIDOSIS TYPE I

This severe disorder is very similar to Hurler disease, the main difference being that signs are usually apparent at birth and there is no excess mucopolysaccharide in the urine. It has been described in the past under various names such as familial neurovisceral storage disease and generalised gangliosidosis (Landing *et al*, 1964; O'Brien *et al*, 1965; Grossman and Danes, 1968).

Inheritance. It is of autosomal recessive inheritance, many instances of two or more affected sibs with normal parents having been reported (Gonatas and Gonatas, 1965; Sacrez *et al*, 1967).

Frequency. The population incidence is not known but the disorder is extremely rare. It is usually apparent at birth or becomes so very early in infancy.

Clinical and radiographic features. The signs are similar to the Hurler syndrome in that there is a general failure to thrive with retardation of development. Patients have the same coarseness of features seen in that syndrome with an enlarged tongue, hepatosplenomegaly and stiff joints. In some 50 per cent of cases there is a cherry-red macular spot to be seen with the ophthalmoscope, and this is not a feature of the Hurler syndrome.

The radiographic signs are similar to the mucopolysaccharidoses with widened ribs and clavicles, a reduced anteroposterior diameter of the vertebrae on lateral view, with the typical broad hook-like appearance in the lower thoracic and upper lumbar spine. The long bones however, are different from the Hurler syndrome in that there is excessive periosteal bone formation (cloaking). In some cases the shafts are very wide and straight, with no diaphyseal modelling. In later infancy, if the child survives, there is over-constriction of the shafts of the long bones.

The short bones of the hands and feet show the bullet shaped failure of modelling seen in the mucopolysaccharide disorders, together with pointed bases of the 2nd to 5th metacarpals.

Differential diagnosis. GM₁ gangliosidosis type I is differentiated from Hurler disease by its earlier onset, periosteal cloaking and the absence of mucopolysaccharide in the urine. Mucolipidosis II (I-cell disease) is almost identical clinically and radiologically with GM₁ gangliosidosis type I, and can only be differentiated on laboratory investigations. The other mucolipidoses are of later onset and both clinically and radiographically less severe.

Progress and complications. Most infants with GM₁ gangliosidosis type I die of respiratory insufficiency in the first few weeks of life and very few survive beyond the second year.

Laboratory investigations. The specific enzyme defect in GM₁ gangliosidosis type I is β galactosidase and this deficiency can be found in many tissues (brain, kidney, liver, spleen, skin, visceral organs, leucocytes and also in the urine and in cultured fibroblasts).

MUCOLIPIDSOSIS II (I-cell disease)

This is also a very severe mucolipidosis, clinically and radiographically similar to GM₁ gangliosidosis type I. The signs of both diseases are apparent at birth and include the marked periosteal cloaking of long bones.

Mucolipidosis II is probably also of autosomal recessive inheritance, but no specific enzyme defect has yet been found. A number of lysosomal enzymes are deficient and the ultrastructure of cultured fibroblasts shows membrane-bound inclusions within lysosomes (Hanai, Leroy and O'Brien, 1971).

The prognosis is poor, most children dying in late infancy or early childhood from cardiac and respiratory failure (Leroy *et al*, 1971).

OTHER MUCOLIPIDOSES

Several other lipid storage diseases have been described but, in general, the 'dysostosis multiplex' is only mild, and other clinical findings are also less marked than in mucolipidosis II and GM₁ gangliosidosis type I. The one most likely to have significant skeletal findings is mucolipidosis III, formerly called pseudo-Hurler polydystrophy (Maroteaux and Lamy, 1966; Melhem *et al*, 1973). This rare disease is probably of autosomal recessive inheritance. It is not manifest until after the second year of life, and thereafter is only slowly progressive. The non-specific enzyme changes are similar but not identical to those in mucolipidosis II.

REFERENCES

Gonatas, N. K. & Gonatas, J. (1965). Ultrastructural and biochemical observations on a case of systemic late infantile lipidosis and its relationship to Tay–Sachs disease and gargoylism. *Journal of Neuropathology and Experimental Neurology*, **24**, 318.

Grossman, H. & Danes, B. S. (1968). Neurovisceral storage disease: roentgenographic features and mode of inheritance. *American Journal of Roentgenology*, **103**, 149.

Grossman, H. & Dorst, J. (1973). The mucopolysaccharidoses and mucolipidoses. In *Progress in Paediatric Radiology*, **4**, Intrinsic Diseases of Bones, 495. Karger, Basel.

Hanai, J., Leroy, J. & O'Brien, J. S. (1971). Ultrastructure of cultured fibroblasts in I-Cell disease. *American Journal of Diseases of Children*, **122**, 34.

Landing, B. H., Silverman, F. N., Craig, J. M., Jacoby, M. D., Lahey, M. E. & Chadwick, D. L. (1964). Familial neurovisceral lipidosis. *American Journal of Diseases of Children*, **108**, 503.

Leroy, J. G., Spranger, J. W., Feingold, M., Opitz, J. M. & Crocker, A. C. (1971). I-cell disease. A clinical picture. *Journal of Pediatrics*, **79**, 360.

Maroteaux, P. & Lamy, M. (1966). La Pseudo-polydystrophie de Hurler.[1] *La Presse Médicale*, **74**, 2889.

Melhem, R., Dorst, J. P., Scott, C. I., Jr, McKusick, V. A. (1973). Roentgen findings in mucolipidosis III (Pseudo-Hurler polydystrophy). *Radiology*, **106**, 153.

O'Brien, J. S., Stern, M. B., Landing, B. H., O'Brien, J. K. & Donnell, G. N. (1965). Generalised gangliosidosis. *American Journal of Diseases of Children*, **109**, 338.

Sacrez, R., Juif, J. G., Gigonnet, J. M. & Gruner, J. E. (1967). La maladie de Landing ou idiotie amaurotique infantile précoce avec gangliosidose généralisée, de Type GM1. *Pédiatrie*, **22**, 143.

Spranger, J. (1969). Mucopolysaccharidoses and mucolipidoses. *Annals of Radiology*, **12**, 981.

Spranger, J. & Wiedemann, H. R. (1970). The genetic mucolipidoses. Diagnosis and differential diagnosis. *Humangenetik*, **9**, 113.

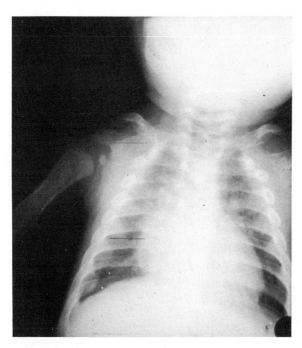

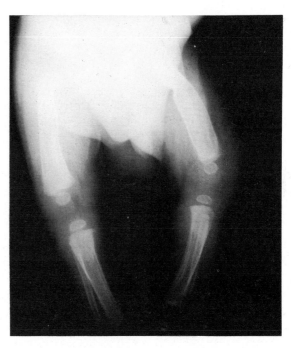

Fig. 49.1   (J.T.) GM$_I$ Gangliosidosis Type 1. Broad ribs and clavicles, wide humeral shaft. (G.O.S.)

Fig. 49.2   (J.T.) Periosteal cloaking, lower limbs. (G.O.S.)

The sphingolipidoses are the third group of inherited storage diseases so far identified, but unlike the mucopolysaccharidoses and the mucolipidoses, they have little general effect upon the skeleton. Those so far described include Gaucher disease, Niemann-Pick disease, metachromatic leucodystrophy, Fabry disease and lactosyl ceramidosis, but only Gaucher disease has significant radiographic findings.

GAUCHER'S DISEASE

This is an inherited storage disease principally affecting the spleen, in which accumulations of gluco-cerebroside are found in large reticulo-endothelial cells deposited throughout the skeleton and liver, as well as the spleen and other organs. These cells, and the disease, were first described by Gaucher (1882) and later reports have been by Herndon and Bender (1950), Hsia, Naylor and Bigler (1959) and Herrlin and Hillborg (1962).

The skeletal manifestations are osteoporosis, bone destruction by Gaucher cells and bone infarction and necrosis.

Inheritance. Gaucher disease is of autosomal recessive inheritance: there are many reports of affected sibs with normal parents. Wiedemann and Gerken (1964) were able to find Gaucher cells in the heterozygote parents and sibs of patients with Gaucher's disease.

Frequency. In general this is an extremely rare disease but it is relatively common amongst Ashkenazi Jews. There is an acute infantile form, rapidly fatal, and without skeletal manifestations, but the age of onset is more usually in young adult life and the disease has a more chronic course.

Clinical and radiographic features. In the early stages the presenting signs are of weakness, anaemia and splenomegaly. Later, enlargement of the liver, pulmonary and skeletal infiltration occur and pathological fractures are common. When radiographic evidence of skeletal involvement is present, there are bone symptoms of pain and swelling over the joints.

Radiographic signs are initially those of chronic marrow disease with widening of the marrow cavity and osteoporosis. This often asymmetrically affects the pelvis and the femoral and humeral shafts and is due to resorption of bone adjacent to the Gaucher cells. Larger areas of bone destruction occur later showing as irregular cyst-like lesions. There is often some modelling defect of the long bones with an expanded 'flask-shaped' metaphyseal region, and there may be periosteal new bone formation.

One of the most characteristic features of Gaucher's disease is infarction of bone, which occurs typically in the femoral and (nearly as often) humeral heads as well as in the diaphyses of the lower limb bones. The subarticular necrosis is manifested by zones of sclerosis and radiolucent defects in the head of the femur or humerus, and the head flattens as the necrotic process progresses.

Pathogenesis. Gaucher's disease is a storage disease caused by reduced activity of gluco-cerebrosidase, and the reticulo-endothelial cells filled with gluco-cerebroside accumulate not only in the spleen but in the liver, haemopoietic skeleton, lymphoid tissue and sometimes also in the lungs and central nervous system. These Gaucher cells are unique in appearance. They are large, often multinucleated, with a wrinkled cytoplasm, non-vacuolated and pale-staining. There is a strong acid phosphatase reaction.

Laboratory investigations. Diagnosis is made by finding the characteristic Gaucher cells on marrow puncture, though rarely spleen or liver biopsy may be needed. Blood cell investigations are normal unless hypersplenism is well developed, in which case there will be anaemia, thrombocytopenia and leucopenia. The serum acid phosphatase is raised.

Treatment. There is no specific treatment for this slowly progressive disease, though splenectomy may be indicated for hypersplenism. The pathological fractures may cause problems of treatment due to their slow rate of healing.

REFERENCES

Gaucher, E. (1882). *De l'Epithélioma primitiv de la rate*. Thèse de Paris.
Herndon, C. N. & Bender, J. R. (1950). Gaucher's disease: cases in 5 related Negro sibships. *American Journal of Human Genetics*, **2**, 49.
Herrlin, K. M. & Hillborg, P. O. (1962). Neurological signs in a juvenile form of Gaucher's disease. *Acta Paediatrica Scandinavica*, **51**, 137.
Hsia, D. Y., Naylor, J. & Bigler, J. A. (1959). Gaucher's disease. *New England Journal of Medicine*, **261**, 164.
Wiedemann, H. R. & Gerken, H. (1964). Gaucher cells in healthy relatives of patients with Gaucher's disease. *Lancet*, ii, 866.

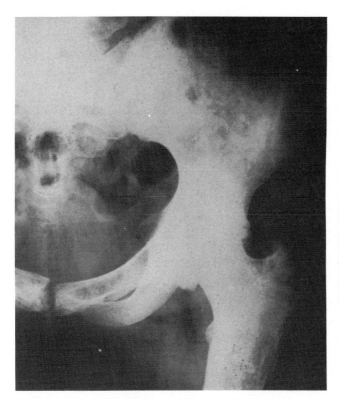

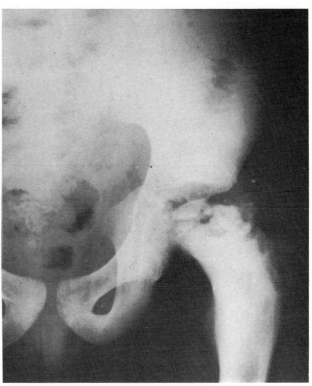

Fig. 50.1 (B.C.) Multiple cyst-like areas in the upper part of the femur and pelvis. (H.A.T.F.)

Fig. 50.2 (D.B.) Infarction and necrosis of the femoral head, a typical sign in Gaucher's disease. (H.A.T.F.)

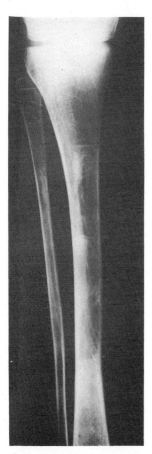

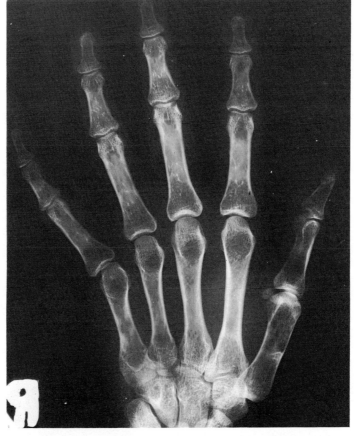

Fig. 50.3 The metaphyseal region is expanded and there is some osteoporosis and also areas of infarction of the tibial shaft. (H.A.T.F.)

Fig. 50.4 (B.C.) The hand shows similar areas of patchy osteoporosis and cyst-like areas. (H.A.T.F.)

51 Homocystinuria

This is an inherited disorder of amino-acid metabolism characterised by body disproportion and frequently accompanied by mental retardation, dislocated lenses, disordered modelling of long bones and osteoporosis occurring in the child or young adult.

It was first described in 1962 both by Carson and Neill, and by Gerritsen, Vaughan and Waisman. More recent reviews of the disorder are by Cusworth and Dent (1969) and by Schedewie (1973).

Aetiology and inheritance. Homocystinuria is of autosomal recessive inheritance. A family survey of 20 sibships was carried out by Schimke *et al* (1965), who demonstrated the expected 1:4 risk to sibs. Carson and Carré (1969) described two forms of the disorder—one in which there was no response to treatment with pyridoxine and one in which excess pyridoxine was needed. Both forms were of autosomal recessive inheritance. The deficient or defective enzyme in homocystinuria is cystathionine synthetase. This enzyme catalyses the formation of cystathionine from homocystine, and its lack leads to homocystine in the urine. Homocystine and cystine are chemically similar and both give a reddish purple colour in the cyanide-nitroprusside test of urine. This simple test is useful for screening purposes; urine giving a positive reaction can then be further examined chromatographically or by electrophoresis to differentiate between cystine and homocystine.

Homocystinuria is one of the inborn errors of metabolism in which the enzyme defect can be detected antenatally in an affected foetus by culturing cells grown from amniotic fluid after the 14th week of gestation. Parents who each carry the abnormal gene cannot be detected with certainty, but once they have had a child with homocystinuria the high risk to later born children is recognised and subsequent pregnancies can be screened to detect the disease in the foetus.

Frequency. The population incidence is not known but this is a rare disorder. The sexes are equally affected. The disease becomes apparent at any time during childhood, with mental retardation and ectopia lentis being the commonest presenting signs. Mild cases may be discovered incidentally at any time of life.

Clinical and radiographic features. Between half and two-thirds of these individuals are mentally retarded though none is very severely so. A second common feature of the disease is dislocation of the lens, which is usually bilateral and develops before the age of 10 years. The general appearance and height of these patients may be entirely normal but many show body disproportion, with the head to pubis measurement being less than pubis to heel, and with an arm span that exceeds the height. In the past, these patients have been confused with the Marfan syndrome, not only because of body disproportion, but because the two diseases also have in common a narrow, high arched palate, frequent scoliosis and deformity of the chest (pectus excavatum or carinatum).

Radiographic signs are variable, there being little of note in some patients with homocystinuria. One characteristic feature is a generalised osteoporosis, manifested most obviously by flattened or biconcave vertebrae. Compression fractures and collapse of vertebrae can occur even in childhood.

In the long bones there is widening of the metaphyses with general failure of modelling, most obvious around the knee joint. Epiphyses may be larger than normal and at the upper end of the femur the femoral neck may be convex along the upper border, instead of showing the usual concave line.

Arachnodactyly is not so common as in the Marfan syndrome, though somewhat long fingers and toes have been noted. A comparison of homocystinuria and the Marfan syndrome was reported by Brenton *et al* (1972).

Differential diagnosis. The disorder with which homocystinuria is most likely to be confused is the Marfan syndrome, but this should be clearly distinguished by dominant inheritance, aortic aneurysm, lack of osteoporosis and infrequent cases of mental retardation. Firm diagnosis of homocystinuria is made by detecting homocystine in the urine.

Progress and complications. Mental retardation and the development of scoliosis, which may be severe, have already been noted, as well as osteoporosis with the risk of compression fractures of vertebrae.

A serious developing complication in homocystinuria is the risk of thrombosis in arteries or veins (Gibson, Carson and Neill, 1964), which is likely to be precipitated by surgery and the subsequent immobilisation. The cause of this thrombotic tendency is not known but it may be due to abnormal stickiness of the platelets, caused by the presence of homocystine in the blood (Barber and Spaeth, 1969).

Treatment. Treatment is possible in homocystinuria with pyridoxine or a low protein diet, but although homocystine may disappear from the blood and urine, it is not certain that the patient benefits clinically from this. However, there may be some protection from the thrombosis which can be a lethal complication (Barber and Spaeth, 1967).

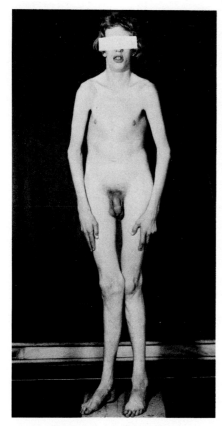

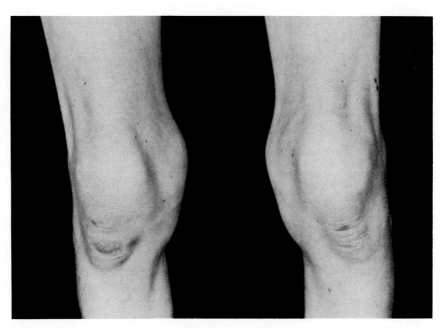

Fig. 51.2 (P.K.) Characteristic enlargement of the knees, particularly in the region the medial femoral condyles. (Courtesy of Dr D. Brenton, London.)

Fig. 51.1 (S.McF.) Body disproportion with the head to pubis measurement being less than pubis to heel. Bony enlargement of the knees is characteristic. (Courtesy of Dr D. Brenton, London.)

REFERENCES

Barber, G. W. & Spaeth, G. L. (1967) Pyridoxine therapy in homocystinuria. *Lancet*, **i,** 337.

Barber, G. W. & Spaeth, G. L. (1969). The successful treatment of homocystinuria with pyridoxine. *Journal of Pediatrics*, **75,** 463.

Brenton, D. P., Dow, C. J., James, J. I. P., Hay, R. L. & Wynne-Davies, R. (1972). Homocystinuria and Marfan's syndrome. *Journal of Bone & Joint Surgery*, **54B,** 277.

Carson, N. A. & Neill, D. W. (1962). Metabolic abnormalities detected in a survey of mentally backward individuals in Northern Ireland. *Archives of Diseases in Childhood*, **37,** 505.

Carson, N. A. J. & Carré, I. J. (1969). Treatment of homocystinuria with pyridoxine. *Archives of Diseases in Childhood*, **44,** 387.

Cusworth, D. C. & Dent, C. E. (1969). Homocystinuria. *British Medical Bulletin*, **25,** 42.

Gerritsen, T., Vaughan, J. G. & Waisman, H. A. (1962). The identification of homocystine in the urine. *Biochemical and Biophysical Research Communications*, **9,** 493.

Gibson, J. B., Carson, N. A. & Neill, D. W. (1964). Pathologic findings in homocystinuria. *Journal of Clinical Pathology*, **17,** 427.

Schedewie, H. (1973). Skeletal findings in homocystinuria: a collaborative study. *Paediatric Radiology*, **1,** 12.

Schimke, R. N., McKusick, V. A., Huan, G. T. & Pollack, A. D. (1965). Homocystinuria. Studies of 20 families with 38 affected members. *Journal of the American Medical Association*, **193,** 711.

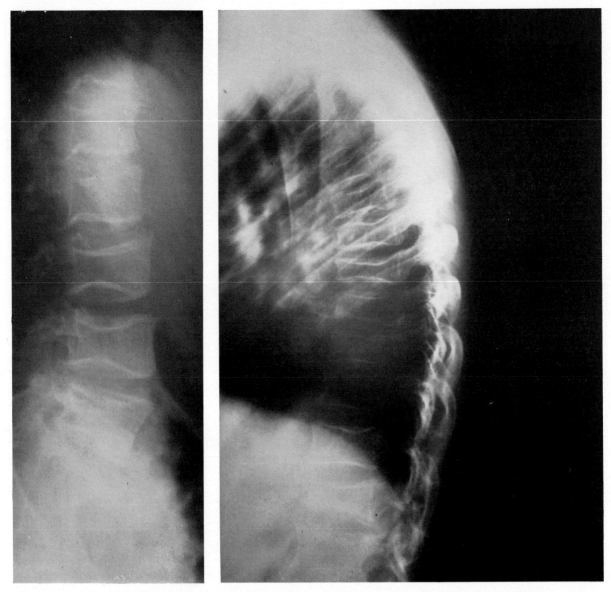

Figs 51.3 & 51.4 (F.McI. & J.C.) Osteoporosis even in young adults is a feature of this disease. The vertebrae may be biconvex or show a more general platyspondyly. (Courtesy of Dr D. Brenton, London.)

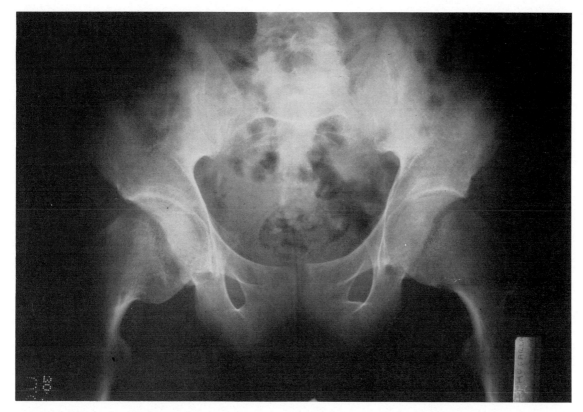

Fig. 51.5 (S.McF.) The femoral necks are thicker than normal and convex along the upper border. (Courtesy of Dr D. Brenton, London.)

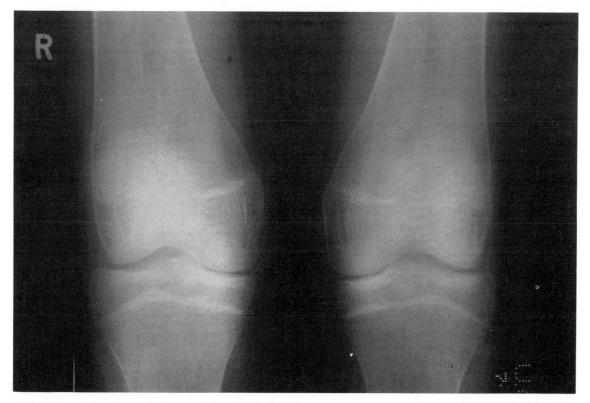

Fig. 51.6 (F.McI.) There is some widening of the metaphyses with general failure of modelling. (Courtesy of Dr D. Brenton, London.)

52　Histiocytosis X
Eosinophilic granuloma : Hand–Schüller–Christian and Letterer–Siwe disease

The disorders of the reticulo-endothelial system now called histiocytosis X include diseases formerly described as separate entities—eosinophilic granuloma, Hand–Schüller–Christian disease and Letterer Siwe disease.

All are characterised by proliferation of histiocytes with secondary storage of cholesterol in them, and in the more chronic stages this is accompanied by fibrosis and scarring. The diseases seem to be inflammatory in nature rather than neoplastic. Eosinophilic granuloma is the least severe of the three, presenting often as a single localised skeletal lesion which heals spontaneously in the course of 12 to 18 months. Hand–Schüller–Christian disease is of moderate low grade severity with multiple lesions in the liver, spleen and skeleton. Letterer Siwe disease is an acute fulminating disorder occurring in young infants, which in rare cases can revert to the more moderate Hand–Schüller–Christian type. It is clear that the three diseases are related and indeed probably illustrate only different degrees of severity of the same disorder; however they are here described separately.

Inheritance. Eosinophilic granuloma and Hand–Schüller–Christian disease are always sporadic. Letterer Siwe disease has been reported on many occasions in more than one sib and in both of identical twins (Rogers and Benson, 1962; Omenn, 1965; Juberg, Kloepffer and Oberman, 1970), and it may therefore be of autosomal recessive inheritance in some instances.

Frequency. All three disorders are extremely rare. Males are affected more frequently than females. The age of onset is variable during childhood or adolescence, Letterer Siwe disease occurring at the earliest age, usually under 2 years.

EOSINOPHILIC GRANULOMA

Eosinophilic granuloma presents as a tumour of bone usually during the first two decades of life. In some 65 per cent of cases there is a solitary skeletal lesion frequently affecting a 'flat' bone (pelvis, skull or vertebrae). However, there may be several lesions and any bone may be involved, the ribs and major long bones more frequently than other bones of the extremities. Pathological fractures occur, and non-osseus lesions, particularly pulmonary, have been reported. Lesions can form rapidly and then regress.

On radiography the affected bone shows a small, circumscribed translucent area with bevelled edges, usually circular or oval and perhaps containing a small sequestrum. There is not usually any sclerosis of the surrounding bone. Involvement of a vertebra results in the characteristic vertebra plana, which is usually associated with an adjacent soft mass of affected tissue.

It is remarkable that these extremely flat vertebrae, reduced to perhaps one-fifth the normal height, can repair spontaneously within a matter of 1 to 2 years, regaining an almost normal radiographic appearance.

In the long bones, the eosinophilic granuloma lesion is usually in the diaphysis and provokes considerable endosteal and, to a lesser extent, periosteal reaction. The epiphysis is only very rarely involved.

The differential diagnosis is from chronic osteomyelitis, tuberculosis and bone tumour, and biopsy may be needed to differentiate them. In eosinophilic granuloma there are usually no abnormalities on blood examination.

HAND–SCHÜLLER–CHRISTIAN DISEASE

In this more severe form of histiocytosis X there is a generalised body disturbance with hepatosplenomegaly and lymphadenopathy. Growth and sexual development are retarded. The lytic lesions in the skeleton are much larger than in eosinophilic granuloma, are multiple and sometimes destructive of large areas of bone such as the floor of the skull. Involvement of the skull and pituitary fossa led to a triad being described of skull defects, diabetes insipidus and exophthalmos, though in fact this combination of signs is rare (Murray and Jacobson, 1971). The sharply outlined, round osseous defect has a punched out appearance, and various lesions of different size may be seen, particularly in the skull. They are unlike the defects of myelomatosis, being larger and fewer in number.

The prognosis is variable, depending upon the age of onset and number of lesions: the younger the child and the greater the number of lesions, the more serious the prognosis.

LETTERER SIWE DISEASE

This is the most severe form of histiocytosis X, and is usually an acute fulminating disorder. The onset is in infancy and the presenting features are of an ill child with fever, anaemia, bleeding from mucous membranes or other sites, and frequently with a rash and sores. The liver and spleen are much enlarged, pulmonary lesions are present and may predominate: indeed there may be no skeletal lesions at all in the most acute cases. When present, the osteolytic areas are multiple and usually poorly defined.

There may be some response to corticosteroid therapy and on occasion this severe disease reverts to the more moderate Hand–Schüller–Christian type. Confirmation of the diagnosis is obtained from biopsy of the skin or lymph nodes which show the typical histiocytes common to this group of diseases.

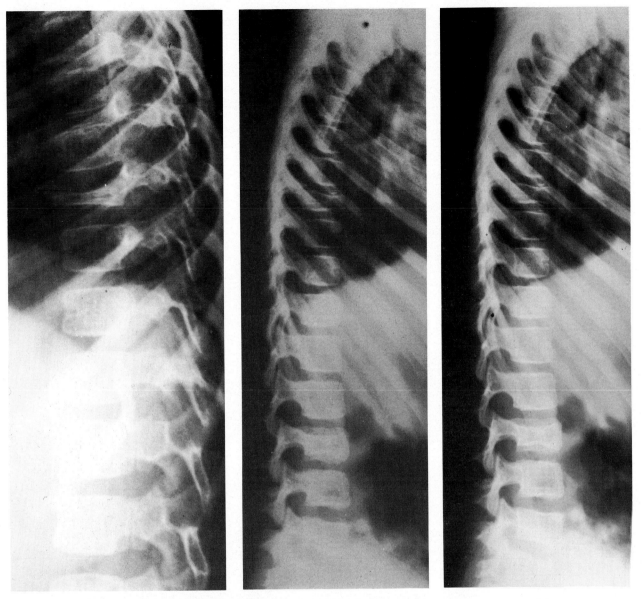

Figs 52.1, 52.2 & 52.3   (T.H.) Vertebra plana due to eosiniphilic granuloma. This deformity is reversible, and may heal within one to two years. (H.A.T.F.)

REFERENCES

Christian, H. A. (1919). *Contributions to Medical and Biological Research.* New York: Hoeber, **1**, 390.

Hand, A. (1893). *Archives of Pediatrics*, **10**, 673.

Juberg, R. C., Kloepffer, H. W. & Oberman, H. A. (1970). Genetic determination of acute disseminated histiocytosis X (Letterer–Siwe syndrome). *Pediatrics*, **43**, 753.

Letterer, E. (1924). *Frankfurt Zeitschrift für Pathologie*, **30**, 377.

Murray, R. O. & Jacobson, H. G. (1971). In *The Radiology of Skeletal Disorders.* Churchill Livingstone (Edinburgh).

Omenn, G. S. (1965). Familial reticuloendotheliosis and eosinophilia. *New England Journal of Medicine*, **273**, 427.

Rogers, D. L. & Benson, T. E. (1962). Familial Letterer–Siwe disease: report of a case. *Journal of Pediatrics*, **60**, 550.

Schüller, A. (1915). *Fortschritte auf dem Gebiete der Roentgenstrahlen*, **23**, 12.

Siwe, S. (1933). *Zeitschrift für Kinderheilkunde*, **55**, 212.

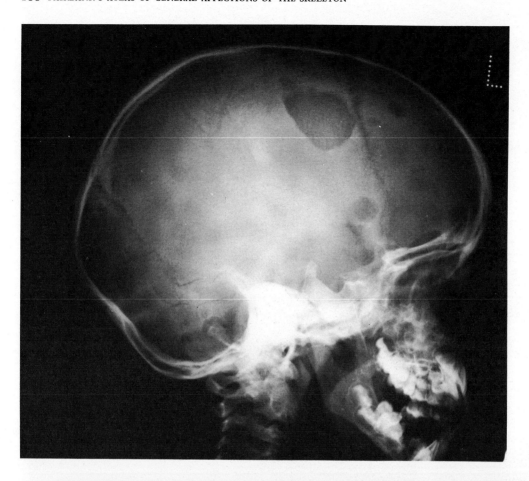

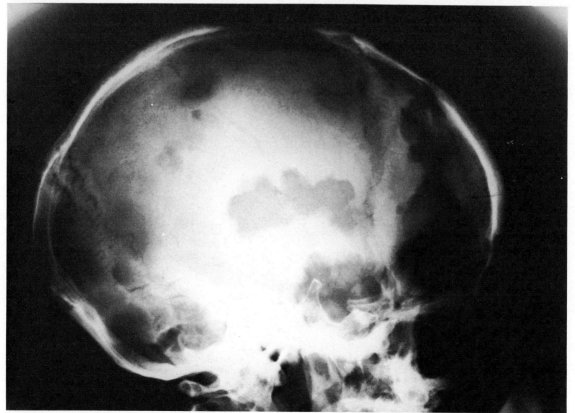

Figs 52.4 & 52.5   (M.M.) A more severe form of histiocytosis X, with large areas of bone destruction in the skull. 7½ years has elapsed between these two radiographs. The lesions are sharply outlined with a punched out appearance and there are many different sizes. (Courtesy of Dr T. D. Hawkins, Cambridge.)

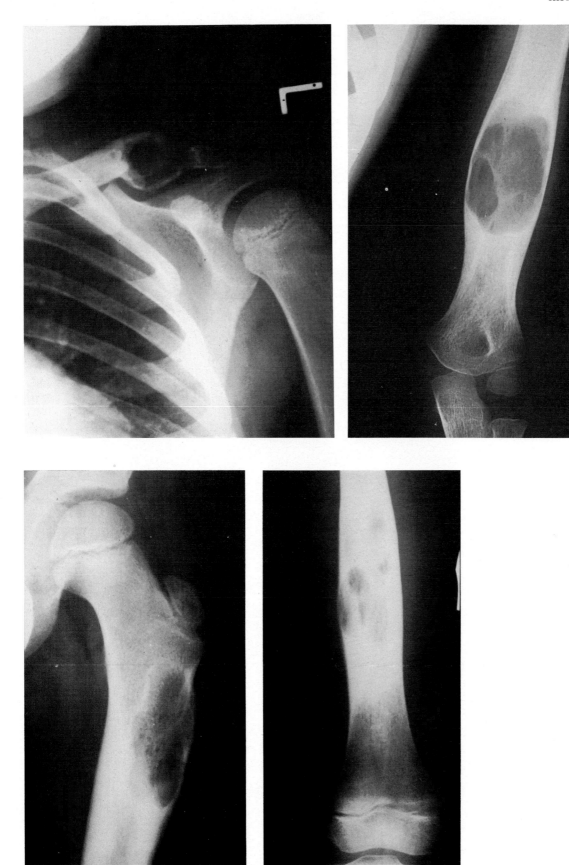

Figs 52.6, 52.7, 52.8 & 52.9   (M.M.) Examples of lytic lesions in the clavicle, humerus and femur of the same patient. (Courtesy of Dr T. D. Hawkins, Cambridge.)

SECTION IV

METABOLIC BONE
DISEASE

53 Metabolic Bone Disease with Hypercalcaemia

HYPERPARATHYROIDISM

It is many years since the association between the parathyroid glands and bone disease was first described, and by 1934 Albright and other authors had established that in fact accompanying renal disease was rather more common than bone disease. With the introduction of biochemical screening in clinics it has now become clear that only some 10 to 20 per cent of all patients with hyperparathyroidism have any radiographic signs of bone involvement. There are recent reviews of the subject by Fourman and Royer (1968) and Paterson (1974).

Aetiology and inheritance. In the great majority of cases parathyroid disease is associated with a single (occasionally double) benign adenoma of the gland. In some instances the overaction of the gland is due to primary hyperplasia, and more rarely still to carcinoma.

Occasionally, hyperparathyroidism presents as a familial disorder (both dominant and recessive inheritance has been reported), in which case the cause is usually primary hyperplasia of the chief cells, though some cases are associated with multiple endocrine neoplasia.

Frequency. The population frequency of hyperparathyroidism is not known but screening of a clinic population gives an incidence of about 1 per 1,000 (Boonstra and Jackson, 1971). However, few of these patients had symptoms suggestive of parathyroid disease. Females are affected two or three times as commonly as males, the excess numbers being due to those women who develop the disease in the postmenopausal period. Hyperparathyroidism may become apparent at any time of life but it is commonest after the third decade.

Clinical and radiographic features. The clinical features of hyperparathyroidism are associated with the accompanying hypercalcaemia, the renal consequences of this, and with the bone disease, which is present in only perhaps one tenth of patients.

Symptoms of hypercalcaemia include general malaise, thirst, polyuria, anorexia, nausea, vomiting, and constipation. Patients frequently complain of muscle pains and weakness and may have ataxia. The renal disease is accompanied by changes in the distal tubules and patients pass large volumes of hypotonic urine. The disturbance of calcium balance leads first to microscopic calcification in the kidney and subsequently nephrocalcinosis may be seen on radiography. Finally, larger calculi develop with the attendant problems of urinary obstruction, pyelonephritis and secondary hypertension.

There are few bone symptoms in hyperparathyroidism though occasionally there is some pain. Severely affected bones become bent and deformed and pathological fractures occur. An occasional clinical feature is 'pseudo-clubbing' of the fingers associated with resorption of the terminal phalanges.

One of the main radiographic features in hyperparathyroidism is subperiosteal bone erosion, mainly affecting the radial side of the necks of the phalanges but also found in the clavicle, ulna, femoral neck and along the superior surface of the ribs. Bone cysts are another characteristic feature, and these may be true haemorrhagic cysts or so-called brown (giant cell) tumours, which appear cyst-like on radiographs. In patients with severe and long-standing disease there is also generalised osteoporosis with some patchy sclerosis. The radiographic appearance of the bone cysts and tumours is not specific for hyperparathyroidism, but by the time an individual has such advanced disease other signs of parathyroid overaction will be apparent.

The skull often has a mottled appearance and, again, areas of bone resorption can be seen giving the characteristic picture of the 'pepper pot' skull.

Among the complications of hyperparathyroidism are joint disorders, which include simple secondary osteoarthritis due to limb deformity following fractures, and in chronic cases crystal synovitis may develop, both true gout and pseudogout (chondrocalcinosis), with the radiographic feature of calcification in hyaline cartilage.

Pathology of bone lesions. The pathology of the bone lesions is indicated by the name, osteitis fibrosa cystica. It is said that the lesions are more severe in areas where the normal turnover of bone is most active—such as the vertebrae, phalanges and at the ends of the long bones. There is increased activity by fibroblasts with deposition of excess fibrous tissue in the bone marrow. Areas of bone resorption and regeneration may be seen in close proximity but overall the main feature is of bone loss. The cystic lesions may be filled with mucus or a brown fluid and are probably haemorrhagic in nature. Less often giant cell tumours form, sometimes at several sites, and these may be histologically indistinguishable from the solitary osteoclastomas unassociated with hyperparathyroidism. Malignant change can occur in these brown tumours, but it is of rare occurrence.

Both the small areas of bone resorption under the periosteum and the 'brown tumours' heal, albeit slowly, after parathyroidectomy.

Clinical chemistry. The serum calcium is very nearly always raised in hyperparathyroidism and the serum phosphorus usually low. In some cases the serum alkaline phosphatase is also raised. Patients may have a mild metabolic acidosis.

Differential diagnosis. Simple bone cysts and other bone tumours are differentiated by reason of their solitary nature, hyperparathyroidism being a generalised disease. Polyostotic fibrous dysplasia usually has an earlier age of onset, it is frequently asymmetrical, is accompanied by skin pigmentation and the clinical chemistry is normal.

Progress and complications. Untreated hyperparathyroidism is a lethal disease, death being due either to acute hypercalcaemia with dehydration and death in anuria or resulting from the renal disease, calculi and infection.

Treatment. The treatment of established hyperparathyroidism is surgical, with removal of the hyperplastic or adenomatous glands. Surgery is indicated if the serum calcium is markedly raised and bone or renal disease, or one of the associated diseases of hyperparathyroidism, for example peptic ulcer, is present.

DISEASES ASSOCIATED WITH HYPERPARATHYROIDISM

It seems that there is an increased incidence of peptic ulcer amongst patients with hyperparathyroidism (Pyrah, Hodgkinson and Anderson, 1966) and the condition of multiple endocrine adenosis has also

been reported. However, in this latter case the parathyroid disease tends not to be severe, and these patients usually have no skeletal manifestations.

SECONDARY HYPERPARATHYROIDISM

The parathyroid glands respond with hyperplasia and increased output of parathyroid hormone to hypocalcaemia of any cause—thus secondary hyperparathyroidism is found in many patients with vitamin D deficiency rickets and osteomalacia, renal tubular disease, and particularly in renal failure. The most valuable radiographic evidence of the condition is subperiosteal erosion of bone in the phalanges. Secondary hyperparathyroidism usually remits when the primary disorder is treated.

TERTIARY HYPERPARATHYROIDISM

This is the term used to describe patients with secondary hyperparathyroidism (usually following one of the malabsorption syndromes or renal failure) in whom an autonomous parathyroid adenoma develops, and the condition is thus characterised by hypercalcaemia (Davies, Dent and Watson, 1968). Tertiary hyperparathyroidism with hyperplasia of the parathyroid glands is an increasing problem in patients with renal failure treated with regular haemodialysis.

REFERENCES

Albright, F., Aub, J. C. & Bauer, W. (1934). Hyperparathyroidism. A common and polymorphic condition as illustrated by seventeen proved cases from one clinic. *Journal of the American Medical Association*, **102**, 1276.
Boonstra, C. E. & Jackson, C. E. (1971). Serum calcium survey for hyperparathyroidism: Results in 50,000 clinic patients. *American Journal of Clinical Pathology*, **55**, 523.
Davies, D. R., Dent, C. E. & Watson, L. (1968). Tertiary hyperparathyroidism. *British Medical Journal*, **3**, 395.
Fourman, P. & Royer, P. (1968). *Calcium metabolism and the bone*. Oxford: Blackwell.
Paterson, C. R. (1974). *Metabolic Disorders of Bone*. Oxford: Blackwell.
Pyrah, L., Hodgkinson, A. & Anderson, C. K. (1966). Primary hyperparathyroidism. *British Journal of Surgery*, **53**, 245.

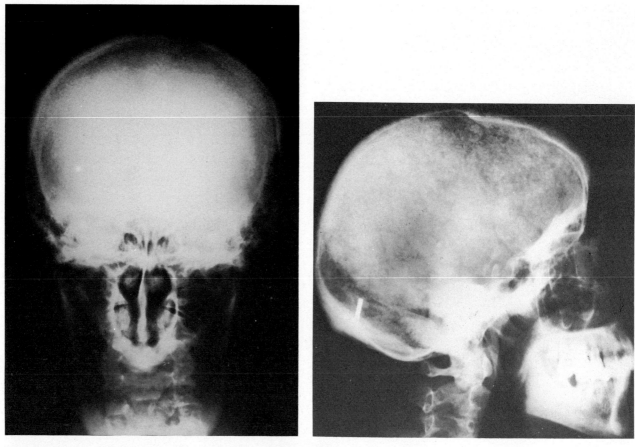

Figs. 53.1 & 53.2 (K.T. & D.P.) Mottling of the skull with areas of bone resorption. (A.H.)

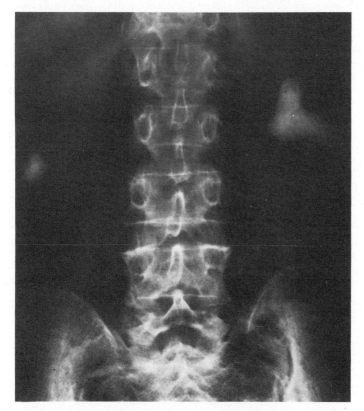

Fig. 53.3 (M.M.) Hyperparathyroidism associated with renal calculi. (Courtesy of Mr J. C. Chalmers, Edinburgh.)

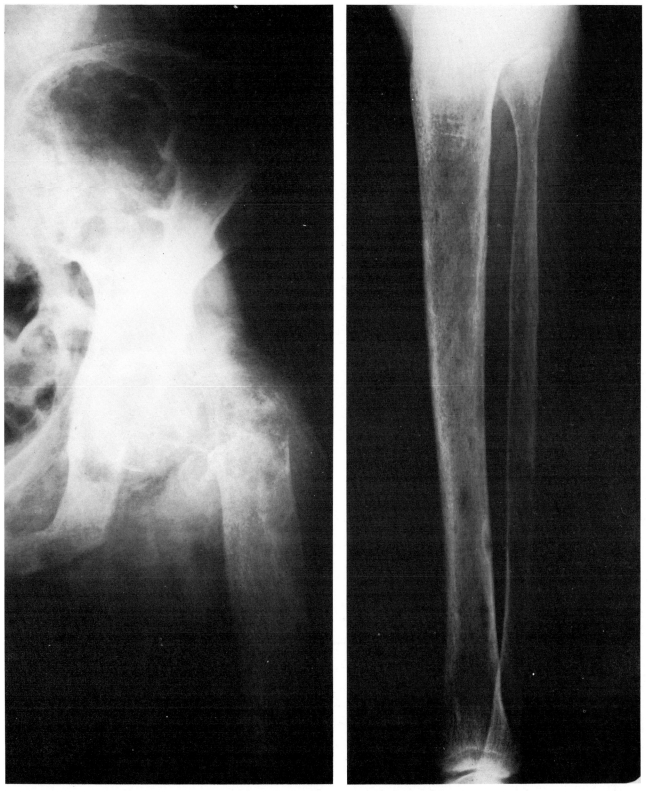

Figs 53.4 & 53.5   Patchy areas of bone loss in the ilium, femur and tibia, with a pathological fracture of the trochanteric region. (H.A.T.F.)

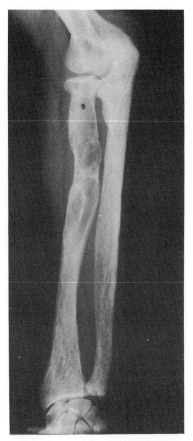

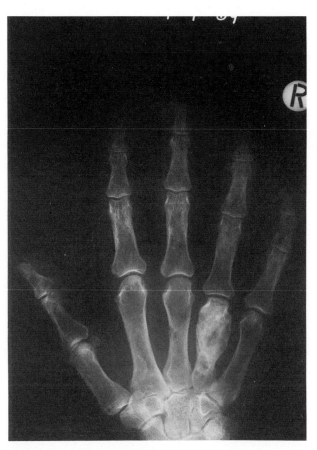

Fig. 53.6 (M.P.) Cystic lesion involving the radius with generalised patchy sclerosis. (H.A.T.F.)

Fig. 53.7 (M.M.) Cystic lesion involving the 4th metacarpal and subperiosteal erosions in several of the phalanges. (Courtesy of Mr J. C. Chalmers, Edinburgh.)

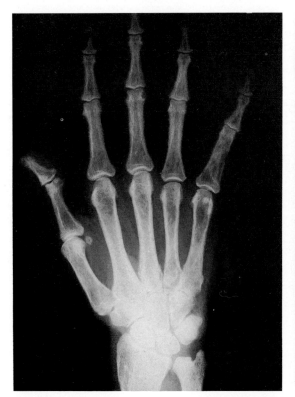

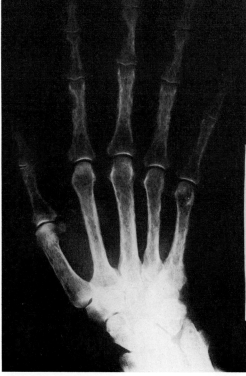

Figs 53.8 & 53.9 (K.T. & L.B.) Early and late signs of hyperparathyroidism in the hands, with sub-periosteal erosions, some resorption of terminal phalanges. (A.H.)

VITAMIN D POISONING

Poisoning from excessive doses of vitamin D is not uncommon. In the past this vitamin was given for a variety of conditions such as rheumatoid arthritis, tuberculosis and chilblains, without there being any real evidence for its value in these diseases. The toxic features of hypercalcaemia due to excessive doses of the vitamin were described by Anning *et al* (1948). At present vitamin D in large doses is used only in the management of hypoparathyroidism, in the 'vitamin D resistant' rickets and sometimes in uraemic osteodystrophy.

Control of vitamin D therapy is difficult because requirements vary from patient to patient and also in the same patient at different times; thus serum calcium estimations are a necessary part of therapy, in order that hypercalcaemia may be detected early. Paterson (1974) notes that toxic signs have seldom been described with doses of less than 1 mg (40,000 iu) per day.

A potential source of danger to the public is the vitamin D fortification of foods. Seelig (1969 and 1970) has noted that in children it has proved difficult to find any level of vitamin D fortification which will consistently prevent both rickets and hypercalcaemia.

Clinical and radiographic features. The presenting signs of vitamin D poisoning are those of hypercalcaemia, with general malaise, weakness, anorexia, vomiting, thirst and polyuria. Abdominal pain and diarrhoea are frequent. The time of onset of symptoms is variable, having been reported within a week or so of starting treatment, or only after many years.

The late complications are nephrocalcinosis, renal failure and ectopic calcification in various sites.

On radiography dense metaphyseal lines are seen, similar to those of lead poisoning, although sometimes there is a more generalised osteosclerosis. In severe cases osteoporosis occurs due to the continued loss of calcium.

Clinical chemistry. The serum calcium is increased but the degree is variable. The serum phosphorus and serum alkaline phosphatase are occasionally low, but more usually normal. Urinary excretion of calcium is increased.

Treatment. This consists of reducing the vitamin D intake, and avoiding vitamin D rich foods and undue exposure to sunlight.

VITAMIN A POISONING

Chronic vitamin A poisoning is rare, though Ruby and Mital (1974) note that it was known, long before vitamin A was discovered, in Arctic explorers who became ill after ingesting polar bear liver. It was Rodahl and Moore (1943) who isolated vitamin A as the toxic factor in the liver.

Skeletal changes are uncommon but transient demineralisation, a wide epiphyseal line and metaphyseal irregularities have been reported. Pathological fractures are uncommon. The patient described by Ruby and Mital (1974) with a 12 year follow up had scoliosis, flexion contractures of the knees and hips, short stature and leg length discrepancy, indicating perhaps premature closure of some epiphyses. The metaphyses were widened and cupped with misshapen epiphyses.

Treatment. This consists of reducing the vitamin A intake.

REFERENCES

Anning, S. T., Dawson, J., Dolby, D. E. & Ingram, J. T. (1948). The toxic effects of calciferol. *Quarterly Journal of Medicine*, **17**, 203.
Paterson, C. R. (1974). In *Metabolic Disorders of Bone*. Oxford: Blackwell.
Rodahl, K. & Moore, T. (1943). The Vitamin A content and toxicity of bear and seal liver. *Biochemical Journal*, **37**, 166.
Ruby, L. K. & Mital, M. A. (1974). Skeletal deformities following chronic hypervitaminosis A. *Journal of Bone & Joint Surgery*, **56A**, 1283.
Seelig, M. S. (1969). Vitamin D and cardiovascular, renal and brain damage in infancy and childhood. *Annals of the New York Academy of Sciences*, **147**, 537.
Seelig, M. S. (1970). Are American children still getting an excess of vitamin D? *Clinical Pediatrics*, **9**, 380.

IDIOPATHIC HYPERCALCAEMIA OF INFANCY

It is likely that this is a syndrome including several different disorders, having in common a general failure to thrive, with hypercalcaemic symptoms of thirst and polyuria, and radiological signs of osteosclerosis.

It was first described by several authors in 1952 (Lightwood, 1952; Payne, 1952; and Fanconi et al, 1952). Since then two main forms of the disease have been differentiated, mild and severe. The former was particularly common in Great Britain and was possibly related to excessive vitamin D intake, perhaps in certain infants with unusual sensitivity to calcium and vitamin D (Paterson, 1974). Skeletal radiographs are usually normal in the mild form, which is therefore not described further here.

SEVERE FORM (FANCONI-SCHLESINGER TYPE)

Aetiology and inheritance. The cause of idiopathic hypercalcaemia is quite unknown. In most cases there is no apparent genetic factor. However, it has been described in monozygous twins, and in sibs, so possibly some cases may be of autosomal recessive inheritance (Manios and Antener, 1966; Dupont et al, 1970). The disorder is frequently present at birth and the possibility of maternal vitamin D intoxication has been explored, but there is no firm evidence to support this theory.

Frequency. This is a rare disorder. Fraser et al (1966) estimated 1 in 150,000 births. The sexes are equally affected. The symptoms in some cases are present at birth but in others the infant appears normal for the first few months of life and the disease develops between the third and sixth months.

Clinical and radiographic features. The main symptoms are of failure to thrive, with symptoms of hypercalcaemia, that is anorexia, vomiting, constipation, thirst and polyuria. In severe cases there is mental retardation and a characteristic facial appearance ('elfin' face, or 'pekinese' face). The forehead is bulging and the ears pointed and low set. The odd appearance of the face, however, is not usually noticed until after the onset of the hypercalcaemia. Frequently there are congenital cardiovascular anomalies, including supravalvular aortic stenosis, coarctation of the aorta, or stenosis of other systemic or pulmonary arteries. The hypercalcaemia is sometimes associated with hypertension (Coleman, 1965). Dental anomalies are common, with absent or small teeth.

Radiological signs are striking, with extensive osteosclerosis usually shown as a banded area within the metaphysis, though sometimes there is a more generalised sclerosis of the long bones. Sclerotic bands also frame the vertebral bodies, and occur in the pelvis, shoulder girdle, ribs and base of the skull. Some patients develop bowing of the long bones and there may be failure of modelling of the metaphyseal area.

Renal calcification may be extensive, as well as calcification in other tissues such as the lungs.

Differential diagnosis. This is from other sclerotic bone lesions, in particular osteopetrosis, heavy metal intoxication, hypervitaminosis A and D (this latter perhaps being given as treatment for rickets). However, the overall clinical picture and raised serum calcium should differentiate these conditions.

Progress and complications. The prognosis of infants with the severe form of the disease is poor and many die within the first few years of life. The cause of death is usually renal failure, or as a result of their cardiovascular anomalies. Those who survive are mentally retarded.

Dupont and colleagues noted that the hypercalcaemia lasts for up to 4 years, but eventually becomes normal, even without treatment. However, by this late stage the physical and radiological signs may be irreversible.

Treatment. This is dietary, with a diet containing a minimum of calcium and vitamin D, the latter being further reduced by avoiding exposure to sunlight. Corticosteroids are of value in the emergency treatment of an acutely hypercalcaemic child.

REFERENCES

Coleman, E. N. (1965). Infantile hypercalcaemia and cardiovascular lesions. *Archives of Disease in Childhood*, **40**, 535.

Dupont, B., Dupont, A., Bliddal, J., Holst, E., Melchior, J. C. & Ottesen, O. E. (1970). Idiopathic hypercalcaemia of infancy: The elfin face syndrome. *Danish Medical Bulletin*, **17**, 33.

Fanconi, G., Girardet, P., Schlesinger, P., Butler, N. & Black, J. (1952). Chronische Hyperkalzämie, kombiniert mit Osteosklerose, Hyperazotaemie, Minderwuchs und kongenitalen Mißbildungen. *Helvetica Paediatrica Acta*, **7**, 314.

Fraser, D., Kidd, B. S. L., Kooh, S. W. & Paunier, L. (1966). A new look at infantile hypercalcaemia. *Pediatric Clinics of North America*, **13**, 503.

Lightwood, R. (1952). Idiopathic hypercalcaemia in infants with failure to thrive. *Archives of Disease in Childhood*, **27**, 302.

Manios, S. G. & Antener, I. (1966). a study of vitamin D metabolism in idiopathic hypercalcaemia of infancy. *Acta Paediatrica Scandinavica*, **55**, 600.

Paterson, C. R. (1974). In *Metabolic Disorders of Bone*. Oxford: Blackwell.

Payne, W. R. (1952). The blood chemistry in idiopathic hypercalcaemia. *Archives of Disease in Childhood*, **27**, 302.

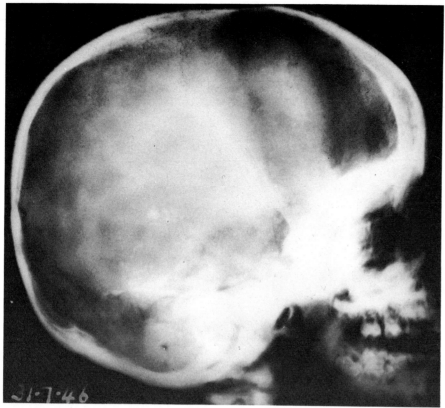

Fig. 53.10   (C.R. aged 19 months.) The osteosclerosis of the vault and base of the skull is striking. (H.A.T.F.)

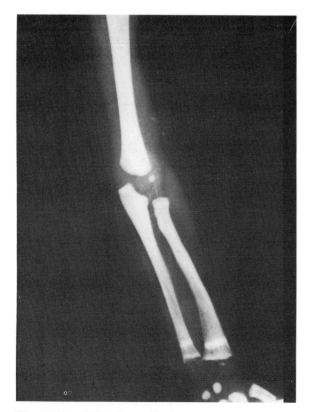

Fig. 53.11   (C.R.) Generalised osteosclerosis of the humerus but at the lower end of the radius and ulna there is a banded area of sclerosis within the metaphysis. (H.A.T.F.)

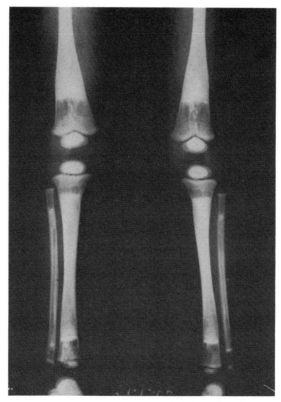

Fig. 53.12   (C.R.) Some general failure of modelling of the metaphyses as well as the sclerotic bands. (H.A.T.F.)

RICKETS AND OSTEOMALACIA

True rickets and osteomalacia are caused by a deficiency of vitamin D, whether dietary together with lack of sunlight, resulting from malabsorption, or due to defects of vitamin D metabolism. The terms 'rickets' and 'osteomalacia' are also traditionally used to describe some of the clinical and radiographic features of the renal tubular disorders and those of severe renal disease and uraemia, although in these instances the pathophysiology is different and there is no evidence to implicate vitamin D. However rickets, osteomalacia and uraemic osteodystrophy are together the commonest causes of hypocalcaemia, and since the radiographic features are similar all three groups are considered together in this chapter. Various specific causes of rickets and osteomalacia are not considered in detail but for convenience they are listed in Table I. Recent reviews of the subject have been by Fourman and Royer (1968), Dent (1970), Smith (1972) and Mankin (1974).

AETIOLOGY
VITAMIN D DEFICIENCY
RICKETS AND OSTEOMALACIA

Nutritional. Lack of vitamin D in the diet may occur at any time of life from the neonatal period (it has even been identified on prenatal radiographs) to old age. Paterson (1974) points out that vitamin D deficiency only occurs in individuals who have *both* a dietary lack of the vitamin *and* inadequate exposure to ultraviolet light. This means that it is commoner in high latitudes, in areas where there is heavy atmospheric pollution and (in the northern hemisphere) between the months of January and April.

Premature infants are particularly at risk since they take insufficient milk to provide an adequate amount of vitamin D. Rickets in the neonatal period is likely to be due to a maternal deficiency of the vitamin. Nutritional rickets in infancy, childhood and adolescence is still seen amongst the white population of overcrowded northern cities, when mothers fail to take advantage of welfare foods, or when perhaps the family is living on the north side of multi-storey blocks of flats where the effort of getting the infant out-of-doors is beyond the mother (Evreux, 1962). However, it is particularly the immigrant population in northern cities who are at risk of developing rickets, where additional factors to diet include skin pigmentation and the tradition of confining girls to the house. Also Preece et al (1973) have shown that Asian immigrants to Britain have lower levels of 25-hydroxycholecalciferol in the serum than do European

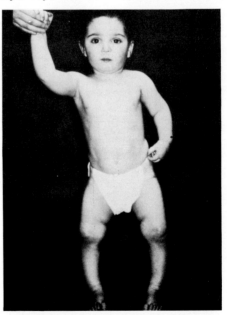

Fig. 54.1   An Indian immigrant to Scotland with nutritional rickets. (P.M.R.)

controls. Rickets in infancy and childhood is, however, a problem throughout the world wherever poverty and overcrowded living conditions are found (Ford *et al*, 1972; Holmes *et al*, 1973).

Vitamin D deficiency in adults (osteomalacia) is particularly likely to occur during pregnancy and

---

TABLE I

CAUSES of RICKETS and OSTEOMALACIA

I. VITAMIN D DEFICIENCY
    Nutritional
    Malabsorption
    (partial gastrectomy
    coeliac disease,
    pancreatic disorders)
    Metabolic defects
    (Renal disease, liver disease,
    anticonvulsant therapy, pseudo-
    vitamin D deficiency rickets)

II. RENAL TUBULAR DISORDERS
    (Phosphorus depletion and acidosis)
    Familial hypophosphataemia
    Cystinosis
    Hereditary tyrosinaemia
    Wilson disease
    Neurofibromatosis
    Metabolic acidosis
    Ureterosigmoidostomy

III. URAEMIC OSTEODYSTROPHY ('renal rickets')
    Undialysed
    With regular haemodialysis

lactation, when there are increased requirements for the vitamin, and again amongst those races which by tradition keep their women confined to the house. The osteomalacia of elderly women of all races is usually nutritional in origin and is not an uncommon disease (Chalmers *et al*, 1967).

Malabsorption. Malabsorption rickets and osteomalacia are associated with many diseases, for example steatorrhoea, pancreatic disease, coeliac disease, Crohn's disease, or in association with obstructive jaundice (vitamin D requires bile salts for its absorption), and there are many factors other than vitamin D contributing to the calcium deficiency. Osteomalacia also occurs after partial gastrectomy, although the reason for this is not clear.

Metabolic defects. Rarely vitamin D deficiency is caused by defective production of 1,25-dihydroxycholecalciferol. This is the probable cause of rickets in some instances of renal and liver disease, and in that produced by long term anti-convulsant therapy for epilepsy (Schmid, 1967; Dent *et al*, 1970; Adair, 1975).

The disease pseudo-vitamin D deficiency rickets belongs with this metabolic group. It is of autosomal recessive inheritance and the clinical and radiographic features are identical with nutritional rickets, but there is no response to physiological doses of the vitamin (Dent, Friedman and Watson, 1968). The disorder is likely to be due to a defect in the hydroxylation of 25-hydroxycholecalciferol to the 1,25-dihydroxycholecalciferol, since it improves rapidly when small doses of the latter are given (Arnaud *et al*, 1970; Balsan and Garabedian, 1974).

acidosis, or associated with the latter only. The bone changes resemble those of true rickets and osteomalacia, but there is no evidence that the underlying defect is due to vitamin D deficiency.

Familial hypophosphataemia is the commonest of the disorders formerly referred to as 'vitamin D resistant rickets'. It is of X-linked dominant inheritance; thus there is a preponderance of female patients who pass the disease on to half their children, while the male patients (who are more severely affected) only pass the disease to their daughters. There is impaired resorption of phosphorus from the renal tubules and this can be detected during the first year of life. Signs of rickets become apparent usually between 2 and 5 years of age, although the severity and age of onset is variable and the disease may not be recognised until adult life. Individuals are of short stature with typical rachitic deformities, but the other clinical features of nutritional rickets (pain, weakness and tetany) are not features of this disease.

Renal tubular acidosis may occur as a primary anomaly with the bone changes of rickets or osteomalacia. The mechanism for this is not fully understood but it is possible that the acidosis promotes excessive phosphorus excretion. It is thought that this is the cause of the rickets or osteomalacia which follows ureterocolic anastomosis.

Cystinosis (formerly called the Fanconi syndrome) also belongs in this group of renal tubular disorders with phosphorus depletion and acidosis. It is of autosomal recessive inheritance and characterised not only by rachitic changes but by the deposition of crystals of cystine in many tissues.

URAEMIC OSTEODYSTROPHY

The aetiology of rickets or osteomalacia associated with chronic renal disease is complicated by many factors which contribute to the disturbance of calcium metabolism (Wills, 1971). The probable mechanisms involved are shown in Figure 54.2. The three elements of the bone changes seen are: rickets or osteomalacia, osteitis fibrosa associated with secondary hyperparathyroidism, and osteosclerosis sometimes accompanied by ectopic calcification. Those patients with chronic renal failure who are on regular haemodialysis have, in addition, a reduction in the calcified bone mass.

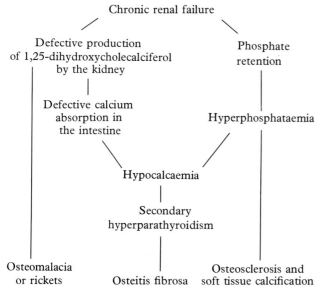

Fig. 54.2 The probable mechanism involved leading to the bone changes in uraemic osteodystrophy. (Courtesy of Dr C. Paterson, University of Dundee.)

RENAL TUBULAR DISORDERS
(Phosphorus depletion and acidosis)

There are a number of renal tubular disorders associated with phosphorus depletion together with

CLINICAL AND RADIOGRAPHIC FEATURES

The clinical features of both rickets and osteomalacia are a consequence of the hypocalcaemia, and which signs appear depend upon the age of onset.

In *infancy* convulsions, tetany or laryngeal spasm, may be the presenting sign. In *older infants* and in *childhood* the first signs are likely to be pain and deformities due to the bending of softened bone and enlargement of bone ends, particularly at the wrists, knees and ankles. Other rachitic features are well known: changes in the costochondral junctions cause the 'rickety rosary', frontal bossing of the skull develops, Harrison's sulcus is caused by softening of the ribs, a groove appearing at the point of attachment of the diaphragm. Bending of the lower limb long bones results in genu valgum or varum.

Late rickets and osteomalacia usually present with bone pain and muscular weakness, and patients often have a characteristic waddling gait. Clinical examination reveals bone tenderness, which may be very severe. The presenting sign of rickets and osteomalacia at any age may be a fracture, and Chalmers *et al* (1967) have noted that green-stick fracture occurring in an adult appears to be unique to osteomalacia. Other symptoms of hypocalcaemia may be a feature of osteomalacia, though tetany only rarely develops. Paresthesiae of the hands and feet may occur, also bradycardia and hypotension. Chronic hypocalcaemia leads to the mental changes of anxiety and depression.

On radiography the characteristic signs of rickets are seen at the ends of long bones, where the epiphyses are widened and separated from the metaphyses by an indistinct, cupped line. Epiphyses are late in appearing and bone is poorly calcified; thus long bones are frequently bent from the weakness of the excessive osteoid. Fractures are also common and there may be accompanying subperiosteal bone formation.

The signs of healing rickets are characteristic in that a dense line of mineralisation appears in the region of metaphyseal cartilage, separate from the metaphysis and subsequent mineralisation then continues between this line and the metaphysis. A ring of calcification, reminiscent of scurvy, may develop around the epiphyseal centres. Healing is complete within a few months of starting treatment, although the frontal bossing of the skull and lower limb deformities may persist to adulthood in severe cases.

The radiographic changes in osteomalacia are usually quite distinctive. Cortical bone is thin but the main features are pseudo-fractures or 'Looser's zones'. These consist of bands of decalcification either right across, or affecting only one side of a bone. They are frequently symmetrical, and the commonest sites are the ribs, the superior and inferior pubic rami and the upper end of the femur. In addition to pseudo-fractures, patients may have genuine fractures, and these too may be symmetrical (Chalmers, 1968). In some patients with osteomalacia the vertebrae have the biconcave shape more typical of osteoporosis, and a few also develop early signs of secondary hyperparathyroidism, resulting from chronic hypocalcaemia, with subperiosteal erosions, particularly in the phalanges.

The radiographic changes of rickets and osteo-

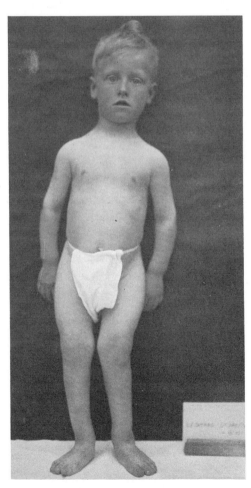
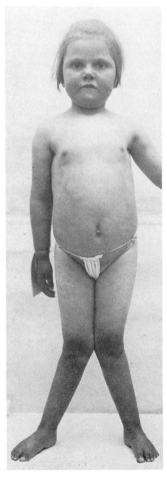

Fig. 54.3 (L.S.) A 7 year old boy with rickets associated with familial hypophosphataemia. (H.A.T.F.)

Fig. 54.4 (S.) 9 year old girl with coeliac rickets. (H.A.T.F.)

malacia associated with the *renal tubular defects* are similar to those of vitamin D deficiency. In *uraemic osteodystrophy* there is a wider range of radiographic findings because the balance of rickets or osteomalacia, secondary hyperparathyroidism and osteosclerosis will vary from one patient to another. There is a general loss of bone density with widening of the epiphyseal regions and associated in children with slipping of epiphyses. The metaphyses are not cupped, as in other forms of rickets. There is subperiosteal resorption of bone in the phalanges and elsewhere, resulting from the secondary hyperparathyroidism, and in some cases these changes affect many bones and are very severe. When osteosclerosis is present this mainly affects the skull, with thickening of the calvarium, maxilla and mandible. The vertebrae may show sclerosis in the upper and lower parts, giving a striped or 'rugger jersey' appearance.

The other feature observed on radiography in chronic renal disease is ectopic calcification, found chiefly along the arteries and in the soft tissues around joints. More rarely it may be seen in subcutaneous tissue, the lungs, kidneys and elsewhere.

Some patients with chronic renal disease on regular haemodialysis develop progressive rarefaction of bone together with pain and fractures (Ritz et al, 1973; and Simpson et al, 1973). The reason for this is not clear, as it appears to be more common in some centres than in others.

PATHOLOGY

The main feature of rickets and osteomalacia is the accumulation of excessive quantities of uncalcified bone matrix (osteoid). In rickets, the growth cartilage is grossly abnormal with failure of calcification, irregular invasion by blood vessels and failure of resorption of that cartilage which does calcify. Proliferation of cartilage cells continues, so that the epiphyseal plate as a whole becomes abnormally wide. Chronic hypocalcaemia leads to secondary hyperparathyroidism and this is accompanied by hyperplasia of these glands.

REFERENCES

Adair, I. V. (1975). Anticonvulsant osteomalacia. *Journal of the Royal College of Surgeons of Edinburgh*, **20**, 380.
Arnaud, C. D., Maijer, R., Reade, T., Scriver, C. R. & Whelan, D. T. (1970). Vitamin D dependency: an inherited postnatal syndrome with secondary hyperparathyroidism. *Pediatrics*, **46**, 871.
Balsan, S. & Garabedian, M. (1974). 1,25-dihydroxycholecalciferol: effect in rachitic children. In *Endocrinology* 1973 ed. Taylor, S. London: Heinemann.
Chalmers, J., Conacher, W. D. H., Gardner, D. L. & Scott, P. J. (1967). Osteomalacia—a common disease in elderly women. *Journal of Bone & Joint Surgery*, **49B**, 403.
Chalmers, J. (1968). Osteomalacia: a review of 93 cases. *Journal of the Royal College of Surgeons of Edinburgh*, **13**, 255.
Dent, C. E., Friedman, M. & Watson, L. (1968). Hereditary pseudo-vitamin D deficiency rickets. *Journal of Bone & Joint Surgery*, **50B**, 708.
Dent, C. E. (1970). Rickets (and osteomalacia) nutritional and metabolic. *Proceedings of the Royal Society of Medicine*, **63**, 401.
Dent, C. E., Richens, A., Rowe, D. J. F. & Stamp, T. C. B. (1970). Osteomalacia with long-term anticonvulsant therapy in epilepsy. *British Medical Journal*, **4**, 69.
Evreux, R. (1962). Le rachitisme dans les grands ensembles. *Revue d'hygiène et de médicine sociale*, **10**, 175.
Ford, J. A., Colhoun, E. M., McIntosh, W. B. & Dunnigan, M. G. (1972). Rickets and osteomalacia in the Glasgow Pakistani Community 1961–71. *British Medical Journal*, **2**, 677.
Fourman, P. & Royer, P. (1968). *Calcium metabolism and the bone*. Oxford: Blackwell Scientific Publications.
Glorieux, F. H., Scriver, C. R., Reade, T. M., Golman, H. & Roseborough, A. (1972). Use of phosphate and vitamin D to prevent dwarfism and rickets in X-linked hypophosphataemia. *New England Journal of Medicine*, **287**, 481.
Holmes, A. M., Enoch, B. A., Taylor, J. L. & Jones, M. E. (1973). Occult rickets and osteomalacia amongst the Asian immigrant population. *Quarterly Journal of Medicine*, **NS42**, 125.
Mankin, H. J. (1974). Rickets, osteomalacia and renal osteodystrophy, Part I. *Journal of Bone & Joint Surgery*, **56A**, 101.
Paterson, C. R. (1974). *Metabolic Disorders of Bone*. Oxford: Blackwell Scientific Publications.
Preece, M. A., Ford, J. A., McIntosh, W. B., Dunnigan, M. G., Tomlinson, S. & O'Riordan, J. L. H. (1973). Vitamin D-deficiency among Asian immigrants to Britain. *Lancet*, **i**, 907.
Ritz, E., Krempien, R., Mehls, O., Malluche, H., Stroebel, Z. & Zimmerman, H. (1973). Skeletal complications of renal insufficiency and maintenance haemodialysis. *Nephron*, **10**, 195.
Schmid, F. (1967). Osteopathien bei antiepileptischer Dauerbehandlung. *Fortschritte der Medezin*, **85**, 381.
Simpson, W., Kerr, D. N. S., Hill, A. V. L. & Siddiqui, J. Y. (1973). Skeletal changes in patients on regular haemodialysis. *Radiology*, **107**, 313.
Smith, R. (1972). The pathophysiology and management of rickets. *Orthopaedic Clinics of North America*, **3**, 601.
Wills, M. R. (1971). *Biochemical consequences of chronic renal failure*. Aylesbury: Harvey, Miller & Medcalf.

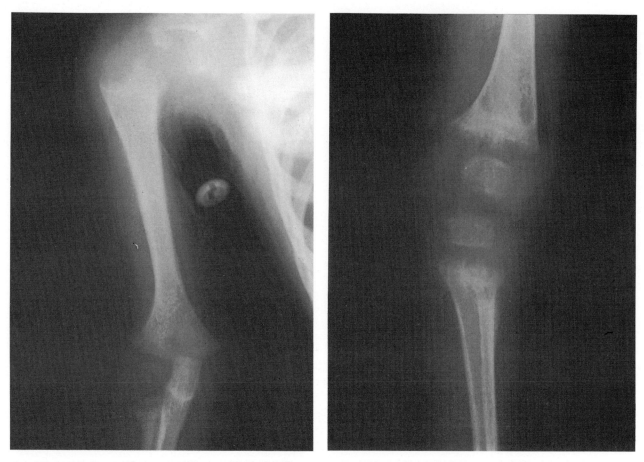

Figs 54.5 & 54.6 (R.W.) Characteristic rachitic changes at the ends of long bones in a 21 month old child. The epiphyses are much widened, late, and there is cupping of the metaphysis with an indistinct edge. (H.A.T.F.)

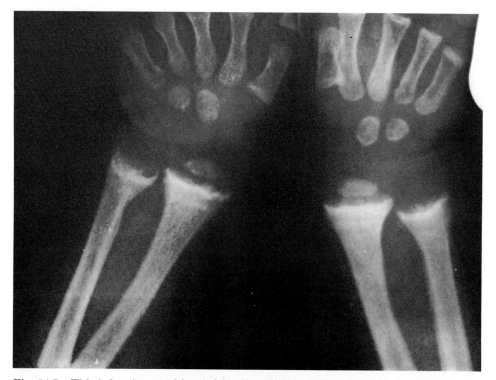

Fig. 54.7 This infant has nutritional rickets in which healing has started. The cupping is still apparent but there is a dense line of mineralisation. (Courtesy of Dr D. McC. Gregg, Cambridge.)

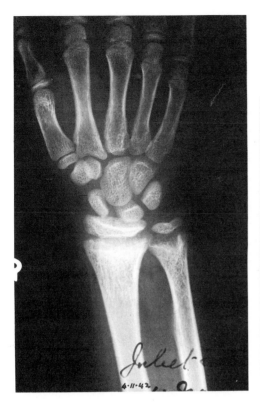
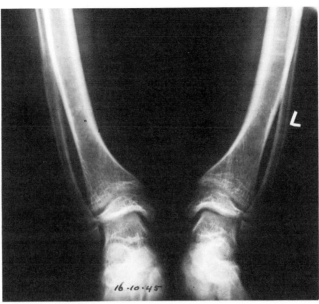

Figs 54.8 & 54.9   (J.S.) Familial hypophosphataemia and rickets in a 5 year old child. The epiphyses are widened and there is bending of bone. (H.A.T.F.)

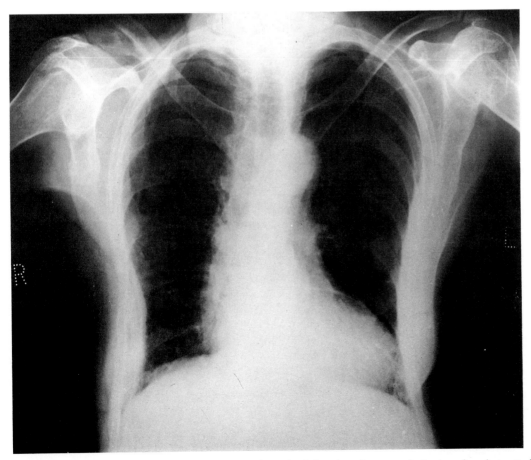

Fig. 54.10   (E.B.) The distinctive bell-shaped thoracic deformity of osteomalacia, in a female treated for years with anticonvulsant therapy. (A.H.)

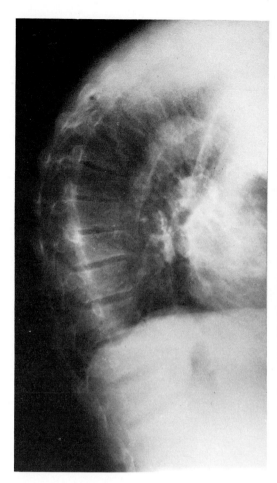

Fig. 54.11   The platyspondyly and thoracic kyphosis typical of osteo-malacia. (A.H.)

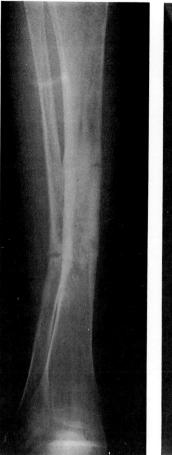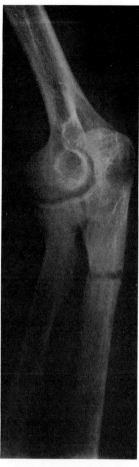

Figs 54.12 & 54.13   (McI.) The cortex of the bone is thin in this patient with osteomalacia and pseudo-fractures are seen in the tibia, fibula and ulna. (H.A.T.F.)

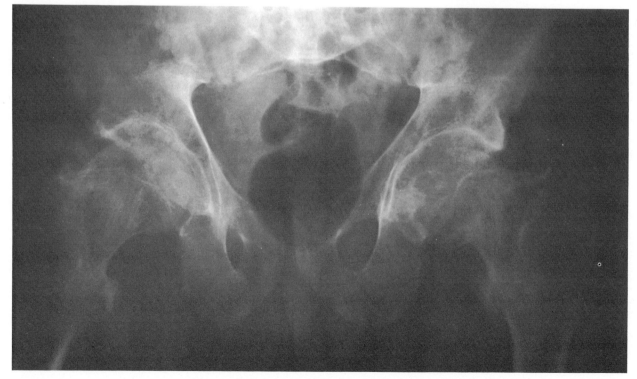

Fig. 54.14   (McI.) Deformed pelvis of osteomalacia with a Looser's zone in the trochanteric region. (H.A.T.F.)

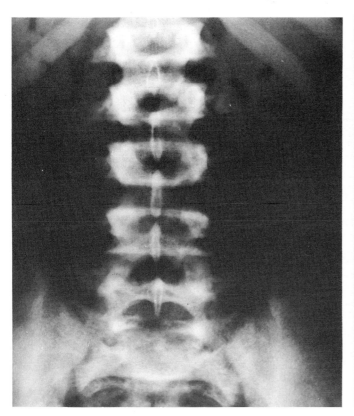

Fig. 54.15 Sclerosis in the upper and lower parts of the vertebral bodies, a feature of uraemic osteodystrophy. (A.H.)

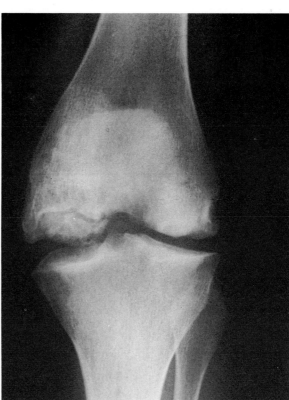

Fig. 54.16 (T.H.) 13 year old female with massive necrosis in the lower femur associated with renal transplantation; three months haemodialysis and immunosuppressive drugs. (A.H.)

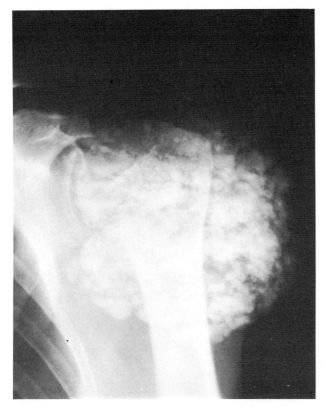

Fig. 54.17 (W.S.) Massive ectopic calcification in the region of the shoulder joint in a patient with chronic renal disease. (Courtesy of Dr D. B. Evans, Cambridge.)

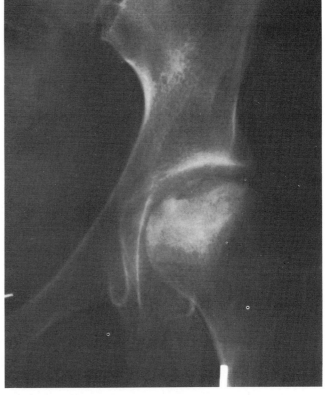

Fig. 54.18 (T.H.) Necrosis of the head of the femur. (Same patient as Fig. 54.16.) (A.H.)

HYPOPARATHYROIDISM AND PSEUDOHYPOPARATHYROIDISM

Hypoparathyroidism is a rare disorder associated with a defect either in parathyroid hormone secretion or in the tissue response to the hormone (pseudo-hypoparathyroidism). The defect in hormone secretion is most usually caused by surgical damage to the glands or their blood supply during neck (particularly thyroid) surgery but hypoparathyroidism can exist, though very rarely, as a separate entity. It may be associated with a polyendocrine deficiency or as an isolated phenomenon. Both these forms are familial, probably of autosomal recessive inheritance, and it is likely there is also an autoimmune element in the aetiology (Paterson, 1974).

The clinical features of hypoparathyroidism are those of hypocalcaemia, though indeed many patients have no symptoms at all. There are no bone symptoms connected with the disease but Gibberd (1965) noted areas of bone sclerosis on radiography, especially in children; in general, however, there are no skeletal findings in hypoparathyroidism and the subject is not discussed further here.

PSEUDOHYPOPARATHYROIDISM

This is a syndrome in which there is a hormone-resistant hypocalcaemia, short stature, obesity, and a round head and face. It is sometimes associated with mental retardation and shortening of the (usually third and fourth) metacarpals.

It was first described by Albright et al (1942) and since then there have been many reports (Garceau and Miller, 1956; Mann, Alterman and Hills, 1962; Geominne, 1965; and Spranger, 1969).

Inheritance. There have been a number of families reported with more than one generation affected and Spranger suggests the disorder is of X-linked dominant inheritance in view of the 2:1 female to male ratio. However, Weinberg and Stone (1972), described father to son transmission and in this instance the disorder must have been of autosomal dominant inheritance. Cederbaum and Lippe (1973) have described a family in which there was autosomal recessive inheritance.

Frequency. The disorder is extremely rare. Females are affected one-and-a-half to twice as often as males. The age at which it becomes manifest is variable, some cases being discovered only incidentally.

Clinical and radiographic features. These individuals are of short stature, obese and with a characteristic round face. Symptoms of hypocalcaemia may appear at any time during infancy or childhood, but Spranger, Langer and Wiedemann (1974) note that these features usually subside with

the cessation of growth, but recur during pregnancy or during other states of increased calcium need. Thus, the characteristic signs of hypocalcaemia (tetany, epilepsy, cataracts, subcutaneous and other ectopic calcification particularly of the basal ganglia, together with mental retardation) may all be features of the syndrome. The hands are usually short and stubby, or there may just be evidence of shortening of one or more metacarpals.

On radiography of the skull, thickening of the calvarium is seen and calcification of the basal ganglia may be present. The only other skeletal feature usually present is shortening of the third and fourth metacarpals and some of the phalanges, due to premature fusion of epiphyses, and the latter may be cone-shaped. The feet show similar changes.

Subcutaneous or other ectopic calcification should be looked for and other features sometimes present are hypoplasia or failure of the teeth to erupt and a short ulna with a curved radius.

Clinical chemistry. The blood changes are those of hypoparathyroidism with hypocalcaemia and hyperphosphataemia. There is unresponsiveness of tubular phosphate reabsorption with infused parathyroid hormone, and no increase of urinary secretion of adenylic kinase following injection of the hormone. In the past a condition called 'pseudo-pseudo-hypoparathyroidism' was reported in which the signs and symptoms were identical with those of the originally described Albright form of the disease, but the serum calcium was normal. However, it is now thought that these are only variants of the same disease, individual patients on occasion being normocalcaemic (Jancar, 1965).

Differential diagnosis. The fully developed syndrome of pseudohypoparathyroidism is unlikely to be mistaken for any other disease. The metacarpal shortening may be seen in the Turner syndrome (XO) or sometimes as an isolated feature, sporadic or of autosomal dominant inheritance. Ectopic calcification is seen in many disorders but none of these have the other features of pseudohypoparathyroidism.

Progress and complications. The main complications of this disease are related to the hypocalcaemia, particularly the tetany and epilepsy. In some instances the parathyroid glands become hyperplastic and secondary hyperparathyroidism with radiographic evidence of subperiosteal bone resorption may develop. The final height of these patients is between 114 and 160 cm (3'9" to 5'3").

Treatment. The treatment is as for hypoparathyroidism, that is, vitamin D. Not only does this relieve the tetany and epilepsy but mental development becomes more normal and, provided treatment is instituted early, it is likely that growth is improved (Alterman and Leiber, 1965).

REFERENCES

Albright, F., Burnett, C. H., Smith, P. H. & Parson, W. (1942). Pseudo-hypoparathyroidism: example of 'Seabright-bantam syndrome'; report of 3 cases. *Endocrinology*, **30**, 922.
Alterman, S. L. & Leiber, A. K. (1965). Albright's hereditary osteodystrophy. *Annals of Internal Medicine*, **63**, 140.

Cederbaum, S. D. & Lippe, B. M. (1973). Probable autosomal recessive inheritance in a family with Albright's hereditary osteodystrophy and an evaluation of the genetics of the disorder. *American Journal of Human Genetics*, **25**, 638.

Garceau, G. J. & Miller, W. E. (1956). Osteochondrodystrophy as a result of or in relation to pseudo-hypoparathyroidism. *Journal of Bone & Joint Surgery*, **38A**, 131.

Gibberd, F. B. (1965). Idiopathic hypoparathyroidism with unusual bone changes and spastic paraplegia. *Acta Endocrinologica*, **48**, 23.

Goeminne, L. (1965). Albright's hereditary poly-osteochondrodystrophy (pseudo-pseudo-hypoparathyroidism with diabetes, hypertension, arteritis and polyarthrosis). *Acta Geneticae Medicae et Gemellolgiae*, **14**, 226.

Jancar, J. (1965). Cerebro-metacarpo-metatarsal dystrophy (pseudo-pseudo-hypoparathyroidism) with chromosome anomaly. *Journal of Medical Genetics*, **2**, 32.

Mann, J. B., Alterman, S. & Hills, A. G. (1962). Albright's hereditary osteodystrophy comprising pseudohypoparathyroidism and pseudo-pseudo hypoparathyroidism, with a report of two cases representing the complete syndrome occurring in successive generations. *Annals of Internal Medicine*, **56**, 315.

Paterson, C. R. (1974). *Metabolic Disorders of Bone*. Oxford: Blackwell.

Spranger, J. W. (1969). Skeletal dysplasias and the eye: Albright's hereditary osteodystrophy. *Birth Defects Original Article: Series 5*, Part 4, 122.

Spranger, J. W., Langer, L. O. & Wiedemann, H. R. (1974). *Bone Dysplasias: An Atlas of Constitutional Disorders of Skeletal Development*. W. B. Saunders Company, Philadelphia, Toronto.

Weinberg, A. G. & Stone, R. T. (1972). Autosomal dominant inheritance in Albright's osteodystrophy. *Journal of Pediatrics*, **79**, 996.

TUBULAR STENOSIS WITH PERIODIC HYPOCALCAEMIA
(Kenny–Caffey Syndrome)

This very rare disease (described by Kenny and Linarelli, 1966; and Caffey, 1967) is characterised by dwarfism, dense long bones with a thickened cortex and reduced width of marrow cavities. It is a cause of hypocalcaemia in infancy, and the low serum calcium, together with hyperphosphataemia tends to recur later in life, particularly during periods of stress.

The disease has been described in a mother and son, and hence is probably of doninant inheritance.

Radiographic signs are apparent in the skull, where the diploic space is absent and there is delayed closure of the fontanelles. In the long bones there is sclerosis of the shafts, but the overall diameter of the bones is reduced. The epiphyses and metaphyses are unaffected.

The complications of the disease are associated with the hypocalcaemia, that is convulsions and laryngeal spasm in infancy, and at a later age carpopedal spasm, tetany and more frequently, paraesthesiae.

REFERENCES

Caffey, J. (1967). Congenital stenosis of medullary spaces in tubular bones and calvaria in two disproportionate dwarfs, mother and son, coupled with transitory hypocalcaemic tetany. *American Journal of Roentgenology*, **100**, 1.

Kenny, F. M. & Linarelli, L. (1966). Dwarfism and cortical thickening of tubular bones. Transient hypocalcaemia in a mother and son. *American Journal of Diseases of Children*, **111**, 201.

55　Metabolic Bone Disease with Bone Loss

OSTEOPOROSIS

In osteoporosis the bone mass is reduced, but what bone remains is of apparently normal structure. It is clear that bone loss is a universal process with ageing, resulting in the so-called 'senile' or 'primary' osteoporosis. 'Secondary' osteoporosis is the term used when there is some additional, sometimes well recognised, cause superimposed on this ageing process. The skeletal manifestations of both primary and secondary osteoporosis differ in no way from each other.

BONE LOSS ASSOCIATED WITH AGEING

The fractures associated with thin bones in elderly women are the most obvious manifestation of senile osteoporosis. All individuals lose bone with advancing age, though women to a greater extent and starting at an earlier age (40–50 years) than men (50–60 years). There have been many epidemiological studies of different populations which confirm these observations (Garn, Rohmann and Wagner, 1967; Newton-John and Morgan, 1970; Ellis and Peart, 1972).
Clinical and radiographic features. The only symptoms of osteoporosis are those resulting from fractures which may occur from quite trivial falls or strains, and the most usual sites are the vertebrae, the femoral neck and trochanteric region, and the distal radius. Backache from one or more vertebral compression fractures is common, the symptoms from any one incident lasting some weeks. Loss of height may be noticed and some minor degree of scoliosis or kyphosis is usual.

On radiography the appearance of the thin osteoporotic bone and associated fractures is well known, though the presence or absence of fractures is a poor guide to the bone mass in any individual patient.
Assessment of bone mass. It is likely that some 30 to 60 per cent of bone mass must be lost before it is visible on simple radiography. Innumerable methods of densitometry or measurements of cortical thickness have been devised in an attempt accurately to assess the bone mass in the living patient, but there are many difficulties. Allowance has to be made not only for variable radiographic technique but also for soft tissue effects. For this reason, the methods devised using peripheral bones such as a metacarpal are likely to be more reliable than those for measuring the vertebrae—though it is usually here that the osteo-

porosis is more in evidence (Morgan *et al,* 1967; Oeser and Krokowski, 1963).

Biopsy and histological assessment of bone provides no more reliable information than does radiology and is not therefore indicated. The problem of histological assessment is that results are variable in any one patient, even from different areas of the same bone (Ellis and Peart, 1972).
Pathology. The reasons for loss of bone with ageing are still far from clear. It is likely that several factors contribute, but in view of the more severe loss in menopausal women it is probable that changes in the balance of oestrogens and androgens are the most significant factor. It is well known that inactivity and immobilisation also contribute to osteoporosis, and these may be associated factors in the elderly. Many other theories of the cause of osteoporosis have been put forward, relating for example, to deficiency of vitamin D, fluoride or calcium. It is unlikely that calcium deficiency can be the universal cause of bone loss with ageing, since individuals on diets low in calcium develop increased intestinal absorption of it. If indeed hormonal changes are relevant, the mechanism is still not understood.
Treatment. Management of osteoporosis can only be symptomatic relating to the fractures, since no specific treatment is available for symptomless patients which will restore bone mass or prevent its continuing loss. Many drugs have been tried, for example phosphates, diphosphonates, oestrogen and anabolic steroids, but although these can cause calcium retention there is no evidence that this retained calcium goes into the bones (Riggs *et al,* 1972). Even when the cause of the (secondary) osteoporosis is known, the bone loss is irreversible.

The management of osteoporotic patients should exclude secondary causes of bone loss such as metastatic neoplasm and osteomalacia, and advice should be given relating to the avoidance of trauma and heavy lifting, as well as to the opposite danger of inactivity.

SECONDARY OSTEOPOROSIS

There are many known causes of reduction in the calcified bone mass but their skeletal manifestations are in no way different from those of bone loss associated with ageing. Several of these diseases have been discussed elsewhere in this book and they are only listed here for convenience:

CAUSES OF SECONDARY OSTEOPOROSIS

Endocrine disorders:
Hyperparathyroidism
Hyperthyroidism
Hypogonadism
Glucocorticoid excess (including steroid therapy)

Generalised bone dysplasias:
Osteogenesis imperfecta
Homocystinuria
Idiopathic juvenile osteoporosis
Turner syndrome (XO chromosome anomaly)

Metabolic and other disorders:
Osteomalacia
Vitamin C deficiency
Alcoholism and liver disease
Intestinal malabsorption and partial gastrectomy
Uraemia with regular haemodialysis
Heparin therapy

REFERENCES

Ellis, H. A. & Peart, K. M. (1972). Quantitative observations on mineralized and non-mineralized bone in the iliac crest. *Journal of Clinical Pathology*, **25**, 277.
Garn, S. M., Rohmann, C. G. & Wagner, B. (1967). Bone loss as a general phenomenon in man. *Federation Proceedings*, **26**, 1729.
Morgan, D. B., Spiers, F. W., Pulvertaft, C. N. & Fourman, P. (1967). The amount of bone in the metacarpal and the phalanx according to age and sex. *Clinical Radiology*, **18**, 101.
Newton-John, H. F. & Morgan, D. B. (1970). Osteoporosis: disease or senescence? *Lancet*, **i**, 232.
Oeser, H. & Krokowski, E. (1963). Quantitative analysis of inorganic substances in the body. A method using X-rays of different qualities. *British Journal of Radiology*, **36**, 274.
Riggs, B. L., Jowsey, J., Kelly, P. J. & Hoffman, D. L. (1972). Treatment for postmenopausal and senile osteoporosis. *Medical Clinics of North America*, **56**, 989.

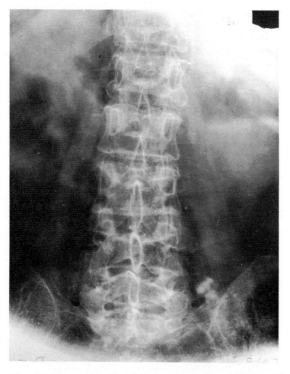
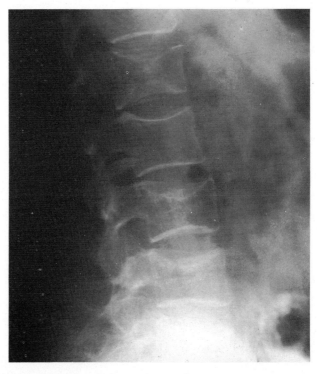

Figs 55.1 & 55.2 The thin bone of osteoporosis with characteristic biconcave vertebrae and compression fractures shown in the lateral view. (H.A.T.F.)

VITAMIN C DEFICIENCY (Scurvy)

This generalised disorder affecting the skeleton and connective tissue is due to lack of vitamin C in the diet. In the growing child there is osteoporosis and characteristic changes in the metaphyses and epiphyses, as well as capillary fragility and bleeding from mucous membrane surfaces and the periosteum. In the adult the only effect on the skeleton is of some bone loss.

Aetiology. Vitamin C is needed for the hydroxylation of proline to hydroxyproline, and without it there is a deficiency of collagen production: thus symptoms and signs arise both in bone and soft connective tissue.

Age of onset. Scurvy is rare in children under the age of 6 months, the child being protected from vitamin C deficiency by its mother during the first few months of life.

Clinical and radiographic features. These infants are usually ill-nourished and may also be suffering from nutritional rickets. In severe cases (and also in cases of adult scurvy), there is spontaneous bleeding from mucous membranes, or haemorrhages from any site. Subperiosteal haematomata form easily and the swelling, severe pain and extreme tenderness are striking and characteristic features of this disease. Pathological fractures and epiphyseal separation frequently occur and are slow in healing.

The radiographic signs in infancy are quite distinctive. There is a so-called 'white line', an area of increased density of the metaphysis immediately adjacent to the epiphyseal plate, and also around the periphery of ossification centres. Apart from this dense white line, there is decreased bone density and the bone cortex is thin. On the diaphyseal side of the metaphyseal white line there is an area of increased translucency (the zone of attrition), and it is in this area of weakened bone that fractures occur from minimal trauma.

Another characteristic radiographic sign of scurvy in childhood is the stripping of loose periosteum from the long bones associated with subperiosteal haemato-

mata. These haematomata are large, extend around the whole shaft of the long bones and layers of calcification develop rapidly in them.

Differential diagnosis. The fully developed picture of scurvy is unlikely to be mistaken for any other disease, but in some cases the battered baby syndrome needs to be considered (though indeed both conditions may be coexistent). A baby subjected to physical maltreatment has perhaps multiple localised lesions rather than a generalised bone disturbance, and although a localised lesion will be painful, he does not suffer from the agonising pain of scurvy. The battered baby syndrome may occur at any age up to about 3 years, whereas scurvy is uncommon before the age of 6 months. On radiography there is no metaphyseal white line, osteoporosis, or zone of attrition. A point of some medico-legal importance is that in a battered baby the skeletal lesions (when there is more than one) may be obviously consecutive, in that one fracture may be fresh and others in different stages of healing; also other signs of physical maltreatment may be apparent.

Infantile cortical hyperostosis is more obviously an inflammatory disorder than scurvy, the child having general malaise, fever, leucocytosis and a raised sedimentation rate. In both disorders there is subperiosteal calcification but in infantile cortical hyperostosis this does not extend as far as the epiphyseal plate.

Congenital syphilis is now of great rarity but in the past was not uncommonly confused with scurvy. In both conditions the ends of long bones are enlarged and tender, there is pseudo-paralysis and subperiosteal new bone formation. However, the osteochondritis of congenital syphilis is not usually seen after the fifth month, whereas scurvy is rare before the age of 6 months. Other syphilitic lesions may be present (Chapter 59) and the diagnosis is confirmed by a positive Wassermann reaction in the mother and child.

Treatment. The treatment of scurvy is specific and consists of giving large doses of vitamin C.

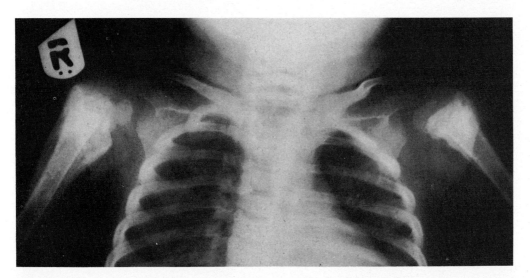

Fig. 55.3 (T.) Infant of 11 months with scurvy. The bone cortex is thin and the upper humerus shows stripping of the loose periosteum and associated calcification of the haematoma. (H.A.T.F.)

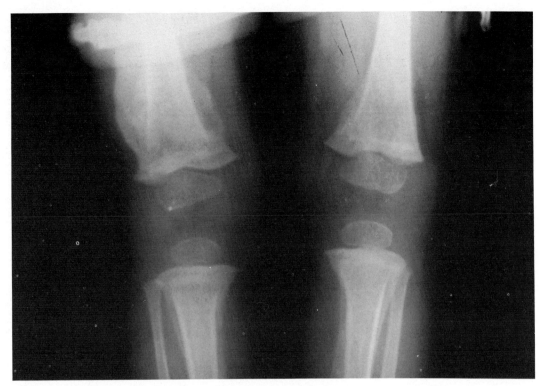

Fig. 55.4 (D.P.) Calcified subperiosteal haematomata are again apparent and there is a line of increased density of the metaphysis immediately adjacent to the epiphyseal plate. (Courtesy of Mr A. G. Apley, Pyrford.)

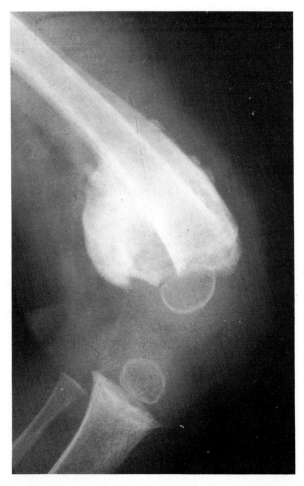

Fig. 55.5 Epiphyseal separation at the lower end of the femur; there is a white line around the epiphyses and calcification of a large subperiosteal haematoma. (Courtesy of Mr A. G. Apley, Pyrford.)

SECTION V

ENDOCRINE DISORDERS

PITUITARY OVERACTION

The skeletal findings associated with an overacting pituitary gland depend on the age at which the disorder develops.

GIGANTISM

Gigantism occurs when the overacting pituitary develops in a child before the epiphyses have closed. In this instance not only is there increased periosteal bone growth but epiphyseal bone formation as well and individuals of 8′ and 9′ tall have been reported. The condition is extremely rare and apart from the increased size, there is little of note in the radiographic appearances.

ACROMEGALY

This is a disorder in which hyperpituitarism develops in the adult, after the epiphyses have joined. It may occur in a young adult but is more likely to develop after the third decade. Since overgrowth of bone cannot occur at the (now fused) epiphyseal plates, the skeletal signs relate to increased periosteal bone growth and affect mainly the skull, mandible, hands and feet.

The onset of the disease is usually insidious, with gradual enlargement of the hands and feet, and sometimes symptoms of severe headache, ocular paresis and paraesthesiae. The enlarged skull with a particularly large mandible are striking and the facial features become heavy and oedematous with thickening of the skin and eversion of the lower lip. The enlarged mandible projects forwards so that normal occlusion of the teeth is impossible. The tongue also enlarges, the voice deepens, and there may be exophthalmos. Other clinical features are an increased anteroposterior diameter of the chest, and thickened clavicles. The enlarged hands and feet are characteristic, particularly the thickening of the terminal phalanges.

On radiography the skull is diffusely thickened, particularly the zygomatic arches and malar bones and there is frontal hyperostosis, prominence of the supraorbital ridges, and a large mandible with a more obtuse angle than normal. The sella turcica may be enlarged due to neoplastic or other pathological changes in the pituitary gland.

In the spine the intervertebral discs are sometimes outlined by new bone on their anterior and lateral surfaces and the bodies of the lumbar vertebrae are concave posteriorly; the spinal canal is not usually encroached upon. The ribs are widened, leading to the increased antero-posterior diameter of the chest (Murray and Jacobson, 1974).

The appendicular skeleton shows increased periosteal bone apposition and surface markings are accentuated. Occasionally there appears to be actual lengthening of bone. Although the total bone width is increased, the cortical thickness is little changed. All bones of the hands and feet are enlarged, and there is tufting of the terminal phalanges.

Clinical chemistry. In acromegaly there is an increased rate of both formation and resorption of bone, but there is no evidence of reduced bone mass and pathological fractures are not a feature (Paterson, 1974). The plasma phosphorus may be high, related to an increased renal tubular reabsorption. Serum calcium is normal or only slightly raised. The urinary calcium is often high and may result in renal calculi.

Progress. The rate of progression of the disease is very variable, and it may remain stationary for years. The principal skeletal complication is secondary osteoarthritis.

PITUITARY INSUFFICIENCY

Deficiency of growth hormone leads to retardation of skeletal maturation, with shortness of stature and failure of fusion of epiphyses, even in adult life. Patients have reduced absorption of calcium from the intestine and reduced urinary calcium excretion. The plasma levels are usually normal.

Apart from the failure of maturation there is little of note to find in the skeleton.

REFERENCES

Duncan's Diseases of Metabolism (1969). 6th Edition. *Genetics and Metabolism*. Ed. Bandy, P. K. & Rosenberg, L. E. W. B. Saunders Company, Philadelphia, London, Toronto.

Murray, R. O. & Jacobson, H. G. (1971). *The Radiology of Skeletal Disorders*. Edinburgh: Churchill Livingstone.

Paterson, C. R. (1974). *Metabolic Disorders of Bone*. Oxford: Blackwell.

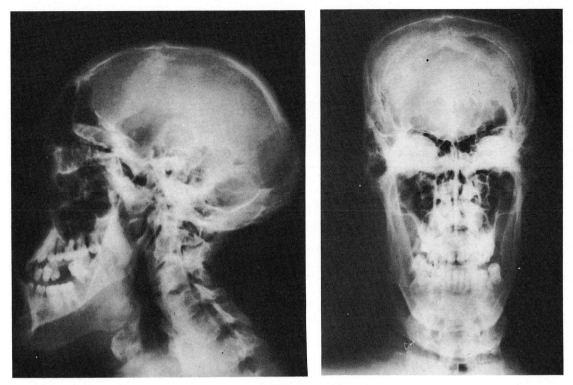

Figs 56.1 & 56.2   (E.E.) The final height of this male with gigantism was 9′3½″. (H.A.T.F.)

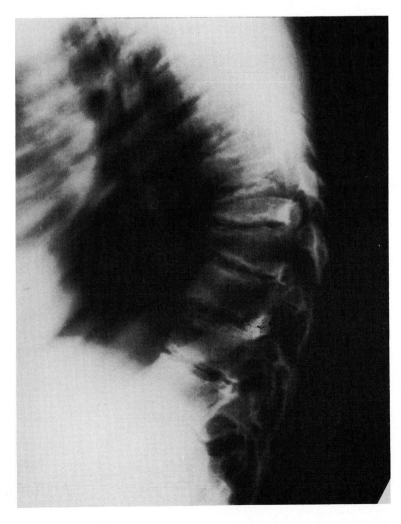

Fig. 56.3   (F.S.) There is mild kyphosis and non-specific epiphisitis in gigantism. (H.A.T.F.)

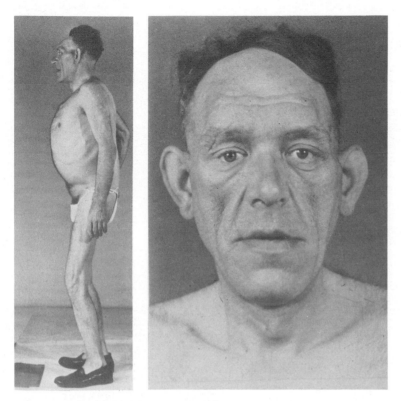

Figs 56.4 & 56.5 (T.J.) The facial features are heavy, the skull large and there is a marked increase in the antero-posterior diameter of the chest. (Male with acromegaly.) (H.A.T.F.)

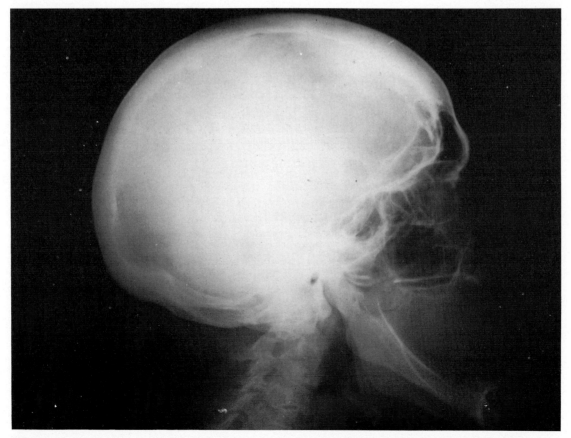

Fig. 56.6 (M.H.) There is diffuse thickening of the skull and a large mandible with an obtuse angle. (Female with acromegaly.) (A.H.)

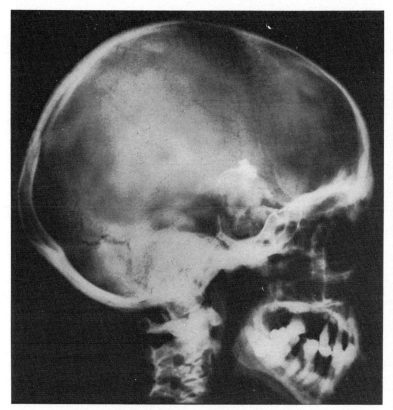

Fig. 56.7 (A.P.) Male aged 46 years with pituitary dwarfism. Enlargement of the pituitary fossa can be seen with a calcified tumour within it. (H.A.T.F.)

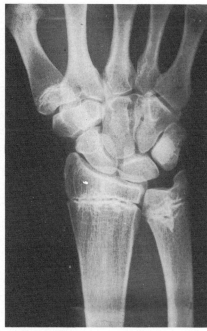

Fig. 56.8 (A.P.) The lower radial and ulnar epiphyses are still not united at the age of 46 years. (H.A.T.F.)

HYPERTHYROIDISM

In hyperthyroidism the principal effect on bone is that of loss; although there is an increase both in bone formation and resorption, the latter is the greater. This fact, however, does not usually contribute to the signs and symptoms of the disease and there are no major radiological features. Pathological fractures are uncommon.

HYPOTHYROIDISM IN CHILDREN

In the hypothyroidism of children (cretinism) there may be severe changes in the skeleton. The insufficiency of thyroid hormones leads to reduction in bone formation and resorption, and there is delay in skeletal maturation with abnormal epiphyses and defective bone modelling.

Aetiology. The defective synthesis of thyroid hormones is not usually genetic in origin, though the rare Pendred syndrome, in which goitre is accompanied by deafness, is of autosomal recessive inheritance.

Age of onset. This is variable: the disease may become apparent in very early infancy or at any time during childhood. The clinical features and radiographic appearances vary with the age of onset and the severity of the disease.

Clinical and radiographic features. The presenting symptoms are of apathy, sluggishness and constipation. The abdomen is large and there is a subnormal temperature and dry skin. Herniae are common. As the child develops it becomes apparent that there is mental retardation, shortness of statute and generalised hypotonia.

On radiography, in the infant there is delayed closure of fontanelles and delayed appearance of all epiphyses, which, when they do appear, are irregular, stippled and fragmented. The long bones show cortical thickening with a narrowed medullary cavity.

In the older child the thickened cranial vault is obvious, and the vertebrae show persistence of the infantile biconvex shape. There is irregularity and failure of development of the anterosuperior part of the vertebrae at the thoracolumbar junction, giving a hook-shaped appearance. The vertebrae are small and angular kyphosis develops at this site. Irregular and retarded epiphyseal ossification is obvious throughout childhood and there may be some increased density in the metaphyseal region.

In the rare case of the adult untreated cretin, the individual is severely dwarfed with scoliosis, persistent, unjoined epiphyses and often severe osteoarthritis due to disorganisation of the articular surfaces.

Pathology and clinical chemistry. The thyroid hormones appear to affect bone cells directly, permitting bone resorption (Vaughan, 1970). There is a reduction in blood flow to bone with reduced formation and resorption.

The serum calcium and phosphorus levels are usually normal. Positive laboratory findings include a low serum protein bound iodine and thyroxin and a decreased I^{131} uptake.

Differential diagnosis. Cretinism can be confused with those skeletal dysplasias which affect the epiphyses, for example, multiple epiphyseal dysplasia, spondylo-epiphyseal dysplasia, cranio-cleido dysostosis and pycnodysostosis. In the young child the hip changes are similar to those of Perthes' disease, or again, to multiple epiphyseal dysplasia. The characteristic hook-shaped vertebrae at the thoracolumbar junction occur in the mucopolysaccharidoses and mucolipidoses. However, cretinism should be readily distinguished on general clinical and laboratory findings, so long as the possibility of a diagnosis of thyroid insufficiency is borne in mind.

Progress and complications. The untreated cretin is severely mentally retarded and dwarfed. Other complications which arise are scoliosis or kyphosis, spondylolisthesis and slipped upper femoral epiphyses (this may be the presenting sign of cretinism developing in later childhood). Some individuals have hypercalcaemia which may lead to metastatic calcification and renal calculi (Adams et al, 1968; Pretorius, 1971).

Treatment. The essential treatment is thyroid hormone. Treatment of skeletal complications is related to the scoliosis, spondylolisthesis, slipped epiphyses and secondary arthritis.

REFERENCES

Adams, P., Chalmers, T. M., Riggs, B. L. & Jones, J. D. (1968). Parathyroid function in spontaneous primary hypothyroidism. *Journal of Endocrinology*, **40,** 467.
Murray, R. O. & Jacobson, H. G. (1971). *The Radiology of Skeletal Disorders*. Edinburgh: Churchill Livingstone.
Paterson, C. R. (1974). *Metabolic Disorders of Bone*. Oxford: Blackwell.
Pretorius, P. J. & Potgieter, M. de J. (1971). Hypothyroidism and hypercalcaemia: report of a cretin showing manifestations of idiopathic infantile hypercalcaemia. *South African Medical Journal*, **45,** 753.
Vaughan, J. M. (1970). *The Physiology of Bone*. Oxford: Oxford University Press.

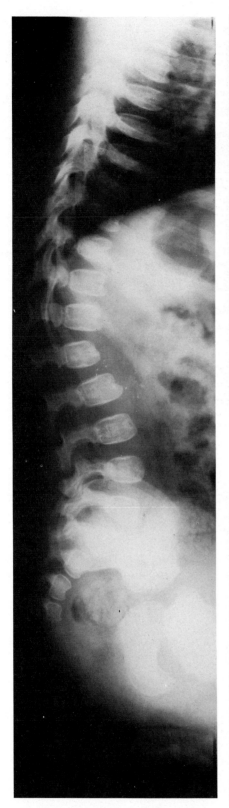

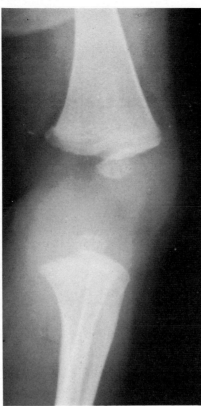

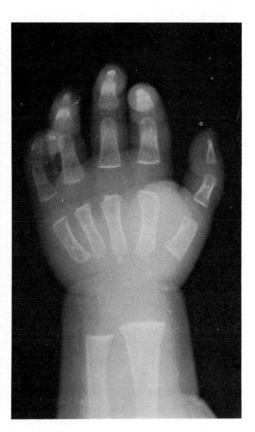

Figs 57.2 & 57.3   (P.R.) Delayed and rather irregular
epiphyses in this 27 month old child. (A.H.)

Fig. 57.1   The thoraco-lumbar kyphos
of cretinism, the broad hook-shaped
vertebrae at this level being similar
to the mucopolysaccharidoses
(H.A.T.F.)

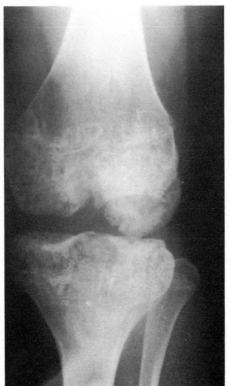

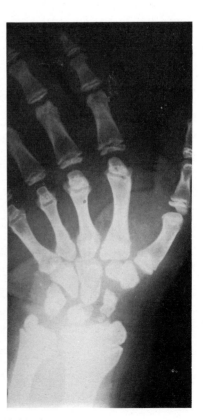

Figs 57.4 & 57.5   (C.C.) Adult untreated cretinism in a
male aged 31 years. He had only intermittent treatment
for a 3 year period in early childhood. The epiphyses are
mottled and still un-united. (A.H.)

58　Adrenals

There are no significant generalised skeletal changes in adrenal insufficiency, whether of the cortex or medulla. Diseases of the latter are only of occasional interest in this connection when a neuroblastoma presents with multiple bone secondaries and no other manifestations.

The adrenal cortex produces a number of steroid compounds of which cortisol and aldosterone, testosterone and oestrogens are the most important. A recent review is by Nabarro and Brook (1975). Only the first of these steroids, if present in excess in the body, produces major generalised skeletal changes. An excess of androgens is the cause of the dwarfism seen in infantile and pre-pubertal hypercorticism, by producing premature fusion of the epiphyses.

The name glucocorticoid was given to cortisol and its synthetic analogues because of their ability to promote gluconeogenesis and raise serum glucose levels.

GLUCOCORTOID EXCESS

Excess of the glucocorticoids may have a variety of causes, such as an adrenal cortical tumour, hyperplasia of the gland following excessive production of corticotrophin by the anterior pituitary, or by therapy with corticosteroids, corticotrophin or similar drugs, and occasionally by tumours elsewhere secreting an ACTH-like peptide.

Pathology and clinical chemistry. Whatever the reason for the glucocorticoid excess, there is an increase in bone resorption and a decrease in bone formation. The action of these steroid hormones is not fully understood, though it is known that the glucocorticoids reduce calcium absorption from the intestine. It is likely also that reabsorption of calcium from the renal tubules is diminished since many patients have hypercalcinuria. The serum calcium is usually normal.

Clinical and radiographic features. The symptoms and signs of this disorder are those of osteoporosis (Chapter 55). Because there is a diminished amount of bone, the presenting sign is often a pathological fracture, most commonly in the thoracic or lumbar spine, so that backache is frequently a symptom. However, backache in these patients is often severe even with no radiological evidence of a vertebral fracture. In addition to osteoporosis, patients who have had long continued corticosteroid treatment may develop collapse of the femoral head as a result of avascular necrosis and degeneration here. This is particularly likely to occur with the high steroid doses given for immunosuppression following renal transplantation. The most obvious radiographic sign is of decreased density of the skeleton, sometimes cortical bone being less affected than trabecular bone. Rarely, enlargement of the pituitary fossa is seen in cases where the glucocorticoid excess is due to a tumour of the pituitary gland.

In infants with adrenal hyperplasia and glucocorticoid excess, their weight is excessive but growth is otherwise retarded. Pathological fractures are frequent and on radiography the bones are seen to be thin and ossification of epiphyses delayed (Darling, Loridan and Senior, 1970).

Following treatment of infants and children with glucocorticoid excess, Paterson (1974) notes that the thin bone previously laid down persists, although the new bone is of normal appearance. In adults there is no evidence that the bone loss is reversible with treatment, or with cessation of steroid therapy.

REFERENCES

Darling, D. B., Loridan, L. & Senior, B. (1970). The roentgenographic manifestations of Cushing's syndrome in infancy. *Radiology*, **96**, 503.
Nabarro, N. & Brook, C. (1975). Diseases of the adrenal cortex. *Medicine*, **8**, 351.
Paterson, C. R. (1974). *Metabolic Disorders of Bone*. Oxford: Blackwell.

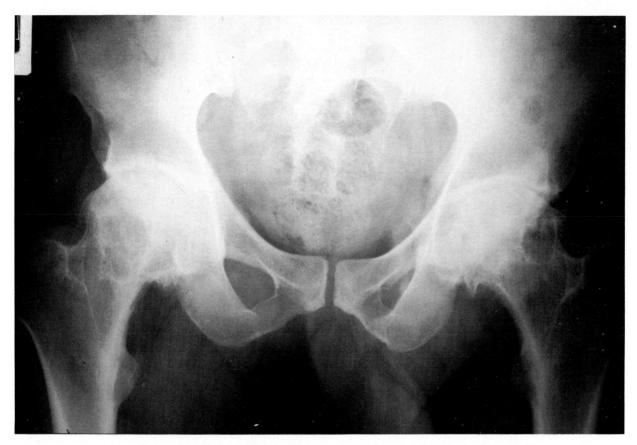

Fig. 58.1 (I.S. aged 43 years.) 10 years of corticosteroid therapy for asthma, resulting in necrosis of the femoral head. (A.H.) (See also Figs 54.16 and 54.18.)

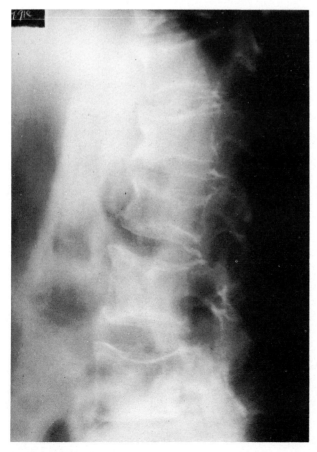

Fig. 58.2 (M.E.) The radiographic signs of glucocorticoid excess and osteoporosis, seen here in the vertebrae. (A.H.)

SECTION VI

INFECTIONS, TOXINS, BLOOD DYSCRASIAS NEOPLASIA AND TRAUMA

SYPHILIS

The importance of syphilis in the field of differential diagnosis of general bone disease has greatly diminished in the last three decades, since early and effective treatment with penicillin has become available and knowledge of the ill-effects of neglect is much greater. The tertiary manifestations of gummata and periostitis are now, even in special clinics, rarely seen.

CONGENITAL SYPHILIS

Aetiology. The disease is transmitted from the mother, who may have been infected before, at the time of, or after conception.

Clinical and radiographic features. The baby suffers from rhinitis (snuffles), rashes and anaemia. The rash is widespread and especially evident around the mouth, where the radiating sores leave behind them the typical scars of rhagades. The eyes and central nervous system are also commonly affected.

Skeletal manifestations are said to be present in 95 per cent of these babies (King and Catterall, 1959) and appear within the first three months of life; by six months of age, with or without treatment, they are improving. There is tender enlargement of the ends of the long bones, the so-called syphilitic epiphysitis, although in fact it is the metaphysis which is chiefly affected. The epiphyseal plate is broadened and irregular leading to the 'saw tooth' appearance of the end of the metaphysis, and the epiphysis may become separated through this region causing pseudo-paralysis. The upper limb is more often affected than the lower, and the manifestations are almost always bilateral. There is some irregular porosis of the shafts and thin periosteal new bone may be laid down, successive layers of this giving an onion-peel appearance. The cortex adjacent to the metaphysis may be eroded, and characteristically this occurs bilaterally at the superomedial aspects of the tibiae (Wimberger's sign). Syphilitic dactylitis, first appearing typically in some of the proximal phalanges, is unusual before the second year of life. Craniotabes is not uncommon, and thickening around the anterior fontanelle—Parrot's nodes—may cause the so-called 'hot cross bun' skull.

Differential diagnosis. In the past the diagnosis of syphilis in infants seen some months after birth might be confused with rickets and scurvy, which were not uncommonly coincident. The radiological appearances of these vitamin-deficiency diseases (which are rarely manifest so early in life) are confusing, the slightly denser line demarcating the saw-toothed end of the metaphysis in syphilis being similar to the so-called 'lattice' in scurvy. Infantile cortical hyperostosis shows a rather similar periosteal reaction and affects the same age group, but this reaction is more extensive and affects the whole diaphysis, other syphilitic manifestations are absent, and serological tests negative. Differentiation from a battered baby is made by the complete lack of manifestations attributable to trauma.

LATE SYPHILIS

Clinical and radiographic features. Bone lesions in the tertiary stage of adult syphilis occur in only a small proportion of cases. Gummata develop in the bone cortices, and in the skull can cause widespread destruction of the vault, nasal bones and hard palate, with ulceration and perforations. In the long bones there may be localised periostitis over the destructive lesions in the cortex, or more commonly a diffuse gummatous periostitis develops, without underlying bone destruction but with a massive laying down of new bone. This characteristically affects the anterior aspect of the middle third of the tibia—it is usually but not always bilateral—causing the so-called 'sabre tibia'. The shaft of the bone, however, is not bowed. In due course the differentiation between the original cortex and the new bone is lost. The bone lesions of late syphilis may cause aching in their early stages, especially at night, but are often symptomless; major sequestration of bone is only seen in the presence of secondary infection. In neuropathic (Charcot) joints however, massive sequestra are a very prominent feature and are part of the complete disorganisation of the joint. Calcification and heterotopic new bone formation are confined to the capsule.

Differential diagnosis. It is in the late bony manifestations that the reputation of syphilis as the great imitator is so well founded; metastatic carcinoma, myeloma, Ewing's tumour and osteosarcoma, multiple tuberculous lesions and chronic osteomyelitis, histiocytosis-X, and the exotic infections of bone have all led to confusion at times. The golden rule remains: the possibility that obscure bone lesions may be syphilitic must never be forgotten.

YAWS

The bony lesions of yaws may start in the secondary stage but are only prominent in the tertiary stage of the disease: they occur in about 20 per cent of patients and are, in general, indistinguishable from the lesions of syphilis. The tendency to periosteal thickening is more marked in yaws, multiple lesions within a single bone are more often seen than in syphilis, and early osteoporosis may lead to true bowing of long bones. Arthritis and contractures of the surrounding soft tissue lead to complete ankylosis of joints, and a remarkable predilection for infection of the nasal processes of the maxillae may produce bulbous swellings known as 'goundou'.

BONE TUBERCULOSIS

The fact that tuberculosis of bone and joint may present with multiple skeletal lesions, irrespective of the presence of pulmonary or renal infection, has been recognised since the causative organism was first discovered. However, such cases have become increasingly rare in highly developed countries during this century, no doubt because public health measures and the relief of poverty and undernourishment have increased the resistance of the population as well as diminishing the means by which infection was spread. Immigration between countries and the apparently lower resistance to the disease indigenous in the Asian, African and some other races are, however, sufficient to ensure that such multiple bone lesions are still occasionally seen.

Clinical and radiographic features. In all ethnic groups males are more commonly affected than females and the systemic illness in patients with multiple skeletal lesions is more severe than in unifocal disease. The thoracic spine, followed by the lumbar spine, in both unifocal and multifocal bone tuberculosis are still the most commonly affected areas (Nicholson, 1974) and in multifocal disease the knee is next most commonly involved. Articular lesions show no special radiological features but clinically the disease is more florid and abscess formation more rapid. The bone lesions are often more destructive and cystic in nature, perhaps showing only a slight periosteal reaction, an expression of the poverty of response by the tissue defences.

Differential diagnosis. If the spine or other joints are involved diagnosis will rarely give rise to difficulty, but where manifestations are confined to bone any disease in which multiple destructive lesions occur must be considered, especially other infections, secondary carcinoma and myelomatosis. Biopsy and culture may be required to ensure early diagnosis of the bacillus.

OTHER INFECTIONS

On occasion almost any infection which can enter the blood stream may produce multiple lesions in the skeleton and the problem of diagnosis is basically no different from that of the single lesion. It suffices that the clinician should be aware that such lesions can occur simultaneously in several bones.

Staphylococcal and streptococcal suppurative osteomyelitis with large abscesses may occur simultaneously in more than one site, particularly in the neonate and in the haemoglobinopathies (Moseley, 1974). These babies may be severely ill from septicaemia, but in other cases the general illness is surprisingly mild. Salmonella and fungus infections of bone, especially blastomycosis, may also occur at multiple sites, as (rarely) can hydatid disease.

REFERENCES

King, A. J. & Catterall, A. D. (1959). Syphilis of bone. *British Journal of Venereal Disease*, **35**, 116.
Moseley, J. E. (1974). Skeletal changes in the anaemias. *Seminars in Roentgenology*, **9**, 169.
Nicholson, R. A. (1974). Twenty years of bone and joint tuberculosis in Bradford. *Journal of Bone & Joint Surgery*, **56B**, 760.

FURTHER READING

King, A. J. & Nicol, C. (1975) *Venereal Diseases* (3rd Edition). Baillière, Tindall and Cassell, London.

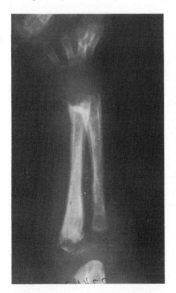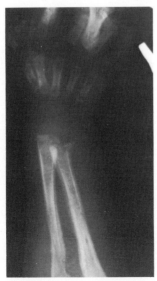

Fig. 59.1 (H.) Congenital syphilis. Separation of lower radial epiphysis through rarified metaphysis with widespread periosteal reaction. (H.A.T.F.)

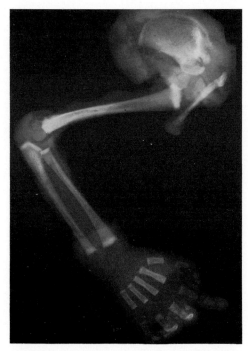

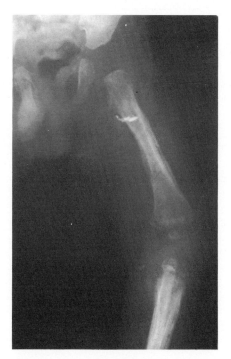

Fig. 59.2 Congenital syphilis. Post mortem specimen from premature stillbirth. Multiple metaphyseal lesions with dense line attributable to bismuth treatment of mother during pregnancy. (Courtesy of Dr D. McC. Gregg, Cambridge.)

Fig. 59.3 Congenital syphilis. Metaphyseal thickening and sclerosis with extensive periosteal reaction. (Courtesy of Dr D. McC. Gregg, Cambridge.)

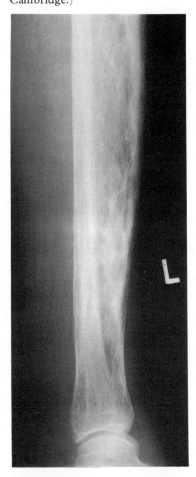

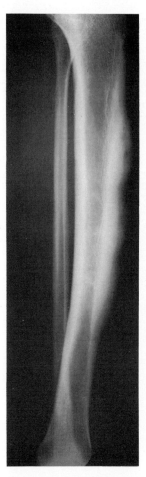

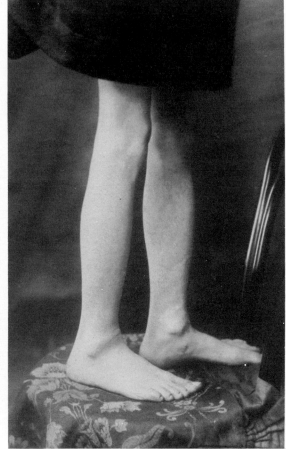

Fig. 59.4 Late syphilis. Sabre tibia. Differentiation of cortex almost disappeared. Note resemblance to Paget's disease. (A.H.)

Fig. 59.5 (above left) Late syphilis. Sabre tibia. Differentiation of periosteal new bone from underlying cortex has disappeared. (A.H.) Fig. 59.6 (above right) Late syphilis. Sabre tibiae. (H.A.T.F.)

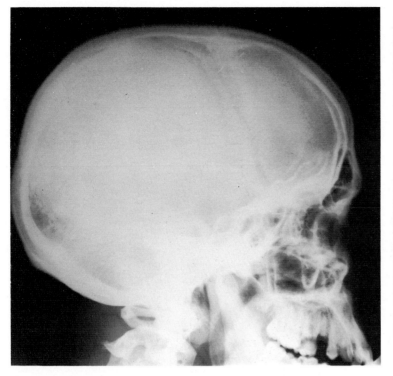

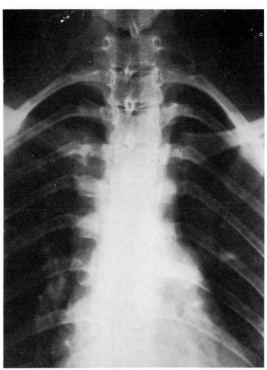

Fig. 59.7 Late syphilis. Showing destruction of nasal bones, thickening of calvarium and spicular periosteal reaction. (A.H.)

Fig. 59.8 Late syphilis. Thickening from periosteal reaction in typical site at inner half right clavicle. (A.H.)

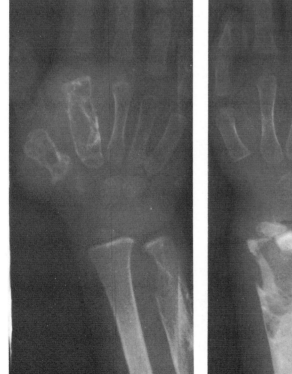

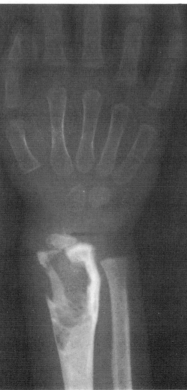

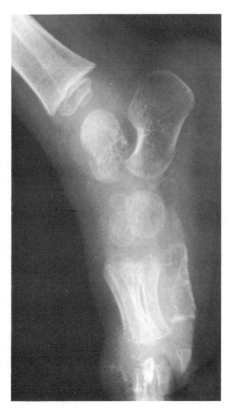

Figs 59.9, 59.10 & 59.11 Multiple tuberculosis. Cystic lesions in metacarpals, radii, metatarsals, talus and os calcis. (Courtesy of Mr A. G. Apley, Pyrford.)

60 Infantile Cortical Hyperostosis

This is an apparently inflammatory bone lesion occurring in young infants, principally affecting the mandible, clavicle or long bones, and self-limiting in nature.

It was first described by Caffey and Silverman (1945) with a fuller review by Caffey (1957).

Aetiology and inheritance. It is likely that there is a genetic factor in this disease since there have been many reports of familial instances, both in sibs and also in members of two succeeding generations (Boyes and Demy, 1951; Gerrard *et al*, 1961; and Van Buskirk, Tampas and Petersen, 1961). Since the disease is self-limiting it is difficult to establish the mode of inheritance but it is likely to be autosomal dominant.

Frequency. The population incidence is not known but it is a very rare disorder. It is occasionally apparent at birth but more usually develops during the first six months of life.

Clinical and radiographic features. The presenting signs may be those of a generalised body reaction, that is fever, irritability and anorexia in the infant; or the first sign may be localised, commonly a painful, firm soft-tissue swelling frequently over the mandible, clavicle or affecting any long bone.

Radiographically in the early stages there is slight periosteal thickening followed by extensive subperiosteal bone formation. Usually more than one area is affected and the large masses of periosteal new bone develop a dense, laminated appearance in and beneath the periosteum. It is unusual for the entire length of the bone to be affected, the subperiosteal reaction not quite reaching the epiphyseal plate. Resorption of the original cortex and widening of the medullary canal with diaphyseal expansion is a feature.

In time (perhaps months later), the excessive masses of new bone resorb, leaving no trace of the earlier disease but there may be residual longitudinal overgrowth and bowing of the affected long bones. A recent review of the radiological findings was reported by Padfield and Hicken (1970).

Differential diagnosis. The main differential diagnoses are from osteomyelitis and the 'battered baby' syndrome. In osteomyelitis signs are more usually confined to one bone and the disorder is progressively destructive, not self-limiting, as in infantile cortical hyperostosis. When more than one bone is affected, not uncommon in neonates, the general reaction may be surprisingly slight. In the 'battered baby' syndrome there will usually be signs of physical maltreatment such as bruises, burns or fractures, these latter perhaps showing different stages of development since there is likely to have been more than one incident of maltreatment.

Congenital syphilis is now of great rarity, but in both disorders there is periosteal new bone formation and it may need to be considered in the differential diagnosis during the first few months of life. In congenital syphilis the osteochondritis cause enlarged and tender areas near the *ends* of the long bones (unlike infantile cortical hyperostosis) and on radiography there is a wide radiolucent area within the metaphysis. The diagnosis is confirmed by a positive Wasserman reaction in the mother and child.

Progress and complications. Infantile cortical hyperostosis may last for weeks or months, but it nearly always regresses ultimately, the bone returning to normal. It is not unknown, however, for some babies to die in the acute phase of the disease and some 25 per cent of cases have a more protracted course with repeated remissions and exacerbations.

Laboratory investigations. The findings are non-specific, there being a leucocytosis, a raised sedimentation rate and occasionally a raised serum alkaline phosphatase.

Treatment. There is no specific treatment for the disease.

REFERENCES

Boyes, J. G. & Demy, N. G. (1951). Infantile cortical hyperostosis: a familial disease? *American Journal of Roentgenology*, **65**, 924.

Caffey, J. & Silverman, W. A. (1945). Infantile cortical hyperostosis: preliminary report on a new syndrome. *American Journal of Roentgenology*, **54**, 1.

Caffey, J. (1957). Infantile cortical hyperostosis: a review of the clinical and radiographic features. *Proceedings of the Royal Society of Medicine*, **50**, 347.

Gerrard, J. W., Holman, G. H., Gorman, A. A. & Morrow, I. H. (1961). Familial infantile cortical hyperostosis. *Journal of Pediatrics*, **59**, 543.

Padfield, E. & Hicken, P. (1970). Cortical hyperostosis in infants: A radiological study of sixteen patients. *British Journal of Radiology*, **43**, 231.

Van Buskirk, F. W., Tampas, J. P. & Petersen, O. S. (1961). Infantile cortical hyperostosis. An enquiry into its familial aspects. *American Journal of Roentgenology*, **85**, 613.

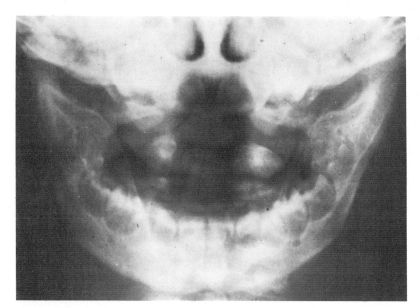

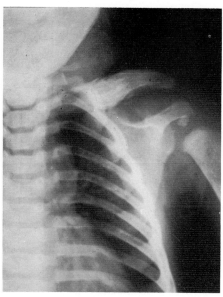

Fig. 60.1 The ramus of the mandible is a characteristic site. (Courtesy of Dr J. Tudor, Cambridge.)

Fig. 60.2 (V.H.) Lesion involving the left clavicle. (H.A.T.F.)

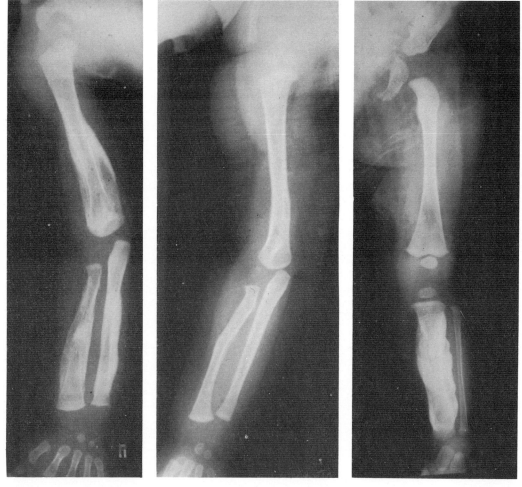

Figs 60.3, 60.4 & 60.5 (H.J.) Extensive subperiosteal bone formation which has almost completely resolved 6 months later (Fig. 60.4). The whole shaft is not involved, the region of the epiphyseal plate remaining unaffected. (H.A.T.F.)

61 Toxins

LEAD, BISMUTH, PHOSPHORUS AND CADMIUM POISONING

Skeletal abnormalities can be caused by the prolonged ingestion of certain toxic elements; of those listed above only lead remains of any importance and even this has greatly diminished in recent years. Neither children with congenital syphilis nor their parents are any longer treated with bismuth—in the past an occasional cause of skeletal manifestations in the newborn. Phosphorus poisoning, outside the fields of war, is extremely rare, both this and lead poisoning having been greatly reduced by their recognition by and the regulations of public health authorities.

Poisoning by lead in adults remains a problem, however, and it is surprising that the largest number of cases occur not in those specifically working in lead or paint production, but amongst ship-breakers and demolition workers on, for example, old bridges, where lead in layer upon layer of paint may be vapourised by oxy-acetylene cutters (Employment Medical Advisory Service Report 1973/74). Lead is now little used in domestic paints or 'lead soldiers' so that small children are less at risk. If poisoning does occur, it is only in children that bone changes develop and the appearances are very similar in lead, bismuth and phosphorus intoxication.

Chronic cadmium poisoning is not seen in children and is listed only because in adults it is a rare cause of osteomalacia secondary to the renal damage produced by this element.

Clinical and radiographic features. In chronic lead poisoning the most important clinical manifestations are anorexia, colicky abdominal pain, constipation, symptoms of anaemia (Barltrop, 1973), and peripheral neuritis, usually, but not always, bilateral and entirely motor in its effects. The upper limbs are affected before the lower and wrist drop is common. The almost pathognomonic blue line on the gums is due to local formation of lead sulphide. Later symptoms may arise from the chronic nephritis and arterial disease which are produced in patients with prolonged poisoning.

Transverse bands of increased density develop in the metaphyses of long bones, particularly in those where growth is most rapid (Murray and Jacobson, 1971). They bear some similarity to the dense lines of arrested bone growth, but tend to be broader and less defined in their margins. The epiphyses and the rate of bone growth are unaffected, although in severe cases there is some interference with metaphyseal modelling. There may be several bands in one metaphysis, those nearer the diaphysis becoming narrower and less well defined. The increased density is thought to be true osteosclerosis, and not due to deposition of the element itself (Park, Jackson and Kadji, 1931). The excess bone is presumably later, to some extent, reabsorbed.

Differential diagnosis. Somewhat similar bands are seen in the metaphyses of children with thyroid deficiency, hypervitaminosis-D, and idiopathic hypercalcaemia of infancy, but the other manifestations of lead poisoning resolve any diagnostic difficulty.

FLUOROSIS

Chronic excessive absorption of fluorine may produce widespread sclerosis in the skeleton, but, except in severe cases, the condition is usually asymptomatic.

Aetiology. Minute quantities of this element are widely distributed in water and plants; between 1 and 2 parts per million are regarded as acceptable in drinking water, and are beneficial in reducing dental caries (though at the cost of mottling of the teeth). In many parts of the world, however, drinking water may have levels far in excess of this, e.g. Lake Rudolph in Central Africa where there are 40 parts per million (Brodie *et al*, 1973). Excessive intake results in the fluorides being selectively deposited in bone. This is aggravated in patients suffering from renal disease or dietary deficiencies, and in whom radiological changes may occur even when the intake of fluorine is not excessive.

Fluorine intoxication also occurs in certain industrial occupations (e.g. amongst cryolite workers) and may be seen in animals grazing in the areas surrounding such works. Animals may be similarly affected in areas of volcanic eruptions, in which fluorine-containing gases may contaminate the pasture.

Clinical and radiographic features. Although osteoporosis may occur—and certainly does in animal experiments in the early stages of poisoning—the bone destruction is accompanied by regeneration, osteosclerosis and extensive osteophyte formation, especially at points of attachment of muscles and ligaments. Experimental X-ray diffraction techniques have suggested that more fluorine is deposited in the outer than the inner parts of the cortex (Jokl and Skinner, 1972). However, the sclerotic changes appear to result from irritation of bone rather than actual fluorine deposition, although there is also evidence of a compensatory hyperparathyroidism (Faccini and Teotia, 1974).

In humans the toxic changes take many years to develop and it is only in the later stages that there are symptoms from increasing joint stiffness, particularly of the spine which may become completely rigid. In one series nearly one half of the cases developed paraplegia (Singh *et al*, 1961).

The final picture is of a diffuse increase in density

of the whole skeleton, though the ribs, spine and pelvis are most obviously affected, accompanied by calcified, then ossified, ligaments. The new bone is rough and irregular in outline with general cortical thickening and no clear differentiation between medulla and cortex. Accompanying the chronic hypercalcaemia, metastatic calcification may be found in the walls of blood vessels and elsewhere. Secondary hyperparathyroidism can result from the renal damage caused by fluorosis, and this may confuse the pathological and radiological findings.

Differential diagnosis. The lack of enlargement of the medullary cavity and the diffuseness of changes differentiate fluorine intoxication from Paget's disease. The degree of osteosclerosis only rarely attains the level seen in osteopetrosis but the radiological changes in myelosclerosis may be very similar. In this condition, however, enlargement of the liver and spleen and haematological abnormalities differentiate the two.

REFERENCES

Barltrop, D. (1973). Interaction of lead with mammalian tissues. *Journal of Bone & Joint Surgery*, **55B**, 423.

Brodie, W., Majale, M., Suleman, S. K. & Church, J. C. T. (1971). Clinical cases: fluorosis of bone. *Journal of Bone & Joint Surgery*, **53B**, 356.

Employment Medical Advisory Service (1973). Report for 1973 and 1974. H.M. Stationery Office.

Faccini, J. M. & Teotia, S. P. S. (1974). Histopathological assessment of endemic skeletal fluorosis. *Calcified Tissue Research*, **16**, 45.

Jokl, P. & Skinner, H. W. C. (1972). X-ray diffraction analysis of fluorine-induced changes in bone mineral. *Journal of Bone & Joint Surgery*, **54A**, 1132.

Murray, R. O. & Jacobson, H. G. (1971). *The Radiology of Skeletal Disorders*, p. 580. Churchill Livingstone: Edinburgh & London.

Park, E. A., Jackson, D. & Kajdi, L. (1931). Shadows produced by lead in X-ray pictures of growing skeleton. *American Journal of Diseases of Children*, **41**, 485.

Singh, A., Jolly, S. S. & Bansal, B. C. (1961). Skeletal fluorosis and its neurological complications. *Lancet*, **i**, 197.

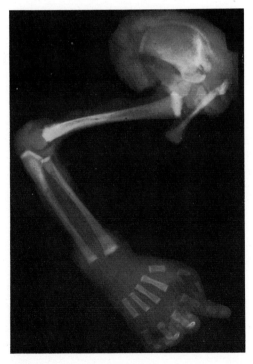

Fig. 61.1 Congenital syphilis. Post mortem specimen from premature stillbirth. Multiple metaphyseal lesions with dense line attributable to bismuth treatment of mother during pregnancy. (Courtesy of Dr D. McC. Gregg, Cambridge.)

There is a group of anaemias found throughout the world, mostly in tropical and sub-tropical areas, which are now recognised as being due to variations in the chemical structure of the haemoglobin molecules within the patient's red cells. This group includes thalassaemia (Cooley's or Mediterranean anaemia) and sickle-cell anaemia. It has for long been known that there are gradations in the severity and in recent years it has been possible to demonstrate that these variations are due to the individual patient's haemoglobin being of more than one type.

Aetiology and inheritance. Every individual inherits a haemoglobin gene from each parent, each gene expressing itself independently. In Great Britain nearly everyone is homozygous for haemoglobin A and the disease does not occur. Individuals who are homozygous for the thalassaemia haemoglobin suffer from thalassaemia major, and if heterozygous from thalassaemia minor. The thalassaemia gene is particularly common in countries around the Mediterranean.

Sickle-cell anaemia can arise either in those homozygous for haemoglobin-S or in a milder form if the patient is doubly heterozygous for haemoglobin-S and haemoglobin-C. Genes for both these haemoglobins are common in tropical Africa, and the S gene is also found in Mediterranean countries, the Middle East and in Southern India. In addition, haemoglobin-S and -C are widespread amongst negroes in the Caribbean and North America, since this population is founded upon slaves brought from Africa. The proportion of abnormal haemoglobin controls the life of the red cell and its liability to early haemolysis. In all the homozygous conditions and many of the heterozygous ones the cell life is markedly shortened, resulting in anaemia. In response to the haemolysis there is marked marrow hyperplasia.

In those patients who carry the sickling trait any reduction in the oxygen tension in the blood leads to a change in shape of the haemoglobin molecule which causes the cell to shrivel, producing a sickle-shaped appearance on a blood film. This occurs particularly where the circulation is sluggish and oxygen tension low. Clotting may then occur and infarcts are produced, most commonly in the spleen but also within bones. It is these two factors, marrow hyperplasia and local infarcts, that produce the skeletal changes. It is important to note, however, that bone infarcts only occur in patients who carry at least one gene for haemoglobin-S.

Clinical and radiographic features. The haemoglobinopathies are symptomless for the first few months of life because of the persistence of foetal haemoglobin, and, apart from the anaemia, other symptoms are relatively minor before the age of 4 years. From this age (in the case of double S sickle-cell disease) joint pains start and there are periodic crises accompanied by pyrexia, malaise and pain elsewhere. This pain is usually due to infarcts and occurs particularly in the abdomen, from splenic infarction, and in the limbs, where hot tender swellings appear, especially in the hands and feet. The liability to such crises is less in the SC-double heterozygous disease, but this combination of genes is particularly liable to produce necrosis of epiphyses, most commonly seen in the head of the femur.

In the later stages of the haemoglobinopathies there is enlargement of the liver and spleen, and in the male attacks of priapism. In thalassaemia major few patients survive till puberty and in all severe forms of the disease there is some general impairment of growth.

Radiographically there is osteoporosis (associated with the marrow hyperplasia) and the collapsed vertebral bodies with bulging intervertebral discs are similar to those seen in senile osteoporosis (Reynolds, 1966). In some vertebrae there is a flat area of increased density in the central part of each depressed end plate, leading to a characteristic 'step deformity'. In the skull there is marked thinning of the outer table, widening of the trabecular pattern of the diploë and, on occasion, the so-called 'hair on end' appearance (Goulding et al, 1959) said to be caused by the overlying periosteal reaction. However, this may occur in other severe anaemias and is probably no more than an exaggeration of the normal vertical striation in the diploë (Moseley, 1974).

In the long bones the marrow hyperplasia may cause thinning and scalloping of the inner side of the cortex, and coarsening of the trabecular pattern. In contrast, bone may be laid down on the inner aspect of the cortex, leading to narrowing of the medullary canal and sometimes the appearance of a 'bone within bone'. In the ribs there is a similar appearance together with cortical erosions, apparently secondary to small infarcts. Almost pathognomonic of thalassaemia is a curious bulbous expansion of the posterior parts of the ribs. In severely anaemic patients the chest radiographs show enlargement of the heart and pulmonary congestion.

The metacarpals and metatarsals, and to a lesser extent the phalanges, show a characteristic finely honey-combed appearance internally, with thinning of the cortex. The original moulding of the shafts is lost so that the two sides are straight and parallel to each other. In other long bones the periosteal reaction may be more obvious, overlying irregular porotic and sclerotic areas, attributable to thrombosis and infarction. The latter process also affects the epiphyses producing, in the head of the femur, an appearance very similar to Perthes' disease but in contrast to this disease the outer third of the capital epiphysis may be spared. Severe involvement of an epiphysis will lead to some shortening of that bone (Middlemiss and Raper, 1966). All the skeletal changes seen in the most severe S-S variety may be found to a lesser degree in the doubly heterozygous forms.

Lastly, patients with bone manifestations are particularly liable to develop osteomyelitis, especially that caused by the salmonella group of organisms. The infection tends to run a chronic course producing only a slight bony reaction. It should be noted that the radiological appearances in the long bones in the haemoglobinopathies, even without infection, may be almost indistinguishable from those of osteomyelitis (Moseley, 1974).

REFERENCES

Goulding, J. S. R., MacIver, J. E. & Went, L. N. (1959). The bone changes in sickle-cell anaemia and its genetic variants. *Journal of Bone & Joint Surgery*, **41B**, 711.

Middlemiss, J. H. & Raper, A. B. (1966). Skeletal changes in the haemoglobinopathies. *Journal of Bone & Joint Surgery*, **48B**, 693.

Moseley, J. E. (1974). Skeletal changes in the anaemias. *Seminars in Radiology*, Vol. 9, No. 3, 169.

Reynolds, J. (1966). A re-evaluation of the 'fish vertebra' sign in hemoglobinopathy. *American Journal of Roentgenology*, **118**, 378.

Weatherall, D. J. (1973). The haemoglobinopathies. *Price's Medicine 11th Edition*, Oxford University Press, London.

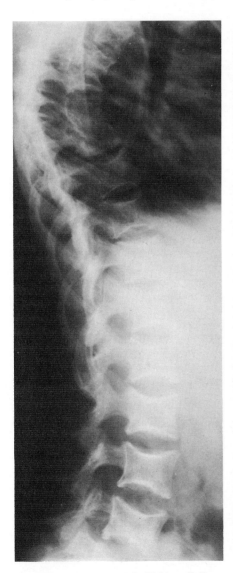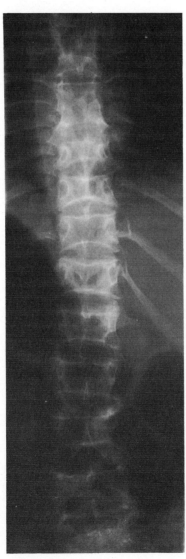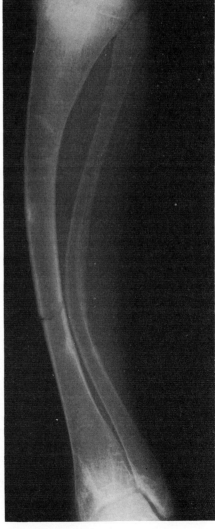

Fig. 62.1 & 62.2 (D.H.) Sickle cell disease. Guyanaian girl aged 15 years. Central collapse of vertebral bodies with bulging discs. Increased density in central part of upper cortex. Two areas of intervertebral fusion in thoracic spine followed infection 5 years before. (A.H.)

Fig. 62.3 (A.T.) Marrow hyperplasia with cortical thinning of tibia with a pathological fracture. Old bowing possibly associated with renal tubular disease. (Courtesy of Mr B. F. Meggitt, Cambridge.)

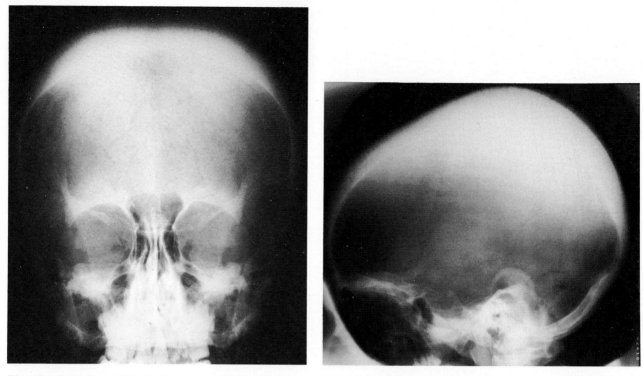

Figs 62.4 & 62.5 (A.T.) Marked thickening of calvarium with vertical striation from hyperplasia of the diploë. In A.P. view the original outer cortex of the vault has disappeared. (Courtesy of Mr B. F. Meggitt, Cambridge.)

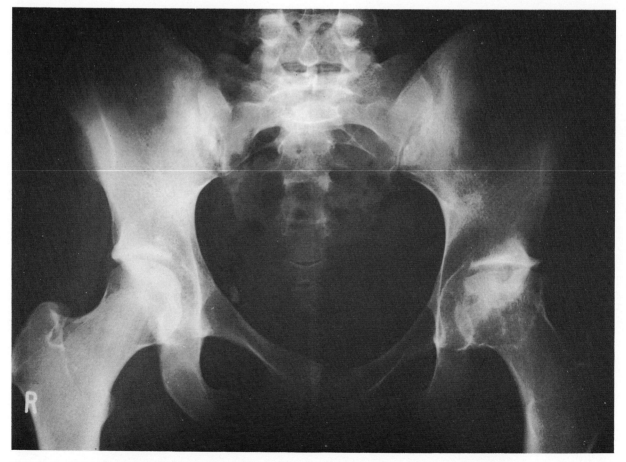

Fig. 62.6 (J.A.) Areas of sclerosis and general irregularity of texture in femoral head from local infarction. (Courtesy of Mr A. G. Apley, Pyrford.)

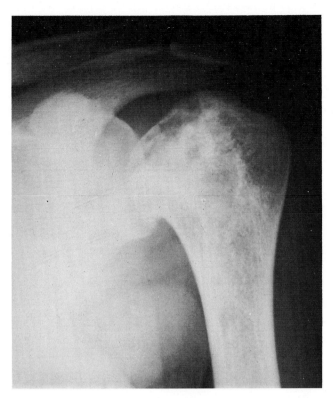

Fig. 62.7 (G.D.) Areas of sclerosis and general irregularity of texture in humeral head from local infarction. (Courtesy of Mr A. G. Apley, Pyrford.)

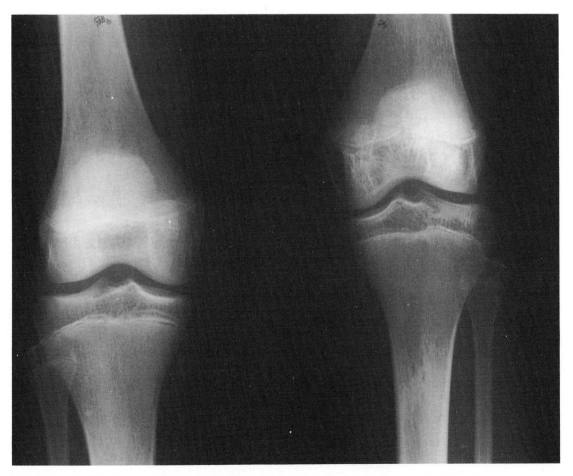

Fig. 62.8 (D.H.) Similar changes in epiphysis of left knee with leg shortening. (A.H.)

63 The Reticuloses
Leukaemias and Lymphomas

In many of the reticuloses skeletal manifestations develop as the bone reacts to the pathologically increased or decreased activity of the marrow cells within it, but in most of them these changes are not of great clinical or diagnostic significance. Only those diseases with widespread bone lesions of diagnostic importance are discussed here (marked with an asterisk on the list below). It is not surprising that there is a general similarity in their skeletal changes, and differentiation on radiography alone is rarely possible.

This classification is based on the work of Dameshek and Gunz (1964).

A. *PRIMARY MALIGNANT DISEASES OF BONE MARROW*
 Acute
  Acute leukaemia★
  Acute erythraemia
 Chronic
  Chronic granulocytic leukaemia★
  Polycythaemia vera
  Essential thrombocythaemia
  Myelofibrosis★

B. *PRIMARY MALIGNANT DISEASES OF LYMPHOID TISSUE*
  Hodgkin's disease★
  Reticulum cell sarcoma
  Giant follicular lymphoma
  Lymphosarcoma
  Burkitt's lymphoma
  Chronic lymphatic leukaemia★
  Myelomatosis★
  Macroglobulinaemia

This classification provides no more than a useful guide since differentiation of these diseases is not always clear-cut, and in time one of them may change its nature, or the manifestations of another in the group may be added. For instance, a patient with lymphosarcoma may also develop chronic lymphatic leukaemia, and one with chronic granulocytic leukaemia almost always eventually develops an acute myeloblastic leukaemia.

ACUTE LEUKAEMIA

This condition results from proliferation within the bone marrow of any of the primitive white cells and the disease is accordingly labelled myeloblastic, monoblastic, lymphoblastic or undifferentiated. Of these, the lymphoblastic type is the commonest with a peak incidence in early childhood; the myeloblastic form is seen at any age, including infancy, and the monoblastic type is the rarest and almost always seen in adults.

Aetiology. There is a proven association with irradiation both in the acute leukaemia and in chronic granulocytic leukaemia (Goldstone and Cawley, 1975). Evidence for this was obtained following the atomic bomb explosions, and also from patients who had undergone radiotherapy for such diseases as ankylosing spondylitis. The evidence is less definite in the case of diagnostic radiation to pregnant women.

There appears also to be a genetic predisposition to both acute leukaemia and chronic lymphocytic leukaemia, a factor absent in the chronic myeloid type. Furthermore, it is known that acute lymphoblastic leukaemia is up to fifty times more common in Down's syndrome (mongolism), a condition in which there is a definite chromosome abnormality (Trisomy 21) (Fairlie, 1973).

Acute myeloid leukaemia can develop following the use of cytoxic drugs for lymphomata, and benzene is also suspect. The possible role of the so-called 'oncoviruses', certain of which are proven causes of leukaemia in animals, is currently under investigation in man.

Clinical and radiographic features. The presenting signs of all types of acute leukaemia are similar, with general malaise, listlessness, easy fatigue, probably due to the accompanying anaemia, and an increased liability to infections. The patients bruise easily, many show purpuric patches and suffer bone pains and joint swellings. The liver and spleen are enlarged in most instances. Palpable, and often visible, lymphadenopathy is usual and may be marked, but it is not invariable. Infiltration of other tissues is common, including the viscera, serous membranes and the central nervous system. Diagnosis depends on findings in the blood films and bone marrow and it is the type of cell revealed rather than just the numbers of them that is significant.

Bone involvement is more commonly seen in lymphoblastic leukaemia than in the other types, and more often in children than in adults. Some degree of generalised osteoporosis is usual in both adults and children.

Skeletal changes occur in about two thirds of children with the disease. A band of osteoporosis may be seen extending across the metaphysis, close to the epiphyseal plate, especially in the lower femora, but this is similar to that seen in other severe illnesses (in adults as well as children) and is not necessarily due to leukaemic infiltration. This reveals itself as more or less discrete lytic areas affecting both the spongiosa and cortex. At first tiny, they may fuse together to produce small ill-defined cysts or streaks without clear-cut walls. More commonly the infiltration spreads widely, producing areas of irregular destruction similar to metastatic deposits, especially in the metaphyses of the upper ends of the femur and humerus. In other instances, a mixture of osteoporosis and bone destruction produces diffuse changes throughout the length of a bone. Subperiosteal infiltration can produce a well-defined layer of periosteal new bone, which may be seen in the ribs as well as in the long bones. Ill-defined sclerotic areas in the metaphyses may be seen, as in myelosclerosis, but the illness is usually too acute to be mistaken for this disease. There may be an even density of one or more of the vertebral bodies. Pathological fractures, rather surprisingly, are not a major feature.

Differential diagnosis. The radiographic appearances of acute leukaemia cannot be distinguished with certainty from those seen in myelomatosis and other reticuloses, nor from carcinomatous metastases. Blood and sternal marrow films, electrophoretic examination of the serum proteins and sometimes biopsy of a lymph node are required, though even these tests do not always suffice to provide a clear differentiation between the reticuloses themselves.

Course and treatment. In the past acute leukaemia, especially in small children, ran a fatal course within a few months. With modern chemography and immunotherapy a complete remission is usually attainable in the lymphoblastic variety (Spiers et al, 1975); relapses are still common but there is an increasing proportion of five year survivals. The prognosis in the other varieties, however, remains very poor.

CHRONIC GRANULOCYTIC LEUKAEMIA

Chronic granulocytic leukaemia is a disease of adult life and the only aetiological factor known is exposure to radiation. The disease presents with general malaise, lassitude and other symptoms of anaemia, purpura and loss of weight; the grossly enlarged spleen may cause local abdominal pain. Enlargement of the lymph nodes is rare, and bone lesions are relatively uncommon and with no characteristic features. Chronic granulocytic leukaemia has a strong tendency to convert to the acute myeloblastic or lymphocytic type in its terminal stages (Glasser and Walker, 1969; Silverstein, Brown and Linman, 1973).

Differential diagnosis. Chronic granulocytic leukaemia can be distinguished from myelosclerosis not only by the appearance of the bone marrow but the finding in some 85 per cent of cases of an abnormal (Philadelphia) chromosome. There is also a reduced alkaline phosphatase content of the granulocytes.

CHRONIC LYMPHATIC LEUKAEMIA

Aetiology. This type of leukaemia is remarkable in that there is no evidence that it ever arises from irradiation: there is however increasing suspicion that it may be viral in origin, and a genetic predisposition may exist (Fairlie, 1973).

Clinical and radiographic features. The disease is very rare under the age of 30 years and it becomes commoner with increasing age. Men are affected twice as often as women.

Chronic lymphatic leukaemia may be discovered incidentally from a routine blood count, but clinically, usually presents with widespread, painless enlargement of lymph nodes or perhaps with repeated respiratory or skin infections. Recurrent attacks of tonsillitis in the elderly should give rise to the suspicion of leukaemia. Purpuric lesions are seen; there is moderate splenic enlargement but no abdominal pain associated with it.

The course of the disease is slow. A haemolytic anaemia commonly develops and there is a strong association with carcinoma in the later stages.

It is this type of leukaemia which most often produces bone lesions in the adult. Progressive osteoporosis is usual and other changes are similar to those seen in acute leukaemia. A sclerotic reaction is rather more often seen, though still rarely, and pathological fractures of long bones or collapse of a vertebral body with or without paraplegia may occur. The skull is not usually so extensively affected as in myelomatosis.

Course and treatment. With appropriate chemotherapy the disease may be kept under control for some years, but death from infection is the usual outcome.

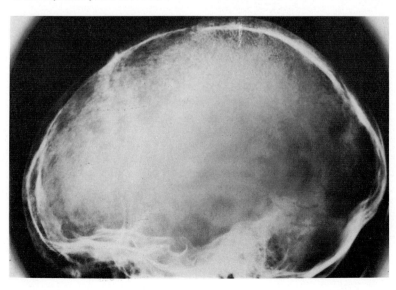

Fig. 63.1 (B.C.) A pepper-pot skull in leukaemia with larger areas of infiltration in the frontal bones. (Courtesy of Dr T. D. Hawkins, Cambridge.)

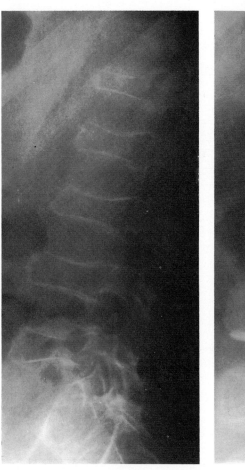

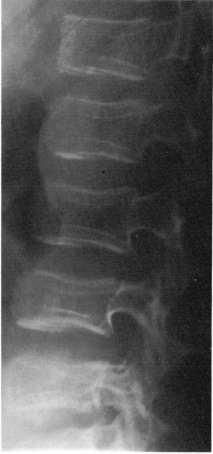

Figs 63.2 & 63.3 (A.S.) Acute lymphatic leukaemia. Infiltration of vertebral bodies with collapse and marked widening of disc spaces. 4 years later, recovery of normal outline leaving 'a bone within a bone' appearance.

Fig. 63.4 (D.F.) Acute lymphatic leukaemia. Diffuse infiltration of vertebral bodies with flattening and in T12 complete collapse. (Courtesy of Professor F. G. J. Hayhoe, Cambridge.)

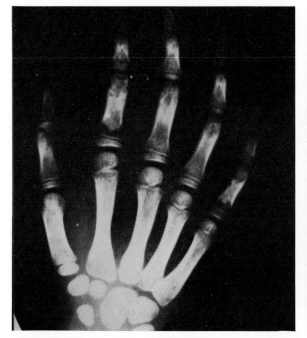

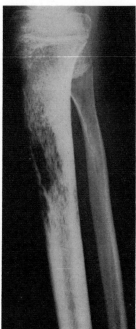

Fig. 63.5 (A.S.) Acute lymphoblastic leukaemia. Spotty osteolytic lesions in phalanges, metaphyseal osteolysis with a thin plate of unaffected bone. (A.H.)

Fig. 63.6 (V.W.) Acute myeloid leukaemia with infiltration of upper tibia. (H.A.T.F.)

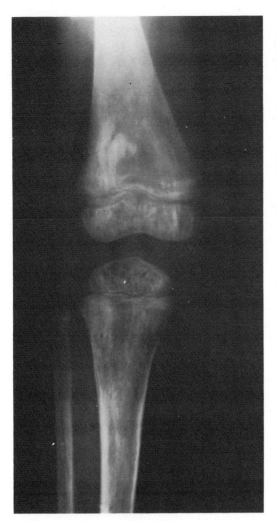

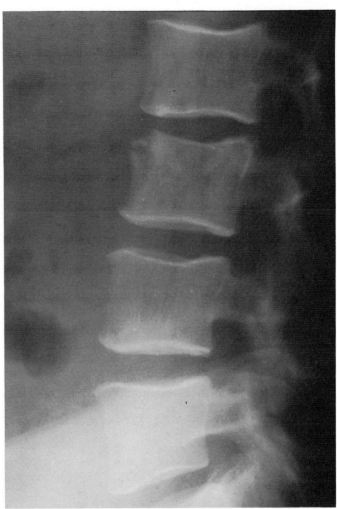

Fig. 63.7 (M.M.) Acute lympho-blastic leukaemia with diffuse medullary infiltration of epiphyses and metaphyses. (H.A.T.F.)

Fig. 63.8 (B.C.) Chronic lymphatic leukaemia with infiltration and collapse of upper surface of L.3. (Courtesy of Dr T. D. Hawkins, Cambridge.)

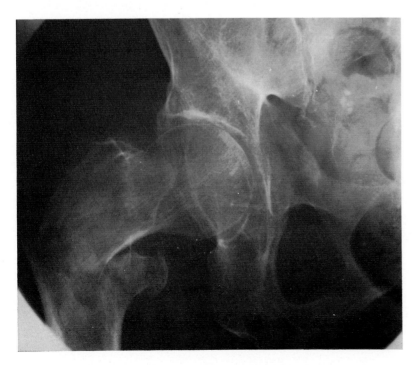

Fig. 63.9 (M.R.) Pathological fracture in chronic lymphatic leukaemia. (A.H.)

HODGKIN'S DISEASE (Lymphadenoma)

This lymphoma is defined as a malignant disease of lymphoreticular tissue and is differentiated from other diseases in the group by the presence of Reed–Sternberg cells.

Aetiology. The cause remains unknown, but because Reed–Sternberg cells are not unique to Hodgkin's disease, sometimes being found in viral infections such as glandular fever, the possibility that Hodgkin's disease may prove to be of viral origin has been strengthened (Order and Hellman, 1972; Wagener and Haanen, 1975). These abnormal cells are perhaps due to an unusual reaction by the host lymphatic system.

Clinical and radiographic features. Hodgkin's disease is commoner in males than females and uncommon in childhood. There are two peaks of incidence, the first at 25 and the second at 70 years of age.

Almost always the patient presents with painless enlargement of lymph nodes, most commonly in the neck, but in the majority of these patients there are already at this time palpable nodes in the axillae and occasionally in the groin as well. They are discrete, of soft rubber consistency, not tender, only rarely with any areas of softening, and may attain a grossly disfiguring size. A mass of enlarged lymph nodes may be easily palpable in the abdomen and splenomegaly and sometimes hepatomegaly may also be a feature.

The disease eventually spreads to almost every tissue of the body; mediastinal lymphadenopathy together with lung infiltration causes a persistent cough, pleural effusion and atelectasis. Obstructive jaundice and ascites may arise in association with the enlarged abdominal nodes. Occasionally paraplegia occurs from infiltration of the spinal theca.

In the earlier stages the patient remains well but subsequently there is general malaise, loss of weight, anaemia, generalised pruritis and at times an undulating pyrexia (the so-called Pel–Ebstein fever).

The radiographic signs are not specific, nor are they invariably outstanding, even when the disease is terminal. Most of the bone lesions are osteolytic but some are sclerotic or there may be a mixture of both types. There may be cortical thickening, or the cortex may be eroded either endosteally or subperiosteally, and the resultant periosteal reaction is occasionally spicular. The bones most frequently affected are the vertebrae, sternum, pelvis, femora, ribs, skull, humeri, scapulae and clavicles. In the long bones lesions usually occur near the proximal ends but the whole of the bone may become involved. In the skull the lesions are osteolytic, multiple and spotty, and rather less sharply cut than those seen in myelomatosis.

Hodgkin's disease is exceptional among the lymphomata in that sclerotic bone lesions are not uncommon, affecting particularly the pelvis and the vertebral bodies. In the spine several adjacent vertebral bodies may be evenly dense without involvement of the intervertebral discs. Sometimes a paravertebral shadow can be seen, and occasionally there is anterior scalloping or erosion of the vertebral bodies due to pressure from neighbouring lymph nodes (Pear, 1975).

Progress and treatment. Early diagnosis, dependent on lymph node biopsy, together with radiotherapy and chemotherapy have greatly improved the prognosis in Hodgkin's disease. Radiotherapy is curative in about 80 per cent of patients where the disease is still localised. At present chemotherapy is no more than palliative. Aids in the diagnosis and accurate localisation of affected nodes prior to radiotherapy are given by lymphangiography, chest tomography, liver and spleen scans, and exploratory laparotomy (Irving, 1975).

In untreated Hodgkin's disease death eventually supervenes from the cachexia associated with widespread disease, intercurrent infections, anaemia or the secondary pressure effects of enlarged lymph nodes.

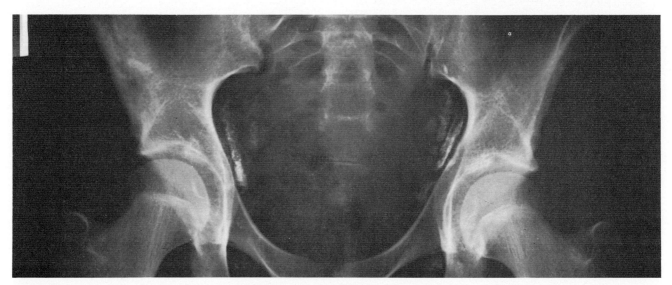

Fig. 63.10   (J.M.) Iliac gland involvement shown by lymphangiography. (Courtesy of Dr T. K. Wheeler, Cambridge.)

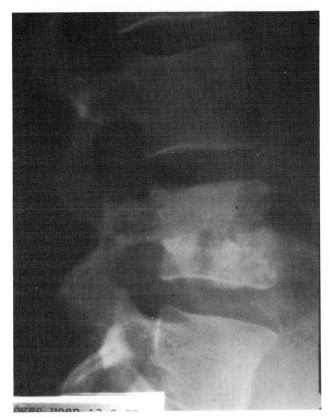

Fig. 63.11 (A.J.) Osteoblastic infiltration of 4th lumbar vertebra. (Courtesy of Professor F. G. J. Hayhoe, Cambridge.)

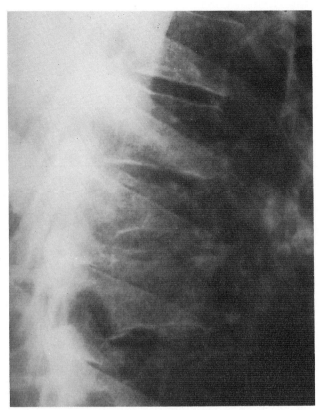

Fig. 63.12 (J.D.) Infiltration and collapse of a mid thoracic vertebra with probable involvement of the body above. (Courtesy of Dr T. K. Wheeler, Cambridge.)

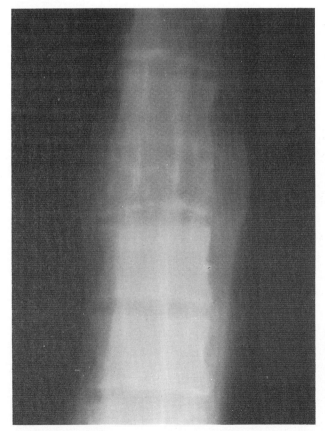

Fig. 63.13 (J.D.) Tomograph showing paravertebral shadow: intervertebral discs unaffected. (Courtesy of Dr T. K. Wheeler, Cambridge.)

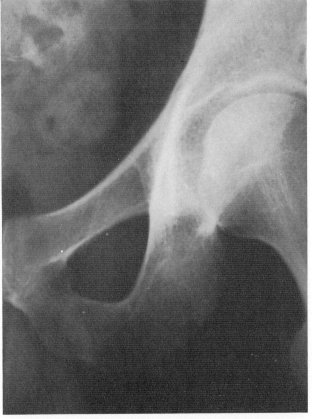

Fig. 63.14 (A.J.) Pelvis showing infiltration of ischium. (Courtesy of Professor F. G. J. Hayhoe, Cambridge.)

MYELOMATOSIS

Myelomatosis is one of a group of diseases in which there is abnormal production of immuno-globulins distinguishable from other hypergamma-globulin-aemias by a characteristic discrete narrow band on electrophoresis. In myelomatosis there is malignant change in the plasma cells of the marrow, and they produce various immunoglobulins, but only in about half the patients is the originally described Bence–Jones protein found in the urine.

Aetiology. The cause is unknown.

Clinical and radiographic features. Myelomatosis is rare before the age of 40 years but thereafter it becomes increasingly common. Males and females are equally affected. The main symptom is of bone pain, particularly in the back. It is unremitting in character, worse at night, unrelieved by posture and is accompanied by bone tenderness, often most readily apparent in the ribs. Pathological fractures are common and notably painful, but they usually heal without difficulty. Other symptoms include pyrexia, abdominal pain, vomiting and constipation. Anaemia is almost constant and patients tend to bleed easily. Lymphadenopathy is not a feature and hepatosplenomegaly, from infiltration with plasmal cells, is usually only moderate in degree. The spinal nerve roots may become involved, particularly in association with vertebral collapse, and paraplegia is not rare. Although the skull is often affected, cranial nerve palsies are not a feature of myelomatosis.

Plasma cells may invade the kidney and renal failure can be fatal quite early in the disease. There is sometimes an association with secondary amyloidosis.

On radiography the typical picture of myelomatosis is of multiple clear, rounded lesions, mostly the size of a pea or less, but occasionally very much larger. Any bone may be affected but lesions distal to the knee and elbow are rare. The bone cortex is eroded from within and there is usually no sclerosis or periosteal reaction, though a bone may be enlarged by the presence of several tumours. Occasionally a lesion is grossly cystic, even expansile, and several such lesions have been found in the same patient. The so-called typical skull, with multiple sharp edged holes is not a constant finding; sometimes there are only a few irregular lytic areas (Meszaros, 1974). The soft tissues may be invaded giving rise to palpable extraosseous tumours and these are most often seen on the skull.

Most patients have a severe generalised osteoporosis, infiltration of marrow, and eventually so severe is the loss of bone that multiple collapsed vertebrae are present in the terminal stages together with pathological rib fractures.

On rare occasions the skeletal lesions are sclerotic or mixed sclerotic and lytic in nature, markedly simulating the appearance of metastases.

Laboratory investigations. The laboratory diagnosis of myelomatosis depends on finding the abnormal immunoglobulins in the plasma and urine, and the infiltration of marrow by plasma cells. Anaemia is usual, but the malignant plasma cells are rarely seen on the blood film. In addition to the hyperglobulinaemia there is a raised serum calcium level and also hypercalciuria. The serum alkaline phosphatase is normal.

Differential diagnosis. The multiple osteolytic lesions of myelomatosis are similar to those of metastatic neoplasm but diagnosis is made on the laboratory findings. Secondary deposits in the lung are almost unknown in myelomatosis, and, in contrast to carcinomatous metastases, the vertebral pedicles are very rarely affected. The osteolytic lesions of myelomatosis in the skull are similar to those of other lymphomata, especially lymphosarcoma and hyperparathyroidism, and histiocytosis X occasionally need differentiation by laboratory investigation.

Progress and treatment. Myelomatosis was previously fatal within a year or so, or much less if kidney involvement had led to early renal failure. The prognosis has been considerably improved in recent years by radiotherapy, intermittent courses of chemotherapy and the use of steroids. These latter are the quickest way of relieving bone pain (Waldenström, 1970).

It should be noted that on occasion a solitary myeloma or plasmacytoma can occur in bone without inevitably progressing to the more generalised disease.

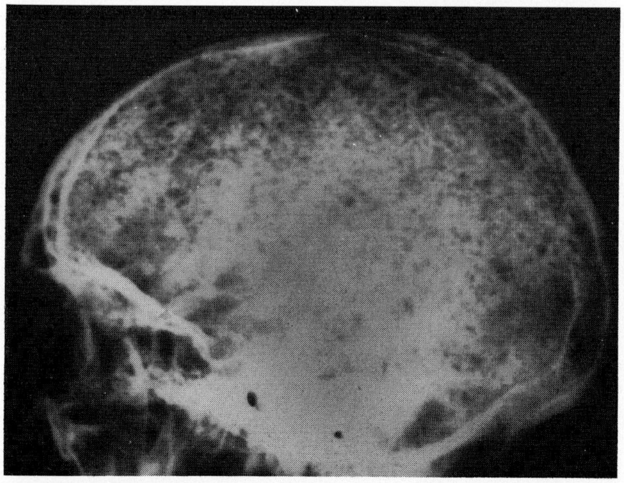

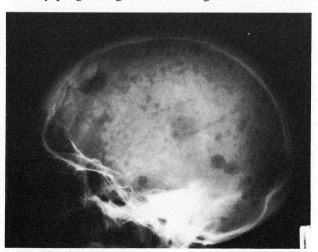

Fig. 63.15 (E.P.) Typical 'pepper pot' skull, with diplöoic widening in the occiput. (H.A.T.F.)

Fig. 63.16 (D.B.) Typical punched out area, some confluent, their margins unclear. (Courtesy of Professor F. G. J. Hayhoe, Cambridge.)

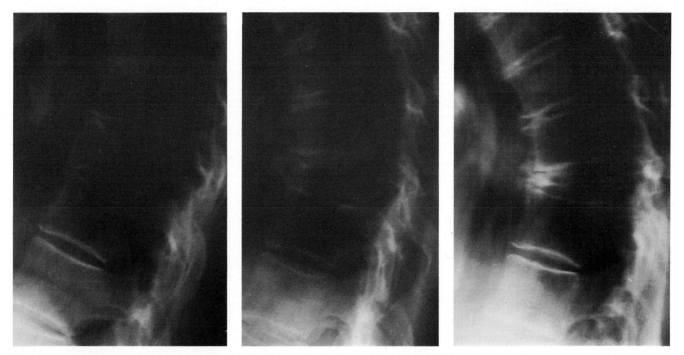

Figs 63.17, 63.18 & 63.19   (M.C.) Progressive collapse of T.10 over 18 month period. (Courtesy of Professor F. G. J. Hayhoe, Cambridge.)

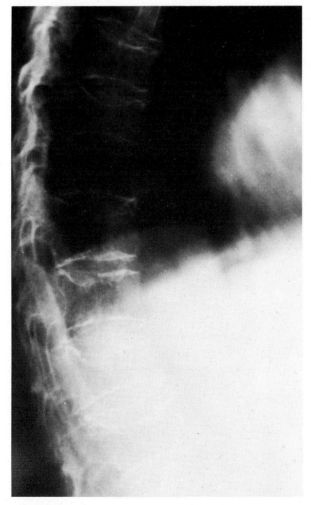

Fig. 63.20   (H.M.) Diffuse infiltration with multiple collapsed vertebral bodies throughout spine. (Courtesy of Professor F. G. J. Hayhoe, Cambridge.)

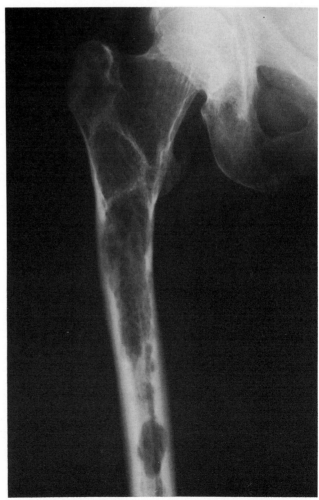

Fig. 63.21   (J.W.) Diffuse medullary infiltration with endosteal erosion by myeloma tissue but no periosteal reaction. (Courtesy of Professor F. G. J. Hayhoe, Cambridge.)

MYELOFIBROSIS AND MYELOSCLEROSIS

There is no clear differentiation between these two since the first commonly progresses to the second, and there is still doubt that either exists as a distinct entity. Dameshek's concept of a 'myeloproliferative syndrome' (quoted by Fairlie, 1973) has much to commend it. Within the marrow the haematopoietic elements are replaced either by fibrous tissue or by new bone, and extramedullary centres of haematopoiesis develop, particularly within the mediastinal lymph nodes.

Aetiology. There are some patients in whom the condition, which is a rare one, appears de novo, and it can then be regarded as a primary proliferation of connective tissue in bone marrow. In most instances, however, it is a secondary condition arising either from other myelo-proliferative diseases, such as polycythaemia vera, essential thrombocythaemia or even myelomatosis, from extensive malignant infiltration of the marrow by metastatic carcinoma cells, or from fibrosis caused by toxins such as radium.

Clinical and radiographic features. Myelosclerosis is a disease of middle age affecting both males and females, and it presents with symptoms of anaemia and abdominal enlargement. This latter is due to massive splenomegaly which is often painful because of infarction and the stretching of the peritoneum. Liver enlargement is only moderate in comparison. Dyspnoea and later congestive heart failure occur, there is marked wasting, and sometimes joint pains from secondary gout. The anaemia is of the leuko-erythroblastic type. In severe cases, diagnostic marrow puncture may have to be replaced by open marrow biopsy.

In about one third of patients skeletal radiographs are either normal or show no more than osteoporosis, and on histological examination there is marked fibroblastic proliferation with only minor haematopoietic changes within the bone itself (Feldman, 1974).

More commonly radiographs show a variable degree of sclerosis with thickening of the endosteum and bony trabeculae, leading to slightly irregular obliteration of marrow cavities and loss of trabecular definition. These changes are most marked in those bones where haematopoiesis is normally active, though the skull is only slightly affected. Although the sclerosis is usually fairly evenly distributed, occasional discrete, denser foci are seen. In the vertebrae increased sclerosis near the end plates may give a 'rugger jersey' effect. Only rarely is there any periosteal reaction, and pathological fractures are unusual.

Differential diagnosis. Widespread skeletal sclerosis with severe splenomegaly is almost pathognomonic of myelosclerosis. Other reticuloses rarely show such marked osteosclerosis. The signs of osteopetrosis present in a younger age group, and the sclerotic bone is both denser and more homogeneous. In fluorosis, ossification of ligament and tendon insertions is characteristic. In the sclerotic metastases of secondary neoplasm and in Paget's disease the sclerosis is more irregular than that seen in myelosclerosis.

Course and treatment. The disease may run an acute course leading to death within a few months, or may last for many years. Early splenectomy may be of value, but treatment with steroids and chemotherapy have both proved disappointing.

REFERENCES

Dameshek, W. & Gunz, F. (1964). *Leukaemia.* 2nd Edition. New York.
Fairlie, G. H. (1973). In *Price's Textbook of the Practice of Medicine.* 11th Edition. London.
Feldman, F. (1974). Myelosclerosis in agnogenic myeloid metaplasia. *Seminars in Roentgenology,* **IX,** 195.
Glasser, R. M. & Walker, R. I. (1969). Transitions among myeloproliferative disorders. *Annals of Internal Medicine,* **71,** 285.
Goldstone A. H. & Cawley, J. C. (1975). Acute lymphatic leukaemia. *Hospital Update,* **I,** 683.
Goldstone, A. H. & Cawley, J. C. (1975). Acute myeloid leukaemia. *Ibid.,* **I,** 719.
Gunz, F. & Baikie, A. (1974). *Leukaemia.* New York: Grune and Stratton.
Irving, M. (1975). The role of surgery in the management of Hodgkin's disease. *British Journal of Surgery,* **62,** 853.
Meszaros, W. T. (1974). The many facets of multiple myeloma. *Seminars in Roentgenology,* **IX,** 219.
Order, S. E. & Hellman, S. (1972). Pathogenesis of Hodgkin's disease. *Lancet,* **i,** 571.
Pear, B. L. (1975). Skeletal manifestations of the lymphomas and leukaemias. *Seminars in Roentgenology,* **IX,** 229.
Silverstein, M. N., Brown, A. L. J. & Linman, J. W. (1973). Idiopathic myeloid metaplasia. *Archives of Internal Medicine,* **132,** 709.
Spiers, A. S. D., Roberts, P. D., Marsh, G. W., Parekh, S. J., Franklin, A. J., Galton, D. A. G., Szur, Z. L., Paul, E. A., Husband, P. & Wiltshaw, E. (1975). Acute lymphoblastic leukaemia; cyclical chemotherapy with three combinations of four drugs (COAP-POMP-CART regimen). *British Medical Journal,* **4,** 614.
Wagener, D. J. T. & Haanen, C. (1975). 'Incubation period' in Hodgkin's disease. *Lancet,* **ii,** 747.
Waldenström, J. (1970). *Diagnosis and treatment of multiple myeloma.* New York: Grune and Stratton.

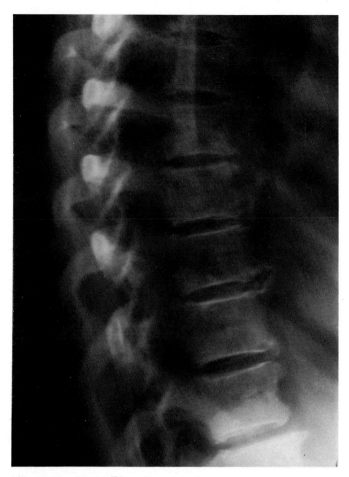

Fig. 63.22 (D.R.) Irregular sclerosis
in vertebral bodies, with osteophytes
and disc degeneration probably
unconnected. (A.H.)

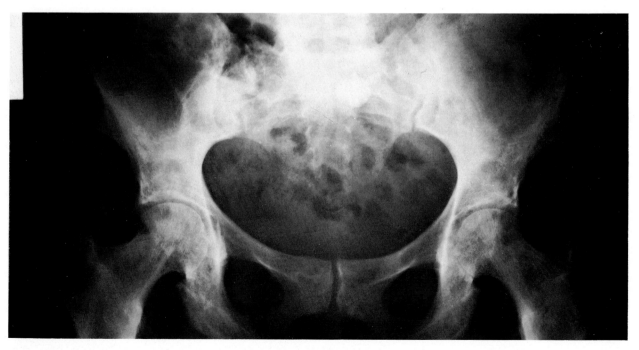

Fig. 63.23 (D.R.) Diffuse irregular sclerosis without periosteal thickening in pelvis and upper femora.
(A.H.)

CYSTIC ANGIOMATOSIS OF BONE

This rare general affection of bone has been well reviewed by Boyle (1972). Although isolated haemangiomata of bone are common, especially in the spine, very few examples of truly generalised angiomatosis have been published (Singh *et al*, 1974). Both blood vessels and lymphatic vessels are involved, and the condition is probably one of multiple hamartomata rather than a true neoplasia. Histologically the cysts are individually benign, though in so far as new lesions develop the disorder could be considered malignant.

Clinical and radiographic features. Almost all patients have presented before the age of 20 years. In infancy the disorder may present with a soft-tissue tumour which in isolation cannot clinically be differentiated from a haemangioma or lymphangioma. In other instances the presenting feature is a pathological fracture; others may be diagnosed incidentally on a chest radiograph. Associated skin naevi have only rarely been reported but viscera may be involved, particularly the spleen.

Radiographs reveal multiple cysts, round or oval in shape, and varying in size from a few millimetres in diameter to the full width of the bone. They are surrounded by a fine ring of sclerosed bone without any associated periosteal reaction. Bone expansion is uncommon, except in the ribs. The bones most often affected are the skull, pelvis, ribs, femora, humeri and scapulae, whereas the peripheral limb bones are less often involved. In the spine, there is multiple involvement of the vertebral bodies, but the vertical striation familiar in the isolated haemangioma of bone is not found. The vertebral bodies may collapse extensively even to the extent of being reminiscent of Calvé's disease. This condition, however, affects a solitary vertebra and is usually due to an eosinophilic granuloma.

Differential diagnosis. Differentiation from hyperparathyroidism, and from polyostotic fibrous dysplasia, in both of which there is more new bone formation, should present no difficulty, but the skeletal changes in some cases of cystic angiomatosis bear a resemblance to those seen in histiocytosis X. However, in the latter condition the punched-out areas in the skull are usually more extensive and without a sclerotic margin; furthermore, the cortical lesions in the long bones show a periosteal reaction not seen in angiomatosis, except sometimes in the ribs. It is from here that biopsy material is best obtained, since histological findings from other sites are not always diagnostic.

Progress. Only those patients with extensive soft part affection, particularly of the spleen, appear to die early and splenectomy has been recommended in those with marked involvement. Radiotherapy does not affect the lesions.

METASTATIC BONE DISEASE

Multiple skeletal metastases only occasionally give rise to a diagnostic problem, but this can occur when a patient presents with bone pain or a pathological fracture; a skeletal survey reveals multiple bony lesions suggestive of metastatic disease, but evidence of a primary tumour is absent.

Bone metastases are caused by cells or groups of cells from a primary growth carried almost invariably in the bloodstream, but chest radiographs do not necessarily show lung metastases also. One explanation of this apparent paradox is that, where metastases are confined to the region of the axial skeleton, spread has occurred via the vertebral venous system which extends from the skull to pelvis. Where metastases of the peripheral skeleton are visible, however, the assumption must be that the malignant emboli have either passed through the lung filter or that micrometastases (invisible on radiography) exist in the lungs, from which further emboli reach the left side of the heart and the systemic circulation.

Routine investigations will usually reveal the site of the primary growth, but confusion can arise with the reticuloses, both leukaemias and lymphomata, with histiocytosis X, multiple tuberculous or simple infective lesions, hyperparathyroidism and occasionally other skeletal diseases. Whenever doubt arises, investigations must include a complete skeletal radiographic survey. It has long been known (Bachmann and Sproul, 1955) that in the spine destruction of 50 per cent of cancellous bone must occur before a metastasis in the vertebral body is visible radiographically, and even when the cortex is involved lesions less than 1·5 cm in diameter may be invisible.

Bone scanning with radioactive isotopes, recently well reviewed by Merrick (1975), greatly improves the detection rate of any lesions where the rate of bone turnover is increased, and these include most metastases. However, the method provides no certain distinction from bone infections, fractures, or indeed any affection, such as Paget's disease, where bone is being destroyed or laid down. Nevertheless it is most valuable in metastatic disease not only for original diagnosis, and therefore for the correct staging of breast carcinoma for example, but also for localisation and in monitoring progress or recurrence. Bone metastases are by no means always multiple when the patient is first seen—in adenocarcinoma of the kidney a metastasis that remains the sole manifestation for a year or two is not very uncommon—and in one series solitary lesions were found in 8 per cent of all scans with ^{18}F, one quarter of them being in the limbs and 11 per cent in the skull (Shirazi, Rayudu and Fordham, 1974).

Biopsy, preferably taken from an actively growing part of the suspect metastasis, may be required, and a histological interpretation may be difficult; if the lesion is a solitary one misdiagnosis as a primary tumour may lead to surgical treatment both futile and disastrous.

Most malignant emboli settle in areas of bone where the blood supply is good but sluggish, that is, in the haematopoietic areas. The spine, ribs, scapulae, pelvis and upper ends of femora and humeri, together with the skull, are more commonly affected than the peripheral skeleton, although no area is safe from attack. The lesions usually start in the medullary cavity and invade the cortex from within, but tumour growth can be so rapid that this differentiation may never be apparent. Metastases may also originate in the periosteum. Cortical destruction is due to erosion of bone by the tumour cells themselves rather than by osteoclasts. The more aggressive the neoplastic process, the less the reactive response and extension into the soft tissues occurs early. More slowly growing metastases, by allowing time for periosteal reaction, may produce apparently expansile lesions, but these are exceptional.

The radiographic appearances depend to some extent upon the primary pathology of the lesion. While the majority of bone metastases are lytic (and this is tue whatever the site of origin of the primary growth), in others there can be considerable reactive bone formation producing the so-called osteoplastic type of secondary growth. This is most commonly seen in metastases from prostatic carcinoma, sometimes from the breast and in the (rare) bony metastases from carcinoma of the stomach. These sclerotic metastases tend to be seen earlier in the disease and to be slower growing than the lytic type. The new bone formed is reactive, not neoplastic as in the case of osteosarcoma. The purely osteoplastic type of bone metastasis is, however, uncommon; it is more usual to see lesions which are both lytic and osteoplastic. Especially with metastases from carcinoma of the breast, lesions which were clearly osteoplastic at an earlier stage may later be seen to have become osteolytic, quite irrespective of any therapy.

Similarly bone metastases may fluctuate in size, and occasionally in a patient some may regress while others advance (Nelson, 1962). Spontaneous regression of both primary tumours and their metastases, although extremely rare, has been recognised to occur for many years, particularly in carcinoma of the breast, chorionepithelioma, adenocarcinoma of the kidney, malignant melanoma, soft tissue sarcomata, carcinoma of the bladder, and carcinoma of the ovary (Smithers, 1962). The mechanism remains obscure; developing homograft immune reactions and naturally occurring changes in hormone levels in the case of hormone-dependent new growths offer possible explanations.

While certain primary growths are notorious for their liability to produce bone metastases—the breast, lung, prostate, kidney and thyroid are particularly so—it must be emphasised that no malignant growth is completely free from this risk, although secondary growths in bone from the skin, other than from melanoma, are very rarely seen.

The age of the patient is a help to diagnosis, pointing towards the likely primary growth. Multiple bony lesions are most commonly attributable to a neuroblastoma in the very young, or to Ewing's tumour in older children. Throughout childhood the acute leukaemias produce diagnostic problems, as can osteosarcomatous secondary growth on rare occasions in adolescents and young adults. The majority of multiple bone metastases, however, appear in middle and old age and derive from carcinomata.

The radiographic appearance may provide a clue to the likely site of the primary growth. For instance, an adenocarcinoma of the kidney or the follicular type of thyroid carcinoma are both particularly liable to produce an expansile bony lesion which may be so vascular that it is pulsatile and has an audible bruit. Such metastases, however, are often isolated or only few in number; radio-iodine studies may reveal activity in thyroid metastases.

With secondary growths, periosteal reaction is usually prominent by its absence, but metastases from the colon, neuroblastomata or, very rarely, from other tumours, may occasionally produce sunray spicules, and are therefore liable to be confused with osteosarcoma. 'Onion skin' layers of periosteal new bone occur very rarely indeed.

Carcinoma of the lung and breast are particularly liable to spread to the spine and osteoplastic lesions in the pelvis may produce the so-called 'piebald' or 'Paget' appearance, although a mixed type of both sclerotic and lytic growth is commoner.

Collapse of the vertebral bodies very commonly occurs, but ballooning of intervertebral discs into the upper and lower surfaces of the vertebral bodies, as seen in osteoporosis, is not a feature of metastatic growth alone. If pathological fracture of the spine occurs in osteoporosis it is almost invariably the upper surface of the vertebral body which is involved. In spinal metastases however, although the upper surface is more commonly affected than the lower, both surfaces may collapse and the vertebral body may 'burst' so that on a lateral radiograph it is seen that the remains of the anterior cortex protrudes in front of the adjacent vertebrae, and a similar posterior protrusion of bone may precipitate an acute paraplegia. The intervertebral disc itself is resistant to malignant invasion, but the pedicles—in contrast to myelomatosis—are often involved.

Prostatic carcinoma is believed to spread most commonly by the prostatic venous plexuses directly into the vertebral system of veins; thus early and extensive involvement of the pelvis and spine may occur. Contrary to what is often taught, the majority of metastases from the prostate are osteolytic in nature but this primary lesion, above all others, is liable to produce osteoplastic lesions. In the pelvis this often gives rise to confusion with Paget's disease, and the spine can mimic the dense vertebral bodies seen in both Paget's disease and the leukaemias. An increase in the tartrate-labile serum acid phosphatase level is almost certain confirmation that the bony lesions are prostatic in origin.

A raised sedimentation rate and serum alkaline phosphatase level commonly occur in patients with widespread skeletal metastases, whatever their origin, and irrespective of whether or no pathological fractures have occurred.

REFERENCES

Bachmann, A. L. & Sproul, E. E. (1955). Correlation of radiographic and autopsy findings in suspected metastases of the spine. *Bulletin of the New York Academy of Medicine,* **31,** 146.

Boyle, W. J. (1972). Cystic angiomatosis of bone. *Journal of Bone & Joint Surgery,* **54B,** 626.

Merrick, M. V. (1975). Review article—Bone Scanning. *British Journal of Radiology,* **48,** 327.

Shirazi, P. H., Rayadu, G. V. S. & Fordham, E. W. (1974). Review of solitary ^{18}F bone scan lesions. *Radiology,* **112,** 369.

Singh, R., Grewal, D. S., Bannerjee, A. K. & Bansal, V. P. (1974). Haemangiomatosis of the skeleton. *Journal of Bone & Joint Surgery,* **56B,** 136.

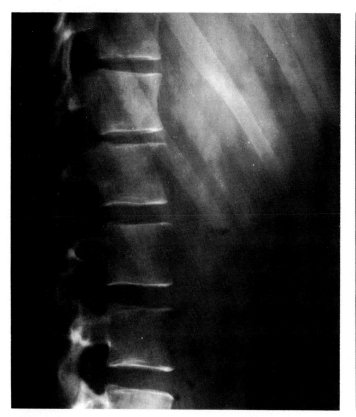

Fig. 64.1 (R.S.) Early diffuse lumbar metastases from carcinoma of bronchus. (A.H.)

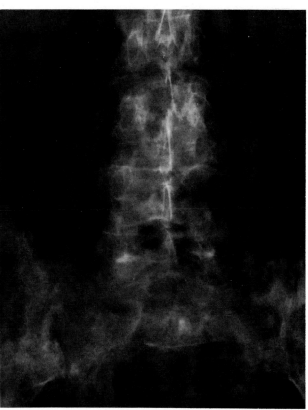

Fig. 64.2 (E.S.) Multiple breast metastases with vertebral collapse and destruction of pedicles. (Courtesy of Dr T. K. Wheeler, Cambridge.)

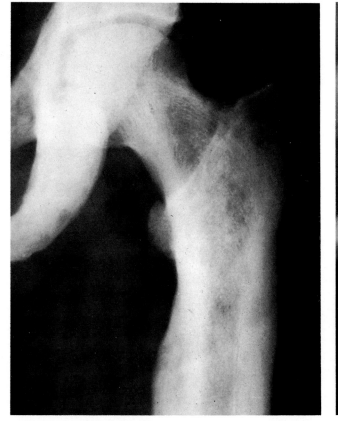

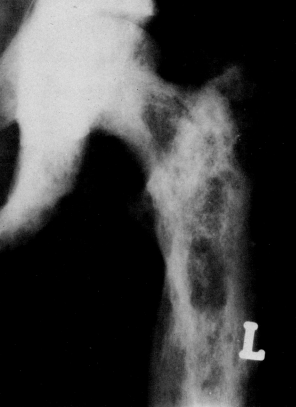

Figs 64.3 & 64.4 (B.C.) Carcinoma of breast metastases, sclerotic in 1967 becoming osteolytic 3 years later. (Courtesy of Dr D. McC. Gregg, Cambridge.)

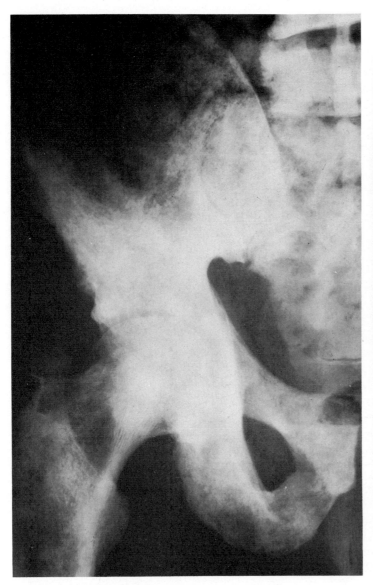

Fig. 64.5 (R.D.) Osteoblastic metastases from carcinoma of prostate. (Courtesy of Dr T. K. Wheeler, Cambridge.)

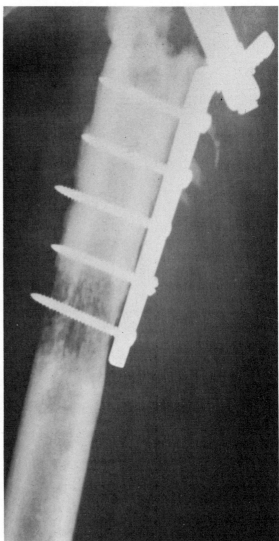

Fig. 64.6 (J.K.) Breast metastases with pathological fractures requiring internal fixation. (Courtesy of Dr T. K. Wheeler, Cambridge.)

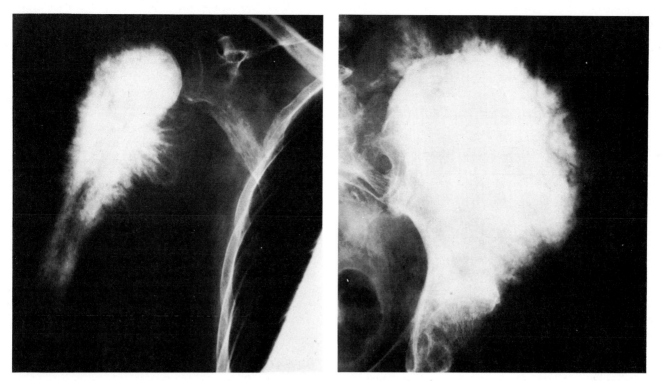

Figs 64.7 & 64.8 (B.D.) Breast metastases showing marked sunray effect in pelvis and humerus although scapula and rib metastases show no such reaction. (Courtesy of Dr D. McC. Gregg, Cambridge.)

65 Hypertrophic Osteoarthropathy

This title covers two separate conditions, a primary variety, genetic in origin, now called 'pachydermo-periostitis' (Chap. 34), and another which is associated with a range of diseases, of which the majority are pulmonary: because the manifestations are apparently identical irrespective of the site of the originating lesions, this variety is now labelled 'secondary' rather than 'pulmonary' as was done in the past.

SECONDARY HYPERTROPHIC OSTEOARTHROPATHY

Aetiology. This condition may occur at any time but is not commonly seen before early middle age. Congenital intra-thoracic lesions are responsible for the few cases reported in children. Chronic lung disease is the commonest cause, particularly bronchiectasis, empyema, primary malignant neoplasm of lung and pleura, and, less often, pulmonary tuberculosis. Carcinomatous metastases in the lung only rarely produce osteoarthropathy, although secondaries from sarcomata and malignant giant-cell tumours may do so. It can also occur with congenital cyanotic heart disease and infective endocarditis, but in these conditions signs are usually restricted to clubbing of the terminal phalanges. A number of other diseases can at times be associated with hypertrophic osteoarthropathy; for example, hepatic cirrhosis, dysentery, pyelonephritis, alcoholism, polycythaemia rubra vera, polyarteritis, steatorrhea, and various extra-thoracic malignant neoplasms have all been incriminated.

Clubbing of the fingers associated with sub-acute bacterial endocarditis has for many years been attributed to multiple capillary emboli, and monomelic changes have been reported distal to an aneurysm in the upper limb. When clubbing is combined with the other changes of hypertrophic osteoarthropathy, however, most discussion centres around a neurogenic or humoral aetiology (Holling, 1967). On the basis that the great majority of organs, diseases of which may manifest hypertrophic osteoarthropathy, receive a nerve supply from the 9th and 10th cranial nerves, Carroll and Doyle (1974) postulate a common afferent arc as an integral and basic part of the causative mechanism. It is well known that rapid relief may follow vagotomy in man (Huckstep and Bodkin, 1958) and this has been reported to occur in the dog also, by Watson (1973). There are, however, many diseases in man with which the condition is associated where some toxic or hormonal change in the circula-tion appears to be the more likely cause (Ginsburg and Brown, 1961).

Clinical and radiographic features. The onset of osteoarthropathy is rapid—a matter of a few weeks—and it can disappear with almost equal rapidity if treatment of the causative lesion is successful. Some degree of clubbing is almost always seen, the toes being affected as well as the fingers; there is hypertrophy of the pulp of the digits, but the terminal phalanges remain unchanged. In the hands and affected limbs there is swelling, warmth and pain, particularly in the region of the joints, which may be thickened and tender. In severe cases there is painful restriction of joint movement, although there is usually little radiographic evidence of arthritis. The wrist and ankle joints are those most liable to be affected. Intense local sweating is not uncommon (Boyle and Buchanan, 1971).

On radiography, the long bones show smooth symmetrical periosteal new bone formation extending over a part or, particularly in the metacarpals and metatarsals, the whole of the shaft, the changes being more or less symmetrical. The process commonly affects the distal parts of the radius, ulna, tibia, and fibula, and less often the proximal and middle phalanges, scapulae, patellae and other bones. If joint changes are present, they are indistinguishable from osteoarthritis.

Differential diagnosis. The primary form of hypertrophic osteoarthropathy, pachydermoperiostitis, is distinguished by its genetic origin, earlier age of onset, soft tissue thickening, skin changes, and roughness of the periosteal new bone. Other conditions sometimes producing marked periosteal thickening in adult life are leukaemia and certain bone tumours. In thyroid acropachy, a rare and late manifestation of hyperthyroidism, the bony changes and clubbing are similar but almost always confined to the upper limbs and accompanied by exophthalmos and pretibial myoedema (Gimlette, 1960; Thomas, Collipp and Sharma, 1973).

Progress and complications. Apart from joint discomfort the condition itself has no effect on life, but severely affected joints may eventually become eroded and osteoarthritic. If the chest or other underlying condition is cured, the bone and soft tissue changes sometimes regress and within a few weeks the clubbing may disappear entirely, only to reappear should the underlying disease recur.

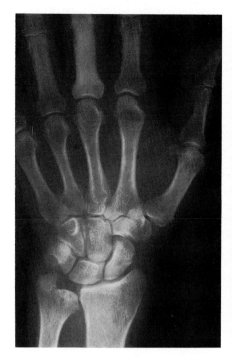

Fig. 65.1 (C.B.) Periosteal reaction, lower radius and ulna with density and thickening of a single phalanx. (Courtesy of Mr A. G. Apley, Pyrford.)

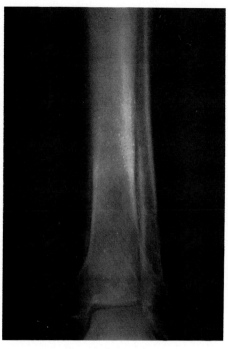

Fig. 65.2 (C.B.) Diffuse, irregular periosteal reaction but ankle joint normal. (Courtesy of Mr A. G. Apley, Pyrford.)

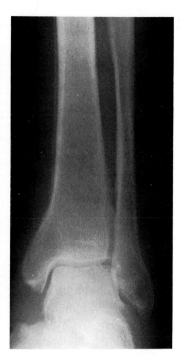

Fig. 65.3 (C.B.) A more limited and smoother reaction: ankle joint normal. (Courtesy of Mr A. G. Apley, Pyrford.)

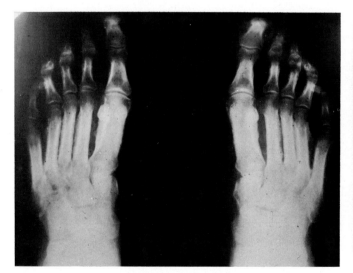

Fig. 65.4 (G.) Diffuse metatarsal involvement. Joints themselves unaffected. (Courtesy of Mr A. G. Apley, Pyrford.)

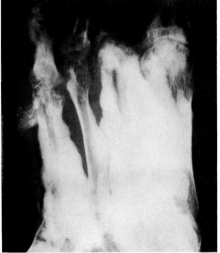

Fig. 65.5 Very severe and irregular metatarsal thickening with degenerative changes in metatarso-phalangeal joints. (Courtesy of Mr A. G. Apley, Pyrford.)

REFERENCES

Boyle, J. A. & Buchanan, W. W. (1971). *Clinical Rheumatology*. Blackwell Scientific Publications, Oxford.

Carroll, K. B. & Doyle, L. (1974). A common factor in hypertrophic osteoarthropathy. *Thorax*, **29**, 262.

Gimlette, T. M. D. (1960). Thyroid acropachy. *Lancet*, **i**, 22.

Ginsburg, J. & Brown, J. B. (1961). Increased oestrogen excretion in hypertrophic pulmonary osteoarthropathy. *Lancet*, **ii**, 1274.

Holling, H. E. (1967). Pulmonary hypertrophic osteoarthropathy. *Annals of Internal Medicine*, **66**, 232.

Huckstep, R. L. & Bodkin, P. E. (1958). Vagotomy in hypertrophic pulmonary osteoarthropathy associated with bronchial carcinoma. *Lancet*, **ii**, 343.

Thomas, J., Collipp, P. J. & Sharma, R. K. (1973). Thyroid acropachy. *American Journal of Diseases of Children*, **125**, 745.

Watson, A. D. (1973). Regression of hypertrophic osteoarthropathy in a dog following unilateral intrathoracic vagotomy. *Veterinary Record*, **93**, 240.

It is becoming increasingly clear that physical mal-treatment of small infants is not uncommon at any level of society, whether by parents, guardians, baby sitters, elder brothers and sisters or other relatives (Griffiths and Moynihan, 1963; Smith and Hanson, 1974).

Clinical and radiographic features. Nearly all these infants are under one year of age, and cases of maltreatment are rare after the age of 3 years, by which time the child is old enough to run out of harm's way. Presenting signs are those of injury, with pain, limitation of movement, swelling and bruising. The examiner should look for signs of physical mal-treatment other than fractures and dislocations, such as bruising, scratching or cigarette burns. Bruising in a child under the age of one year for any reason other than maltreatment is extremely rare. Clinical and radiographic examination of other young sibs may reveal similar findings although sometimes the rest of the family may be deceptively well cared for.

Radiography may show multiple injuries: frac-tures, epiphyseal fracture-separations or joint dis-locations (Helfer and Kempe, 1968). A characteristic feature of injury at this age is that, the periosteum being loose, huge subperiosteal haematomata may form and fracture healing occurs with a massive amount of callus. The subperiosteal haematomata calcify and the hyperostosis (unlike infantile cortical hyperostosis) extends along the whole shaft of the bone to the epiphyseal plate. Residual cortical thickening remains for long periods after the original injury (Caffey, 1957).

A helpful point in the diagnosis of this syndrome is the *consecutive* nature of the lesions—there is un-likely to have been just one incident of physical mal-treatment. Thus one fracture may be fresh; another show a haematoma already calcifying, while a third demonstrates a later stage of healing.

Not surprisingly the mortality is unknown but there is no doubt that in the past many children have died undiagnosed, most commonly from intracranial haemorrhage.

Differential diagnosis. The battered baby syndrome must be differentiated from scurvy, which indeed the infant may also suffer from. Scurvy is rare in the first six months of life, the child still having maternal protection. Bleeding from other sites, the lack of other injuries and the response to vitamin C therapy should differentiate the two, as well as the radio-graphic signs of a 'white line' at the metaphysis and the adjacent zone of attrition.

Infantile cortical hyperostosis is more obviously an inflammatory disorder with a generalised systemic reaction characterised by fever, leucocytosis and a raised sedimentation rate. Radiographically the sub-periosteal calcification does not extend as far as the epiphyseal plate.

In infancy, traumatic lesions near a joint will simulate septic arthritis but this can be distinguished on general clinical grounds and laboratory investiga-tion.

Congenital syphilis is now of great rarity, but in infants up to about five months of age the active osteochondritis causing enlarged and tender areas near the ends of long bones may need to be differen-tiated from the battered baby syndrome. The radio-graphic features of congenital syphilis show a deep radiolucent band *within* the metaphysis, and separa-tion may occur here, not, as in cases of trauma, at the junction of metaphysis and epiphysis. Other radio-graphic signs characteristic of congenital syphilis may be present (Chapter 59) and the diagnosis is con-firmed by a positive Wassermann reaction in mother and child.

The most difficult differential diagnosis of the battered baby is from osteogenesis imperfecta, in those patients who are not severely dwarfed, are without blue sclerotics and have no family history of the condition. It may be impossible to distinguish between the two at the time of injury. It is indeed possible that some infants may fracture more readily than others, without having what is termed 'osteo-genesis imperfecta'.

Treatment. Recognition of the cause of the injuries and removal of the battered child to safety is as important as treatment of the individual fractures. Under no circumstances should the child be allowed to leave hospital or institutional care until the often extremely difficult social and psychological back-ground has been brought under control.

REFERENCES

Caffey, J. (1957). Some traumatic lesions in growing bones other than fractures and dislocations: clinical and radiological features. *British Journal of Radiology*, **30**, 225.

Griffiths, D. L. & Moynihan, F. J. (1963). Multiple epiphyseal injuries in babies ('battered baby' syndrome). *British Medical Journal*, **II**, 1558.

Helfer, R. E. & Kempe, C. H. (Eds) (1968). *The Battered Child*. University of Chicago Press.

Smith, S. M. & Hanson, R. (1974). 134 Battered Children: a medical and psychological study. *British Medical Journal*, **II**, 666.

THE BATTERED BABY 257

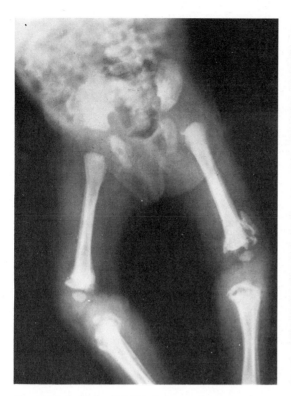 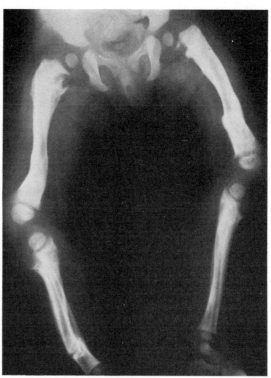

Figs 66.1 & 66.2 (M.Y.) One year between these two radiographs. Fractures shown in various stages of healing; subperiosteal haematomata with calcification extending along the whole shaft of the bone, including the epiphyseal plate. (H.A.T.F.)

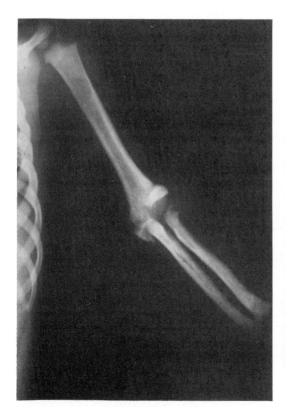 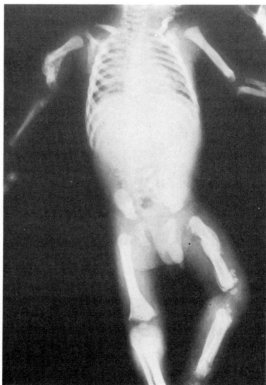

Fig. 66.3 (M.Y.) Same date as Figure 66.2, trauma to elbow and forearm. (H.A.T.F.)

Fig. 66.4 (R.Y. Brother of M.Y.) Same date as Figures 66.2 and 66.3. Multiple fractures involving all limbs in various stages of healing. (H.A.T.F.)

Index

Main references are indicated by bold numerals

Abcess, 227
Achondrogenesis, 21, **26**, 44
Achondroplasia (classical), **20**, 24, 26, 27, 30, 38, 54, 68, 168
Acidosis, renal, 192, 200, **201**
Acid phosphatase, 14, 180, 250
Acromegaly, 118, **216**
ACTH, 222
Adenoma of parathyroid, 192, 193
Adrenal glands, **222**
Ageing, bone loss associated with, **210**
Air cells
　absence of mastoid, 156
　absence of other, 90, 95, 104, 109, 156
Air sinuses
　absence of, 90, 114, 138
　small, 32, 104
Albers-Schönberg disease, **95**
Albright's disease, **138**
Alkaline phosphatase
　high, 32, 91, 114, 115, 122, 138, 192, 230, 250
　low, 44, 78, 197, 239
α-acetyl-glucosaminidase, 168, 172
α-L-iduronidase, 166, 167, 172
Amish community, 30, 38
Amyloidosis, secondary, 244
Anaemia, 40, 90, 91, 115, 180, 186, 226, 232, 234, 238, 239
　Cooley's or Mediterranean, 239
　haemolytic, 239
　sickle-cell, 234
Anarchic development of bone, **126–145**
Aneurysm, 126, 134, 152, 182, 254
Ankylosing spondylitis, 238
Anti-convulsant therapy, 200, 201
Arm span, 152, 182
Arthritis, septic, 256
Arthrogryposis multiplex congenita, 68, 134
Arthro-ophthalmopathy, hereditary progressive, **16**
Asphyxiating thoracic dystrophy, **27**, 30, 64
Asymmetrical bone lesions, 120, 121, 130, 134, 138, 180
Asymmetrical limb growth, 10, 11, 72, 120, 121, 126, 130, 138, 197
Asymmetry of face, 138
Atlanto-axial instability, 20, 60, 68, 169

Battered baby, 79, 212, 226, 230, **256–257**
β-galactosidase, 172, 178
Bismuth poisoning, **232**
Blastomycosis, 227
Blindness, 10, 16, 60, 67, 90, 91, 95, 100, 104, 109, 114, 115, 118, 122, 138, 148, 152, 168, 182, 208

Blood dyscrasias, **234**
Blue sclerae, 78, 79, 86, 114, 256
'Bone within a bone', 90, 91, 234
Brachycephaly, 32, 38
Brachydactyly, 2, 20, 26, 54, 68, 96, 156, 160, 163, 167, 169, 178, 208
Brachyolmia, **48**
Bronchiectasis, 254
Bruising, 78, 79, 238, 256
Buphthalmos, 60
Burkitt's lymphoma, 238

Cadmium poisoning, **232**
Calcification
　ectopic, 10, 134, 160, 192, 197, 198, 201, 203, 208, 233
　sub-periosteal, 34, 178, 202, 212, 216, 226, 230, 254, 256
Calcitonin, 80, 114, 122, 138
Calculi, renal, 192, 193, 216, 220
Calve's disease, 248
Camurati-Engelmann disease, 104, **110**, 114
Capillary fragility, 212
Capital femoral epiphysis, major defects of, 2, 16, 50, 54, 60, 64, 67, 68, 72, 74, 163, 167, 168, 169, 173, 235
Carcinoma
　primary, 192
　secondary, 227, 239, 248–250
Cardiac arrhythmias, 152
Cardiovascular disorders, 28, 30, 120, 122, 152, 166, 167, 168, 169, 198, 254
Carpopedal spasm, 209
Cartilage-hair hypoplasia, 34, **38**
Cataract, 10, 60, 152, 208
Cauliflower ear, 68
Cerebro-hepato-renal syndrome, 10
Charcot (neuropathic) joints, 226
Chemotherapy, 40, 42, 239, 242, 244, 246
Chilblains, 197
Chondrocalcinosis, 197
Chondrodysplasia punctata
　Conradi-Hünermann type, **10**
　severe rhizomelic form of, **10**
Chondro-ectodermal dysplasia (Ellis-van Creveld syndrome), **30**
Chondrosarcoma, 126, 130
Chromosomal anomalies, 10
Cigarette burns, 256
Clavicles
　hypoplasia or absence of, 96, 148, 156, 167
　thickened, 106, 109, 115, 167, 168, 178, 216, 230
Cleft palate, 16, 60, 67, 68

Cleido-cranio-dysplasia, **156**
Clubbing
　of digits, 118, 254
　pseudo-, 192
Clubfoot, 32, 60, 67, 68, 152
Coarse trabeculae, 114, 120, 174, 234
Coeliac disease, 200, 201
Congenital contractural arachnodactyly, 152
Congenital heart defects, 10, 27, 30, 254
Congenital syphilis, 91, 110, 212, **226**, 230, 232, 256
Conradi disease, **10**
Consanguineous parents, 2, 10, 30, 74, 88, 90, 95, 96, 100, 109, 114, 166, 168
Contractures, 2, 10, 20, 30, 32, 67, 68, 72, 88, 114, 134, 152, 160, 166, 167, 168, 169, 197, 226, 234
Convulsions, 44, 201, 209
Cooley's anaemia, 234
Corneal clouding, 60, 74, 166, 167, 168, 169
Coxa valga, 20, 60, 152, 167, 168, 169
Coxa vara, 20, 34, 38, 40, 53, 60, 114, 138, 156
Cranial nerve palsies, 90, 91, 95, 100, 104, 109, 114, 115, 118, 121, 138, 148
Cranial sutures
　delayed fusion of, 96, 156
　widening of, 38, 44
Cranio-cleido dysostosis, 90, **156**, 220
Craniodiaphyseal dysplasia, 91, 100, 104, **109**
Craniometaphyseal dysplasia, 91, **104**, 106, 109, 110
Craniostenosis, 10, 44
Craniotabes, 226
Cretinism, 2, **220**
Crohn's disease, 201
Crystal synovitis, 192
Cubitus valgus, 113
Cushing's disease, 86
Cystathionine synthetase, 182
Cystic angiomatosis of bone, **248**
Cystic lesions of bone, 32, 38, 78, 120, 130, 138, 148, 180, 186, 192, 227, 238, 244, 248
Cystine, 182
Cystinosis (Fanconi syndrome), 200, **201**
Cytoxic drugs, 238

Deafness, 16, 32, 60, 67, 78, 79, 90, 91, 95, 100, 104, 109, 114, 115, 118, 122, 138, 148, 167, 169, 220
Decreased bone density, 44, **78–89**, 114, 120, 203, 210, 212, 222, 238, 239, 240, 244, 246, 249

Delayed union of fractures, 121, 148, 212
Densitometry, 210
Diabetes, 40, 138, 186
Diaphyseal aclasis, 14, **126,** 130, 163
Diaphysis, 100, 106, 109, 110, 113, 114, 115, 118, 126, 130, 167, 169, 178, 180, 186, 226, 230, 232, 254
Diastrophic dwarfism, **68**
1,25-dihydroxycholecalciferol, 201
Diphosphonates, 122, 210
Dislocation (or subluxation)
  of clavicle, 152
  of hand bones, 38
  of hip, 10, 60, 152, 167
  of joints in general, 68, 152, 256
  of patella, 152, 158
  of radial head, 30, 38, 130, 152, 158
  of radiohumeral joint, 126
Down's syndrome (mongolism), 238
Dwarfism
  diastrophic, **68**
  lethal forms of, **26–29**
  metatropic, **64**
  parastremmatic, **72**
  polydystrophic, **168**
  proportionate, 114, 166, 168, 178, 209, 216, 220
  short limbed, 10, 20, 21, 24, 26, 27, 30, 32, 38, 42, 54, 64, 68, 72, 78, 96
  short trunk, 50, 53, 54, 60, 64, 67, 74, 168
  thanatophoric, **26**
Dyggve-Melchior-Clausen disease, **74**
Dyschondrosteosis, 24
Dysosteosclerosis, 91, **95**
Dysostosis multiplex, 166, 178
Dysplasia epiphysealis hemimelica, **14**
Dysplasia epiphysealis multiplex, **2**

Ear deformity, 68
Ellis-van Creveld syndrome, 27, **30**
Empyema, 254
Enchondromatosis, 130
Enchondromatosis with haemangiomata (Maffucci's disease), **130**
Endocrine disorders, 138, 192, 208, 211, **216–223**
  multiple adenosis, 192, 193
Engelmann's disease, progressive diaphyseal dysplasia, 104, **110,** 114
Eosinophilic granuloma, **186**
Epilepsy, 201, 208
Epiphyseal disorders, **2–19**
Epiphyseal dysplasia, multiple, **2,** 220
Epiphyseal fracture separations, 212, 256
Epiphyses
  absent, 26, 60, 169
  cone shaped, 27, 30, 42, 74, 163, 208
  irregular, 2, 14, 16, 27, 50, 54, 60, 64, 67, 68, 72, 74, 142, 167, 169, 182, 226, 234
  mottled, 2, 10, 130, 134, 142, 144, 220
  ringed, 90, 212
Erythraemia, acute, 238
Ewing's tumour, 226, 249

Exophthalmos, 32, 113, 186, 216, 254
Exostoses, multiple, 14, 126, 160

Fabry disease, 180
Facial bones, hypoplasia of, 96
Facial palsy, 104
Familial hypophosphataemia, 200, **201**
Familial metaphyseal dysplasia (Pyle's disease), 104, **106**
Familial neurovisceral storage disease, **178**
Fanconi syndrome, 200, **201**
Fever, 114, 186, 212, 230, 256
Fibrodysplasia ossificans progressiva, **160**
Fibula, long, 24, 38
Fibrous replacement of bone, 88, 138, 148, 192
Flat feet, 152
Fluorosis and heavy metal poisoning, 80, 91, **232–233,** 246
Fontanelles
  delayed closure of, 38, 113, 209, 220
  persistent open, 44, 96
Fractures
  green-stick, 202
  pathological, 14, 44, 45, 78, 79, 80, 86, 90, 91, 95, 96, 106, 114, 120, 121, 122, 130, 138, 148, 180, 182, 186, 192, 197, 202, 203, 210, 212, 222, 239, 244, 246, 248, 249, 250, 256
Fragilitas osseum, **78**
Frontal bones, prominent, 24, 26, 34, 88, 95, 96, 156, 166, 198, 201, 202
Frontometaphyseal dysplasia, 106

Gangliosidosis, generalised, **178**
Gargoylism, **166**
Gastrectomy, 201
Gaucher disease, 172, **180**
Genu recurvatum, 152
Genu valgum, 30, 53, 54, 106, 113, 126, 130, 152, 169, 202
Genu varum, 20, 24, 34, 38, 54, 113, 114, 202
Giant cell tumour, 121, 192, 254
Gigantism, 138, 148, **216**
Glaucoma, 16, 60
Glucocerebrosidase, 172, 180
Glucocorticoid excess, 211, **220**
GM₁ gangliosidosis type I, 167, **178**
Goitre, 220
Gout, 192, 246
Gummatous periostitis, 226

Haemangiomata, 88, 89, 130, 148, 248
Haematomata, subperiosteal, 202, 212, 256
Haemodialysis, 193, 200, 201, 203, 211
Haemoglobin molecules, 234
Haemoglobinopathies, 227, **234–235**
Hair defects, 27, 30, 38, 42, 163
Hallux, short, 160
Hand-Schüller-Christian disease, **186**
Hare lip, 30
Heavy metal intoxication, 198
Heparin therapy, 211

Hepatomegaly, 168, 238, 242, 246
Hepatosplenomegaly, 166, 167, 169, 178, 186, 244
Hereditary osteo-onycho dysplasia, **158**
Hereditary progressive arthro-ophthalmopathy, **16**
Herniae, 78, 152, 166, 167, 168, 220
Hirschsprung disease, 38
Histiocytosis-X, 138, **186,** 226, 244, 248
Hodgkin's disease, 238, **242**
Homocystine, 152, 182
Homocystinuria, 152, **182,** 211
Hunter's syndrome (mucopolysaccharidosis II), **167,** 172
Hurler's syndrome (mucopolysaccharidosis I H), **166,** 167, 168, 169, 172, 178
Hydatid disease, 227
25-hydroxycholecalciferol, 201
Hydroxyproline, 35
Hydrocephalus, 20, 21, 90, 122, 166, 167, 168
Hypercalcaemia, 32, 44, 86, 122, **192–199,** 233
Hypercalcinuria, 222, 244
Hyperparathyroidism, primary, 138, **192,** 211, 232, 244, 248
  secondary, **193,** 201, 202, 203, 208, 233
  tertiary, **193**
Hyperphosphatasia, 110, **114,** 118
  congenita, **114**
  tarda, 100, **114**
Hyperphosphataemia, 208, 209
Hyperpituitarism, **216**
Hyperplastic callus, 79
Hypersplenism, 90, 180
Hypertelorism, 67, 100, 104, 109
Hyperthyroidism, 80, 138, 211, **220,** 254
Hypertrophic osteoarthropathy, **254–255**
Hypervitaminosis A, **198**
Hypervitaminosis D, **232**
Hypocalcaemia, 193, **200–209,** 201, 202, 203, 208, 209
Hypochondroplasia, 21, **24**
Hypogonadism, 211
Hypoparathyroidism, 197, **208**
Hypophosphatasia, **44**
  infantile, **44,** 78
  mild (adult), **44**
Hypothyroidism in children (cretinism), 2, **220**

I-cell disease (mucolipidosis II), 167, 172, **178**
Idiopathic hypercalcaemia of infancy, **198,** 232
  mild form, **198**
  severe form (Fanconi-Schlesinger type), **198**
Idiopathic hypertrophic osteo-arthropathy, **118**
Increased bone density, **90–125,** 130, 134, 138, 142, 144, 197, 198, 201, 209, 232, 234, 249
Idiopathic juvenile osteoporosis, 79, **86,** 211
Immunological defects, 40, 42, 244

Inborn errors of metabolism, **166–189**
Infantile cortical hyperostosis, 110, 114, 212, 226, **230,** 256
Infarction of bone, 180, 234
Infections, **226–229,** 248
  in metaphyseal chondrodysplasia, 38, 42
  prenatal, 10
Intestinal malabsorption, 34, 38, 40, 211
Intracranial haemorrhage, 78, 256
Intracranial pressure, raised, 20, 44, 79, 90, 104, 122, 167
Irradiation, 238, 239

Jansen type of metaphyseal chondro-dysplasia, **32**
Jaundice, obstructive, 201, 242
Jeune's disease, **27,** 64
Joint laxity, 24, 38, 68, 78, 152, 156, 163, 168, 169
  stiffness, 67, 72, 134, 166, 167, 168, 169, 178, 232
Juvenile Paget's disease, **114**

Kenny-Caffey syndrome, **209**
Kniest disease, 64, **67,** 72
Kozlowski type of metaphyseal chondrodysplasia, **42**
Kozlowski type of spondylometaphyseal dysplasia, 42, **53,** 64
Kyphosis, 16, 20, 21, 50, 60, 67, 96, 166, 167, 210, 220

Lactosyl ceramidosis, 180
Laryngeal spasm, 201, 209
Lead poisoning, 197, **232**
Lens, dislocated, 152, 182
Leontiasis ossea, **109**
Lethal forms of short-limbed dwarfism, 21, **26,** 27, 30, 44
Letterer Siwe disease, **186**
Leucocytosis, 212, 230, 256
Leucopenia, 38, 40, 42, 180, 246
Leukaemia, 79, 86, **238–239,** 248, 250
  acute, 86, **238–239,** 249
  acute myeloblastic, 238, 239
  acute myeloid, 238
  chronic granulocytic, 238, **239**
  chronic lymphatic, 238, **239**
  chronic myeloid, **238**
  lymphoblastic, 238, 239
Limb inequality, 10, 11, 72, 120, 121, 126, 130, 138, 197
Loose bodies, intra-articular, 14
Lower segment measurement, 152, 182
Lumbar spine, lordosis, 20, 24, 34, 54, 60
  interpedicular distance, 20, 24, 26, 38, 54, 68
Lymphadenoma, 242
Lymphadenopathy, 186, 238, 242, 244
Lymphangiomata, 130, 148, 248
Lymph nodes, 186, 239, 242, 246
Lymphomata, 238, 244, 248
Lymphosarcoma, 238, 244

Macroglobulinaemia, 238
Maffucci's disease, **130**
Majewski syndrome, **27**

Malignant change, 79, 121, 126, 131, 149, 192
Mandible, defects, 30, 32, 96, 156, 166
Marfan syndrome, 16, 88, **152,** 182
Maroteaux-Lamy syndrome (mucopolysaccharidosis VI), 167, **168,** 172
Maroteaux type of metaphyseal chondrodysplasia, **42**
Marrow, hyperplasia of, 234
  infiltration of, 244, 246
McCune-Albright disease, **138**
McKusick type of chondrometaphyseal dysplasia, 34, **38,** 42
Median nerve palsies, 149
Mediterranean anaemia, 234
Melnick-Needles syndrome, **113**
Melorheostosis, **134,** 138, 142, 144
Mental retardation, 10, 44, 74, 95, 109, 163, 166, 167, 168, 178, 182, 198, 208, 220
Metabolic bone disease with hyper-calcaemia, **192**
  with hypocalcaemia, **200**
  with bone loss, **210**
Metachondromatosis, 130
Metachromatic granules, 166
Metachromatic leucodystrophy, 180
Metal intoxication, 198
Metaphyseal chondrodysplasias, **32–43**
Metaphyseal chondrodysplasia calcificans, 42
Metaphyseal chondrodysplasia, type Jansen, **32,** 34
  type Kozlowski, **42**
  type Maroteaux, **42**
  type McKusick, 34, **38,** 42
  type Peña, **42**
  type Schmid, **34,** 38, 42
  type Spahr, **42**
  type Vaandrager, **42**
  type Wiedemann and Spranger, **42**
  with congenital pancreatic insufficiency and neutropenia, 38, **40**
  with peripheral location, 42
  with thymolymphopenia, 38, **42**
Metaphyseal disorders, **20–47**
Metaphyseal dysostosis, **32**
Metaphyses
  constricted, 168
  cupped, 34, 42, 202
  defective, 44, 60, 86, 96, 104, 169, 226
  flared, 20, 54, 64, 68, 113
  irregular, 32, 40, 53, 54, 64, 238–239
  sclerotic, 38, 40, 142, 198, 239
  stippled, 72
  streaked, 14, 130, 144
  widened, 67, 78, 90, 95, 106, 180, 182
Metastatic bone disease, 120, 210, 226, 238, 239, 244, 246, 248, 249, 254
Metatropic dwarfism, 53, **64,** 67, 72
Microfractures, 78, 120
Micrognathia, 88, 96, 113
Mongolism (Down's syndrome), 238
Monostotic disease, 120, 121, 138
Morquio's disease (mucopolysaccharidosis IV), 16, 50, 60, 64, 67, **168,** 172

Mucolipidoses, 166, 172, **178,** 220
Mucolipidosis II (I-cell disease), 167, 172, **178**
Mucolipidosis III, **178**
Mucopolysaccharidoses, **166,** 172, 178, 220
Mucopolysaccharidosis I-H (Hurler's syndrome), **166,** 167, 168, 169, 172, 178
Mucopolysaccharidosis I-S (formerly mucopolysaccharidosis V), **167,** 172
Mucopolysaccharidosis II (Hunter's syndrome), **167,** 172
Mucopolysaccharidosis III, **168,** 172
Mucopolysaccharidosis IV (Morquio's disease), **168,** 172
Mucopolysaccharidosis VI (Maroteaux-Lamy syndrome), 167, **168,** 172
Multiple endocrine adenosis, 192, 193
Multiple epiphyseal dysplasia, **2,** 10, 16, 50, 54, 220
  Fairbank type, 2
  Ribbing type, 2
Multiple hereditary exostoses, 14, **126**
Muscle weakness, 110, 134, 152, 160, 202
Myelofibrosis, 91, 238, **246**
Myeloma, 226, 244
Myelomatosis, 186, 227, 238, 239, 242, **244,** 246, 250
Myelosclerosis, 233, 239, **246**
Myopia, 16, 60, 67, 152
Myositis ossificans progressiva, **160**

N-Ac-gal-4-sulfatase, 168, 172
Nail-patella syndrome, **158**
Nails, defective, 27, 30, 42, 95, 100, 156, 158
Nasal bridge, depressed, 10, 20, 26, 67, 100
Necrosis of bone, 180, 222, 234
N-heparan-sulfatase, 168, 172
Neoplasia of bone, generalised, **248–250**
  other, 14, 79, 91, 120, 121, 126, 130, 131, 186, 192, 244, 246, 248, 254
Nephritis, chronic, 232
Nephrocalcinosis, 44, 192, 197
Nephropathy, associated with osteolysis, 88
  associated with nail-patella syndrome, 158
Nerve tumours, 148, 149
Neuroblastoma, 222, 249
Neurofibromatosis, **148,** 200
Neuropathic (Charcot) joints, 226
Neutropenia, 38, 40, 42, 180, 246
Niemann-Pick disease, 180
Non-keratan sulphate excreting Morquio's disease, 74

Odontoid process, hypoplasia, 20, 60, 68, 168
Ollier's disease, 14, 32, 42, 126, **130**
Osteitis deformans, **120**
Osteitis fibrosa cystica, 192, 201
Osteoarthritis, secondary, 2, 3, 14, 16, 21, 34, 50, 54, 67, 68, 121, 122, 169, 192, 216, 220, 226, 254

Osteoarthropathy, idiopathic hypertrophic, 118, **254**
Osteoclastoma, 192
Osteodysplasty, **113**
Osteogenesis imperfecta, 44, **78,** 114, 156, 211, 256
  congenita, **78,** 79
  tarda, 78, **79,** 86
Osteolyses, the, **88–89**
  associated with nephropathy, 88
  of hands and feet, **88**
  massive, **88**
Osteolytic lesions, 118, 120, 130, 148, 180, 186, 192, 201, 226, 234, 238, 242, 244, 248, 249, 250
Osteomalacia, 44, 149, 193, **200–203,** 210, 211, 232
Osteomyelitis, 79, 90, 91, 96, 120, 186, 226, 227, 230, 235, 256
Osteopathia striata, **144**
Osteopetrosis, **90,** 95, 96, 104, 134, 198, 233, 246
  congenita, **90,** 91
  tarda, 90, **91,** 95, 106, 115
Osteopoikilosis, **142,** 144
Osteoporosis, 78, 79, 80, 86, 180, 182, 192, 197, 202, **210,** 211, 212, 220, 222, 226, 232, 234, 238, 239, 244, 246, 250
Osteosarcoma, 2, 79, 226, 249
Osteosclerosis, **90–125,** 134, 142, 144, 197, 198, 201, 203, 232, 233, 234, 239, 242, 248, 249

Pachydermoperiostitis, **118,** 254
Paget's disease, 91, 110, 114, **120,** 233, 246, 249, 250
Pain
  abdominal, 197, 232, 239, 246
  in back, 50, 86, 210, 222
  in bone, 110, 114, 120, 122, 134, 180, 203, 212, 226, 230, 234, 238, 244, 248, 256
Palate, cleft, 16, 60, 67, 68
  high arched, 152, 182
Pancreatic disease, 40, 200, 201
Pancytopenia, 40, 90
Paraesthesiae, 202, 209, 216
Paraplegia, 20, 60, 68, 78, 122, 126, 148, 169, 232, 239, 242, 244, 250
Parastremmatic dwarfism, **72**
Parathyroid disease, 192, 197, 208
Parathyroid, hyperplasia of, 203, 208
Parental age, 20, 34, 78, 152, 160
Parrot's nodes, 226
Patella
  absent, 158
  double, 2
  recurrent dislocation of, 152, 158
Pathological fractures. *See* Fractures, pathological.
Pectus carinatum, 38, 64, 152, 168, 169, 182
Pectus excavatum, 79, 152, 182
Pel-Ebstein fever, 242
Peña type of metaphyseal chondrodysplasia, **42**
Pendred syndrome, 220
Peptic ulcer, 193

Periosteal and subperiosteal new bone, 32, 34, 104, 118, 178, 180, 202, 212, 216, 226, 230, 239, 249, 254, 256
Perthes' disease, 2, 38, 163, 220, 235
Pes cavus, 88
Phalanges
  absent or short, 27, 96, 100, 156, 160, 208
  'bone within a bone' appearance, 90, 91
  'bullet-shaped', 167
  constricted, 169
  erosion of, 192, 193, 202, 203
  extra ossification centres in, 67
  osteolysis of, 88
  synostosis of, 160
  syphilitic dactylitis in, 226
  tufting of, 216
Phosphoethanolamine, 44
Phosphorus depletion, 192, 197, 200, 201
Phosphorus poisoning, 232
Pierre Robin syndrome, 16
Pituitary insufficiency, 216
Pituitary overaction, 216
Plasmacytoma, 244
Platybasia, 79, 122, 200
Platyspondyly, 16, 26, 42, 48, 50, 53, 54, 60, 64, 67, 72, 74, 78, 79, 95, 114, 168, 169, 182, 186, 202, 210, 222, 234, 244, 248
Polycythaemia vera, 238, 246, 254
Polydactyly, 26, 27, 30
Polyostotic fibrous dysplasia, 114, 120, **138,** 193, 248
Priapism, 234
Progressive diaphyseal dysplasia (Camurati-Engelmann disease), 104, **110,** 114
Prolapsed intervertebral disc, 21
Pseudarthrosis, 148, 149
Pseudoachondroplasia, 2, 21, **54,** 72
Pseudo-fractures (Looser's zones), 202
Pseudogout, 192
Pseudo-Hurler polydystrophy, **178**
Pseudohypoparathyroidism, **208**
'Pseudo-pseudo-hypoparathyroidism', 208
Pycnodysostosis, 91, 95, **96,** 106, 156, 220
Pyle's disease (familial metaphyseal dysplasia), 104, **106**
Pyrexia, 160, 226, 230, 234, 242, 244

Radioactive isotopes, 249
Radiotherapy, 238, 242, 244, 248, 249
Radius
  curved, 126, 130, 169, 254
  dislocation of head of, 30, 38, 130, 152, 158
Reed-Sternberg cells, 242
Renal calculi or calcification, 192, 193, 198, 203, 216, 220
Renal disorders, 27, 88, 158, 192, 193, 197, 198, 200, 201, 203, 232, 233, 244
Renal tubular disorders, 44, 149, 193, 200, **201,** 203

Reticuloses, the, **238–247,** 248
Retina, detached, 148
Rheumatoid arthritis, 88, 197
Rhinitis, 166, 226
Rib cage, narrow, 26, 27, 64
Ribs, thickened, 106, 109, 114, 167, 178, 216
Rickets, 32, 34, 38, 44, 45, 72, 193, 197, 198, **200–203,** 212, 226

Sabre tibia, 226
Saldino-Noonan syndrome, **27**
Sanfilippo syndrome (mucopolysaccharidosis III), **168,** 172
Scaphocephaly, 166
Scheie synrome (mucopolysaccharidosis I-S), **167,** 172
Scheuermann disease, 16
Schmid type of metaphyseal chondrodysplasia, 24, **34,** 38, 42
Sclerosteosis, **100**
Scoliosis, 10, 21, 32, 42, 53, 54, 60, 64, 68, 72, 78, 79, 96, 113, 114, 148, 149, 152, 156, 166, 169, 182, 210, 220
Scurvy, 202, 211, **212,** 226
Secondary (pulmonary) hypertrophic osteoarthropathy, 118, **254–255**
Sedimentation rate, raised, 212, 230, 250, 256
Sella turcica, enlarged, 166, 216
Short rib/polydactyly syndromes, Majewski and Saldino-Noonon types, **27–28**
Sickle-cell anaemia, **234**
Skin lesions, 10, 42, 79, 88, 95, 118, 120, 122, 134, 142, 186, 216, 248, 249
  pigmentation, 138, 148, 193, 200, 220, 226, 239
  tumours, 148
Skull (*see also* fontanelles and Wormian bones)
  defects of ossification, 44, 156
  'hot cross bun', 226
  increased density, **90–120**
Smallpox, 38
Spahr type of metaphyseal chondrodysplasia, **42**
Sphingolipidoses, 172, 178, **180**
Spina bifida occulta, 156
Spinal cord compression, 20, 60, 68, 78, 122, 126, 148, 169, 232, 239, 242, 244, 250
Spinal stenosis, 21
Splenomegaly, 90, 168, 180, 186, 238, 239, 242, 246
Spondyloepiphyseal dysplasia, 2, 48, **50,** 54, 60, 72, 168, 220
  congenita, 16, 50, **60,** 67
  tarda (X-linked), **50**
Spondylolisthesis, 96, 220
Spondylometaphyseal dysplasia (Kozlowski type), **53,** 64
Steatorrhoea, 201, 254
Steroid compounds, 222
Steroid therapy, 80, 86, 90, 91, 110, 186, 198, 210, 222, 244, 246

Sternal protrusion, 67, 169
Storage diseases, **166–181**
Strabismus, 152
Stubby hands and feet, 2, 20, 27, 38, 54, 60, 68, 96, 156, 160, 167, 169, 178, 208
Sulphoiduronate sulphatase, 172
Subperiosteal erosions, 192, 193, 202, 203, 208, 212
Symphalangism, 68
Syndactyly, 100
Synostosis
    of tibia and fibula, 126
    of radius and ulna, 126
Syphilitic dactylitis, 226
Syphilis, **226**

Tail-like appendage, 64
Talipes equinovarus, 32, 60, 67, 68, 152
Tarso-epiphyseal aclasis, 14
Tarsomegaly, 14
Teeth, defective, 27, 30, 44, 78, 90, 91, 96, 113, 120, 156, 166, 168, 169, 198, 208, 216, 232
Tetany, 201, 202, 208, 209
Thalassaemia (Cooley's or Mediterranean anaemia), **234**
    major, 234
    minor, 234

Thanatophoric dwarfism, 21, **26,** 44
Thorax, increased diameter, 50, 60, 216
    narrow, 26, 27, 28, 64
Thrombocythaemia, 238, 246
Thrombocytopenia, 40, 90, 180
Thrombosis, 182, 234
Thymolymphopenia, 38, 40
Thyroid overaction, 80, **220**
    deficiency, 232
Torticollis, 160
Toxins, **232,** 246
Trauma, **256**
Tricho-rhino-phalangeal syndrome, 126, **163**
Trochanteric hyperplasia, 64, 67
Tuberculosis, 186, 197, 226, 227, 248, 254
Tubular stenosis with periodic hypo-calcaemia (Kenny-Caffey syndrome), **209**
Tumours of bone (*see* neoplasia of bone)
Turner syndrome (XO chromosome anomaly), 208, 211

Ulna, short, 20, 24, 68, 126, 130, 169, 208

Ulnar nerve palsy, 149
Uraemic osteodystrophy, 44, 197, 200, **201,** 203

Vaandrager type of metaphyseal chondrodysplasia, **42**
Vaginal bleeding, 138
Vagotomy, 254
Van Buchem disease, **114**
Varicella, 34, 38
Vertebrae
    'sandwich', or 'rugger jersey', 90, 91, 192, 203
    tall, 152
Viral infections, 239, 242
Vitamin A poisoning, **197**
Vitamin C deficiency (scurvy), 202, 211, **212,** 226, 256
Vitamin D poisoning, **197,** 198
Von Recklinghausen's disease, 147

Wiedemann and Spranger type of metaphyseal chondrodysplasia, **42**
Wimberger's sign, 226
Wormian bones, 78, 95, 96, 156

Yaws, **226**